T0202177

Pasteur's Empire

Bacteriology and Politics in France, its Colonies, and the World

ARO VELMET

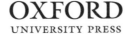

OXFORD
UNIVERSITY PRESS

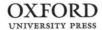

OXFORD
UNIVERSITY PRESS

Oxford University Press is a department of the University of Oxford. It furthers
the University's objective of excellence in research, scholarship, and education
by publishing worldwide. Oxford is a registered trade mark of Oxford University
Press in the UK and certain other countries.

Published in the United States of America by Oxford University Press
198 Madison Avenue, New York, NY 10016, United States of America.

CIP data is on file at the Library of Congress
ISBN 978–0–19–007282–7

1 3 5 7 9 8 6 4 2

Printed by Integrated Books International, United States of America

In memory of Mary Velmet

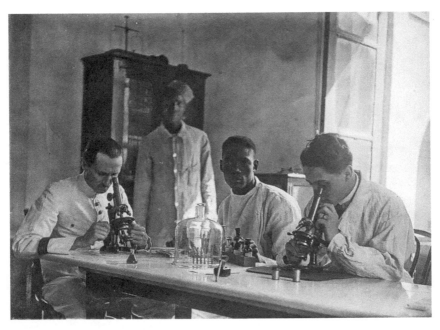

A bacteriological laboratory at a Dakar hospital, early 1930s.
Amicale Santé Navale et Outre-Mer.

Contents

List of Illustrations and Maps

Illustrations

Maps

All maps by Kate Blackmer

Acknowledgments

Much has changed in the world and in the historical discipline since this book began as a doctoral dissertation at New York University in 2013. I came to NYU's Institute of French Studies with an interest in the history of expertise and the use of scientific discourses in politics. At the time, a generation of scholars had reframed the history of France around its relationship to colonialism and highlighted the centrality of race, immigration, and demography in the country's political past. Following a project on French imaginations of colonial beauty and fertility in the "age of depopulation," it made perfect sense to study the history of public health programs and the rise of Pastorian bacteriology. After all, it was hard to read through a single official document on colonial policy without encountering a reference to the vital importance of improving colonial birth rates, public health, and other demographic factors. How did the new laboratory science of bacteriology shape these visions of colonialism?

As is in the nature of research, the focus of this project shifted over time. I realized that, rather than being solely about expertise and discourse, this book was ultimately about imaginations of ecology clashing with actually existing environments. In other words, it was about the different ways experts, administrators, and activists *imagined* the interactions of humans, medical technologies, and microbes, but equally important, it was about the humans, medical technologies, and microbes *themselves*. The book ultimately looks at the politics produced by the increasing chasm between an idea of ecology that portrays humans and microbes as abstracted from any sense of place and local specificity, and a reality that reinforces precisely the opposite. It looks at the scientific, political, and economic forces that make the idea of universalizing abstraction so appealing, and the conflicts generated by the moments when the unpredictable interdependence of tools, microbes, and men make the Pastorian idea fall apart.

Over the years, this project has become both more global and more granular, focusing more on networks extending beyond the French empire, as well as on the nitty-gritty of vaccine engineering, yeast cultivation, and murine biology. These moves were inspired by both intellectual and archival explorations. In terms of theoretical influences, this book owes its greatest debts to Frederick Cooper, Gabrielle Hecht, Ruth Rogaski, and Keith Wailoo. For sheer inspiration, mentorship, and ongoing feedback, Herrick Chapman, Guy Ortolano, and Stefanos Geroulanos deserve infinite credit. Many friends and colleagues at New York University, the University of Oxford, and the University of Southern California have read partial or full drafts of various versions of this manuscript. I cannot thank them enough for their patience, generosity, and sharp feedback. They include, in no particular order, Stéphane Gerson, Frédéric Viguier, Liz Fink, Evan Spitzer, Jessica Pearson, Ian Merkel, Erik Meddles, Sarah Griswold, Alexander Arnold, Larry Wolff, Jane Burbank, Molly Nolan, Myles Jackson, Robyn d'Avignon, and Julie Livingston at NYU; Mark Harrison, Claas Kirchhelle, Martin Conway, and Erica Charters at Oxford; and Paul Lerner, Wolf Gruner, Vanessa Schwartz, and Elinor Accampo at USC. Scholars at other institutions have been no less influential. During my travels I have learned immensely from Eric Jennings, Alice Conklin, Emmanuelle Saada, Guillaume Lachenal, Gilles Pécout, Susannah Wilson, Sarah Easterby-Smith, Albert Wu, Camille Robcis, Tyler Stovall, Kate Brown, Mary Mitchell, Gerard Sasges, Erica Peters, Mitchitake Aso, and Fredrik Meiton.

I have had to navigate archives on four different continents, and the generosity and assistance I have received from local archivists and administrators cannot be overstated. In particular, I would like to thank Daniel Demellier at the Archives of the Institut Pasteur in Paris, André Spiegel at the Institut Pasteur of Dakar, Do Kien at the Vietnamese National University, and Tom Rosenbaum at the Rockefeller Archive Center. Archivists at the League of Nations Archives in Geneva and the National Archives in France, the United Kingdom, Senegal, and Vietnam (Ho Chi Minh City, Dalat, and Hanoi) all deserve credit, as do librarians at the Bodleian Library in Oxford, the Bobst Library in New York, the Bibliothèque Nationale de France, and the Estonian National Library in Tallinn.

This project has benefited from financial support from the Estonian Ministry of Education and Research, the Michel Beaujour Fellowship, the Rockefeller Archive Center, the American Historical Association, the Josephine De Karman Dissertation Fellowship, the Jerrold Seigel Fellowship in Intellectual or Cultural History, the NYU Remarque Institute Fellowship, and numerous other grants and fellowships at NYU, as well as research funding from the University of Oxford and from the University of Southern California. The Wellcome Unit for the History of Medicine and Wadham

College provided me with an academic home at Oxford, and the Department of History at USC (particularly Philip Ethington and Karen Halttunen as chairs, and Dean Peter Mancall) have been very generous in permitting research leaves. In Paris, I was hosted by the École Normale Supérieure, by the Centre de Sociologie de l'Innovation at Mines-ParisTech, and by NYU in Paris. The project leading to this book has received funding from the European Union's Horizon 2020 research and innovation program under the Marie Skłodowska-Curie grant agreement No. 747591.

I have workshopped versions of the argument at the University of St. Andrews, University of Warwick, and the Royal Society in the United Kingdom; at the American University in Paris; at Tallinn University in Estonia; at numerous workshops at NYU; at the HSTM seminar at Oxford; and at annual conferences of the Society for French Historical Studies (United States) and the Society for the Study of French History (United Kingdom). All resulted in excellent comments and vastly improved the final draft.

Academia is nowhere near as solitary as people assume. For all the long conversations, walks, adventures, museum visits, movie nights, and shared glasses of wine, I thank the various communities of researchers I have encountered over the years. In Senegal, I enjoyed the company of Séverine Frison, Lauren Honig, Devon Golaszewski, and Jules Shen. In France, Kit Heintzman, Melissa Anderson, Arthur Asseraf, Sarah Bellows-Blakeley, Alli Cozic-Sova, Maëlig Cozic-Sova, Michelle Kuo, Alexandre Mallard, Vololona Rabehirasoa, Albert Wu, and many others made the stay worthy of la ville lumière. In Vietnam, I had the privilege of meeting Hazel Hahn, Chi Thuc Ha, Jason Picard, Pascal Bourdeaux, and Brynn Hatton. In Switzerland, Anne Burghardt, Ederi Ojasoo, and Peep Mardiste were excellent tour guides. My list of academic friends in Estonia is too long to enumerate, but I thank those who have had to suffer more than enough of my monologues about Indochinese industrial policy: Gustav Kalm, Maarja Kaaristo, Uku Lember, Linda Kaljundi, Riina Raudne, Toomas Lott, Marek Tamm, and Laur Kiik.

At Oxford University Press, Sarah Humphreville, Alexandra Dauler, and Bronwyn Geyer have been excellent, insightful, and responsive editors. Thanks, too, to the anonymous reviewers. Kate Blackmer deserves her reputation: she has produced amazing maps for this book. Tom Rosenbaum at the Rockefeller Archive Center, Michaël Davy at the Photothèque Institut Pasteur, and Robbi Siegel at Art Resource Inc. all helped with illustrations, as did Lori Rogers at the USC Department of History. Thanks to Cambridge University Press and Duke University Press for allowing me to include research originally published in the *Journal of Global History* and *French Historical Studies*. A special thanks to Katherine Marino for her support and advice in the final stages of the book.

I could not have written this book without the support of family, both chosen and inherited, on both sides of the Atlantic. They have celebrated with me in good times and supported me in turbulent times. Eero Janson, Mari Rebane, Erko Sõrmus, Keiu Virro, Paavo Piik, Kertu Moppel, Liina Pääbo, Mariliis Trei, Jackie Palmore, Armin Gollogly, Valeria Tsygankova, Emily Kern, Julia Harte, Timo McGregor, and Michelle Riegman: thank you. Whether visiting pigs in New York, scaling mountains in Poland, cooking vegan delights in Los Angeles, or exploring Ingmar Bergman's legacy in Sweden, Marysia Jonsson has been a source of inspiration, kindness, and laffs. My father, Toomas Velmet, has been a constant presence, across borders and time zones, over Skype, and over countless dinners and sauna sessions. Leelo Valgma's contribution to my well-being is impossible to describe in words.

My mother, Mary Velmet, did not live to see the completion of this book. In late 2015, she was diagnosed with a brain tumor. For several years, as I was completing my work at NYU, I lived in transit between the United States and Estonia and saw my entire family come together in mutual support, love, and resilience. It gave us all strength and brought us closer. I dedicate this book to her memory.

Note on Translations

Most French titles in common usage (i.e. governor-general) have been translated into English. Less common titles or titles without an obvious English equivalent have been left in the French original. When possible, I've tried to retain Vietnamese spellings of names and places, but in some cases French sources have rendered them without the requisite diacritical marks. Place names that have customary English or French equivalents (Hanoi, Saigon) have been rendered in those forms.

Introduction

Technology and Scale in Colonial Politics

At the dawn of the twentieth century, bacteriology and imperialism came to symbolize a new vision of the grandeur of France. A new epilogue, added to the iconic schoolbook of the Third Republic, *Two Children's Journey around France*, in 1905, celebrated the "promising start . . . to the century," first by tracing Louis Pasteur's advances in hygiene, vaccination, and agricultural improvement, and then moving to "the constitution of a new colonial empire, the largest after those of Russia and Britain."[1] As little Jean, the protagonist of the epilogue, learned from his well-traveled uncle, Monsieur Gertal, these two developments were intimately linked. Microbiological studies conducted at the Pasteur Institute of Nha Trang, in Indochina, protected colonizers and indigenous colonial subjects from diseases such as the plague; the institute also conducted agricultural studies that helped make the colony profitable. As this one small laboratory stood in for the glory of the French civilizing mission, one subheading of the epilogue made the moral lesson clear: "France, always generous, shares without limits, its blessings and its aid."[2] The textbook looked at Indochina solely through the lens of a bacteriologists' microscope. What it observed had the potential to change not just the French empire but the world.

This book investigates how the link between bacteriological technoscience and imperial governance was forged, deployed, and negotiated in Third Republic France, its colonies, and the international scientific arena. Historians, depending on their vantage points, have argued that the bacteriological revolution, akin to Schroedinger's cat, simultaneously did not happen and transformed everything.[3] Bacteriology produced new ideas about disease causation, reorganized knowledge around concepts such as "virulence," and led to the development of institutions such as the microbiological laboratory. Yet it also integrated simultaneously with existing sanitary-hygienist models of public health. Hygiene in France, after Pasteur as much as before, meant emphasizing moral regulation, policing living conditions, educating

Pasteur's Empire. Aro Velmet, Oxford University Press (2020). © Oxford University Press.
DOI: 10.1093/oso/9780190072827.001.0001

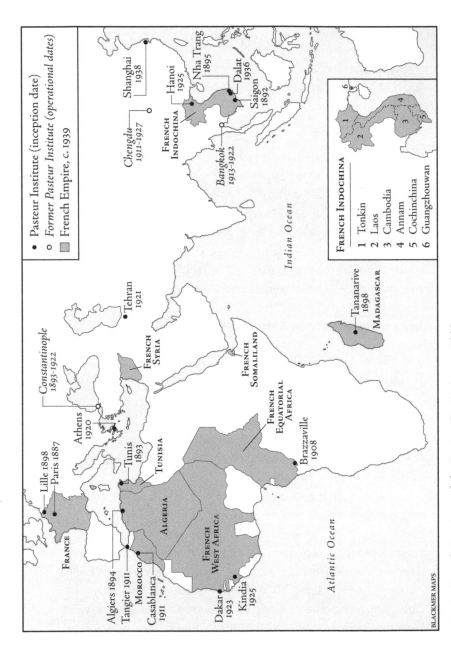

Map 1 French Empire and the Pasteur Institutes, ca. 1939.

Pasteur Institute (inception date)

○ *Former Pasteur Institute (operational dates)*

French Empire, c. 1939

Lille 1898

Paris 1887

FRANCE

Constantinople
1893–1922

Athens
1920

Tehran
1921

FRENCH
SYRIA

Tunis
1893

TUNISIA

Algiers 1894

Tangier 1911

MOROCCO

Casablanca
1911

ALGERIA

FRENCH
WEST AFRICA

Dakar
1923

Kindia
1925

FRENCH
EQUATORIAL
AFRICA

FRENCH
SOMALILAND

Brazzaville
1908

Atlantic Ocean

Indian Ocean

Tananarive
1898

MADAGASCAR

Chengdu
1911–1927

Shanghai
1938

Hanoi
1925

Nha Trang
1895

Dalat
1936

Saigon
1892

FRENCH
INDOCHINA

Bangkok
1913–1922

FRENCH INDOCHINA

1 Tonkin
2 Laos
3 Cambodia
4 Annam
5 Cochinchina
6 Guangzhouwan

BLACKMER MAPS

in sanitary discipline, and other social factors. Only theories of causation changed.

In the imperial world, scholars have shown how Western biomedicine became the basis for a "colonization of the body" or "biomedical citizenship."[4] After the 1880s, scientists and officials used the language of microbial contagion to inscribe new habits on subject populations, while simultaneously marking them as indelibly different from Europeans. Western hygiene, these scholars argue, channeled ever deeper and more invasive forms of imperial power.

The descriptions in *Journey around France* point toward a more complex dynamic. Monsieur Gertal discussed at length the hygienic state of metropolitan France, emphasizing the various moral, social, and medical reforms required to combat tuberculosis, alcoholism, and depopulation. However, in discussing the colonies, Gertal and the children excluded the living conditions of colonial subjects entirely and focused only on the microbiological transformations accomplished with the microscope and the syringe.[5] Rather than governing people, cities, and environments, colonial bacteriology was about the management of microbes. The meaning of French bacteriology changed as it moved from metropole to empire.

In tracing this movement, *Pasteur's Empire* pursues several connected questions. What did bacteriology, as a method, a social community, a technological practice, and a form of government, look like *in motion*, between metropole, different colonies, and international scientific communities? How did local actors respond to and reshape bacteriological reforms? How did bacteriologists see themselves, their mission, their politics, and their ethics as they moved between various sites? What kinds of factors—human and nonhuman, institutional and cultural, material and ideological—shaped the fate of bacteriology and the empire to which it increasingly linked itself?

In France, Louis Pasteur's reputation neared that of a saint. He had discovered the role of bacteria in causing illness (the "germ theory of disease"), improved French viticulture and livestock farming, and invented the rabies vaccine. By his death in 1895, Pasteur had successfully, though after much conflict, reoriented public health officials' understanding of hygiene to include the elimination of germs from the urban environment. In 1887, the scientist founded the Pasteur Institute on rue Dutot (today rue du Docteur Roux, after its famous director), hoping it would propel his research forward into the new century and train generations of new microbiologists—Pastorians—in the methods and ethics of the discipline's founder.[6]

The empire, this book argues, profoundly changed the methods and aims of Pastorian bacteriology; Pastorians then reshaped the empire in turn. This process required work, and the accumulation of resources and allies. When Pasteur's student Albert Calmette founded the first bacteriological laboratory in French Indochina in 1891, he faced immediate opposition from French administrators who feared that Calmette's "humanitarian endeavors" would divert from the more urgent task of "pacifying" the newly acquired colonies. Meanwhile, fellow bacteriologists in Paris, who paid lip service to the role of science in the civilizing mission, betrayed through their skepticism toward many colonial ventures the conviction that *real* research was done in the metropole.

Pastorians—as these students of Pasteur called themselves—ultimately melded their work with France's vision of its empire and embedded themselves in its governance. From 1890 to 1939, Pasteur Institutes spread from Saigon to the rest of Indochina, then to French colonies in North Africa—Algeria, Tunisia, and Morocco—and finally to French West Africa (Afrique Occidentale Française [AOF]) and French Equatorial Africa (Afrique Équatoriale Française [AEF]). Other scientists set up Pasteur Institutes beyond the empire, including in Constantinople, Rio de Janeiro, Athens, and St. Petersburg. Researchers at the institutes did groundbreaking work on the bubonic plague, malaria, typhus, sleeping sickness, and yellow fever, as well as on industrial agricultural methods ranging from treating rinderpest (an infectious disease of ruminants, especially cattle) to inventing new forms of distilling industrial alcohol. While recognizing that much of the Pastorians' overseas work extended beyond colonial borders, *Pasteur's Empire* argues for understanding bacteriology as a specifically *imperial* project.[7] The association of microbes with the civilizing mission created a privileged space where administrators, bacteriologists, and imperial subjects could debate and shape the science.

The "colonial situation" shaped the kinds of research Pastorians pursued; the methods with which they pursued it; their own self-perception as scientists, explorers, and imperial agents; and their power in scientific struggles *outside* the boundaries of Greater France.[8] While public health reformers in metropolitan France, from bacteriologists, to hygienists and sanitationists, talked about health and governance in increasingly socioecological terms, Pastorians in the empire argued for the primacy of the human-microbe interaction and turned to microbiological technologies—principally vaccines, sera, and ferments—as their primary mode of intervention. The central contention of *Pasteur's Empire* is that this shift to the technological management of microbes was not accidental but was structured by colonial context. This Pastorian approach generated its own microbial politics, which scientists, administrators, and colonial subjects could sometimes harness but never fully control. Exploring this new model of microbial management, which I term "pastorization," helps us rethink the history of French imperial rule and places bacteriology at the heart of early twentieth-century experiments in global governance.

Pastorization, a Technopolitical Strategy

Pasteur's empire was a collaborative project, and in the process of construction, what exactly was being built and who the architects were became increasingly unclear. Though Pastorians liked to think they were in charge, the institutions and political aims of colonial bacteriology were shaped by actors both much larger and far smaller than the Pastorian scientist. Colonial administrators, businessmen, colonial subjects, and international scientific bodies, but also microbes, vaccines, syringes, epidemiological surveys, lab animals, and human test subjects all shaped the kinds of politics that pastorization could advance.

The term "politics" means here the assertion and distribution of power among various actors and groups in society. The exercise of political power means, as one common definition would have it, the ability to get a person or a group to do what they otherwise would not do.[9] This definition extends beyond the boundaries of parliamentary or party politics. It includes the material and discursive methods by which experts establish their authority within decision-making bodies and the use of technical knowledge by colonial administrators and business leaders, but also the methods by which colonial subjects exercise agency within their communities and with or against the interests of the colonial state. In short, politics is the process through which one group claims the right to act and to direct the actions of others.

Because actors consciously used bacteriological technoscience to advance political goals, I analyze pastorization as a *technopolitical* strategy.[10] This concept helps to highlight the entanglement of Pastorian politics with microbial life as well as with the various technical and scientific infrastructures that rendered microbes legible and manipulable by humans, a feature that sets it apart from other forms of colonial governance. Specifically, *Pasteur's Empire* develops four dimensions of Pastorian technopolitics: (1) the use of micro-biological technologies to empower or foreclose political choices; (2) the effects of these technologies on constraining political options; (3) the rhetor-ical and spectacular power of microbiological technologies; and (4) the role of technological infrastructures in shaping the masculine ethos of Pastorian science.

First, pastorization provided colonial administrators with seemingly low-cost, "magic bullet" solutions to public health crises. This allowed officials to maintain the hands-off, intermediary-based regime of colonial rule and keep the cost of running public health programs at a minimum. It was also a con-sciously *universal* method, which allowed Pastorians to import technologies from any setting where they could identify a pathogenic microbe, irrespec-tive of differences in social and political conditions. As such, pastorization differed from the metropolitan focus on social medicine, which emphasized local specificity, the built environment, and climate and therefore required both complex local knowledge and substantial investment in public health infrastructure. In other words, pastorization created a pan-imperial scope for public health work, promised to run it on the cheap, and placed Pastorians at its center. This strategy was not unique to the Pastorians—other empires, too, pursued vaccination programs and other "pastorian" interventions. Vector control was standard policy for public health programs in Latin America, sponsored by the American Rockefeller Foundation.[11] Nor was pastorization the only game in the French empire: naval medical officers, Catholic doctors, and visiting specialists all brought their own notions of hygiene into the French colonies, many of them echoing the principles of social hygiene in vogue in Paris, others deriving from a long tradition of tropical medicine. Yet only in the French context did Pastorian interventions become a coherent strategy, with official backing from the Ministry of the Colonies in France and the support of officials on the ground from Saigon to Dakar.

Pastorian technoscience could both open and foreclose political options. In some cases, it justified otherwise contentious colonial reforms in the name of the advanced biotechnological innovation in diverse domains—from labor relations and freedom of association, to questions of race and impe-rial humanitarianism. In Indochina, officials restructured industrial policy and monopolized rice alcohol and opium production, claiming this would help introduce Pastorian fermentation methods and render production safer and more efficient. In the AOF, Pastorian studies on yellow fever vac-cination helped assuage racial conflict created by older methods of epidemic disease containment, which focused on segregation and quarantine. Most often, however, pastorization narrowed the boundaries of public health, particularly compared with models of social hygiene, which could encompass domains ranging from public works to social policy. When confronted with demands for better housing or shorter working hours in the name of disease prevention and hygiene, colonial officials could point to a Pastorian technological solution, a vaccine or serum, as the primary method of defense, and deflect broader demands for social rights in the name of bacteriological expertise. Analyzing pastorization as a technopolitical strategy allows us to foreground the shifting boundaries between technical expertise and overtly political claims-making and observe how administrators, scientists, and colonial subjects challenged each other in this boundary work.[12]

Second, Pastorians designed their technologies for political ends, but they never had full control over the means. The material and biological features of pastorian technoscience set unexpected constraints on human actors. Sometimes, biological and material reality forced Pastorians to make political decisions they would have preferred to avoid. Georges Stefanopoulo's decision to cultivate a yellow fever vaccine in the brains of mice led to serious cases of encephalitis in some test patients and raised the question of who was to be the ideal recipient of such a dangerous vaccine. In other situations, scientific decisions, once they were inscribed into law, fit into supply chains, and built into industrial machinery, locked French officials into decisions that were materially difficult to reverse, even when they proved politically costly. Once rice wine production in colonial Indochina had been "pastorized," it became nearly impossible to return to local production methods, although the product's unsatisfying taste led to political strife across the colony.

Third, the rhetorical importance placed on pastorization, as a universal method and pinnacle of French science, simultaneously empowered and undermined its technopolitical force. The Pastorians' single-minded focus on microbes and humans gave the method its high level of abstraction, attractive to administrators who moved from one colony to another and preferred having their expertise move with them. Pastorization's ambition of universal application, independent of race, environment, or society, made it a powerful representation of the civilizing mission, confirming rhetorically that colonization was, at its heart, a humanitarian project. Yet such a lofty promise was impossible to fulfill, and colonial subjects quickly adopted the language of Pasteur to demand satisfaction their money back. Pastorian methods, which promised to work equally well in Dakar and Da Nang, often failed precisely because such universal models obscured local social, infrastructural, and political obstacles from planners' view. Critics of bacteriological grandeur, whether international rivals or African or Vietnamese activists, could then point to the chasm between the Pastorians' lofty rhetoric and the far more ambiguous reality, demanding concessions. When Pastorians enrolled microbes and technological tools in their political projects, they became dependent on microbial cooperation. Microbes, it turned out, were fickle allies.[13]

Fourth, the scientific practices, technological tools, and politics developed in the empire all shaped how bacteriologists understood their scientific, masculine ethos. Over time, many colonial Pastorians styled themselves not as dispassionate and ascetic laborers but as conquerors committed to capitalism and empire. This ethos, articulated in terms of "virility," "potency," and "regeneration," prescribed new attitudes towards industry, the state, and scientific competitors. Increasingly, colonial Pastorians such as Charles Nicolle and Albert Calmette sought to reorient the Parisian head institute, the affectionately named *maison-mère* along these lines, believing it to provide more opportunities for Pastorian self-actualization as *men*. The politics of bacteriological governance in the colonies reshaped relations within the broader Pastorian network and within the French scientific community at large. Pastorians changed the empire, but in the process, the empire changed them.

The Problem of Scale as Analysis and as Politics

The geographical scope of Pastorian research poses both an analytical challenge and a historical problem. The analytical challenge is: How do we study bacteriology in the age of empire, a process that involved at once the manipulation of microscopic worlds within a single laboratory, interactions with colonial and imperial actors, and movement across the globe, from Nha Trang to New York, Geneva to Guinea? The sheer variety of contexts that demand the historian's attention is staggering. The shape of the Pastorian yellow fever vaccine was determined by the variability of the yellow fever virus when grown in the brains of lab mice; by experimental protocol in a laboratory in Lagos leading to an unexpected infection; by the racial politics of the city of Dakar, which the Pasteur Institute could exploit to jump-start its own research program; by the existence of correspondence networks between Pastorians in Dakar and other bacteriologists in Nigeria, the United States, and England; and by the rivalry between two transnational institutions operating on three continents with different national and epistemological commitments. How should our analysis be structured, so that it does not turn from explanation to itemization?[14] And, then, there is the historical problem, simply put: How did the Pastorians accomplish this?

Both historians of empire and historians of science have long recognized Jacques Revel's call to not assume a single predetermined context into which actors' decisions can be fit, but their ways of attending to the multiplicity of contexts, to the "play of scales," have been different.[15] Historians of empire have recognized the "nation" as an inadequate container, the category requiring explanation, rather than the explanatory frame. They have thus increasingly looked at networks and connections, attending to the movement of people and ideas across borders and territories. These analyses foreground that some boundaries (often imperial) matter more than others, and that cross-border networks are necessarily lumpy and uneven, with some people having more agency in choosing their trajectories, and others being forced to move, or not moving at all.[16] Historians of science, by contrast, tend to zoom in, looking at "centers of calculation"—laboratories, factories, international commissions, where scientists and engineers marshal their allies, whether microbial or intergovernmental, and pull them together into research papers, blueprints, and patents.[17] Historians can then unpack the range of actors and contexts involved in shaping the day-to-day work of a toxicology lab in Senegal or a small group of urban planners in England, showing how a local institution is made by and generative of national, imperial, and global currents.[18]

Pasteur's Empire proposes an alternative approach, one focused on the creation of and movement between multiple centers of calculation. It highlights how the center of Pastorian gravity could shift depending on the projects the scientists were working on, and the circumstances of their work. Moving could have profound political consequences. Alexandre Yersin's suggestions for a plague containment program could be transformed in transit from Hong Kong to Saigon. The parameters of a yellow fever vaccine could change as it moved from Paris to West Africa. The reliability and safety of bacillus Calmette-Guérin (BCG) appeared different when the vaccine was used in Paris or in Indochina.[19] In a number of instances (in particular chapters 1, 3, 5, and 7), therefore, this book centers on the *politics* of mobility.

Our other analytical tool attempts to answer the historical problem: How did the Pastorians acquire this range of mobility? Pastorians did not simply fit themselves into a variety of contexts. Very often, bacteriological research itself *generated* new contexts. As Pastorians integrated themselves in colonial politics, they convinced officials, doctors, experts, and activists of diverse origins that accomplishing their political objectives in any particular colony required working on a microscopic scale while using tools that had a potentially global scope. Pastorians, in short, had a politics of scale. They created ways of seeing microbial life in human politics—the yeast in Indochinese industrial policy, the yellow fever virus in West African race relations— and convinced others that the proper scale for studying these microbes was the empire, and perhaps the world.[20] This study looks at the work done to bring microscopic organisms into human-scale, and indeed imperial-scale, politics whether by the Pastorians themselves (chapter 2) or by rival actors using the language of biomedicine (chapters 5 and 6). In other instances, it investigates how scientists reframed colonial problems such as political stability (chapter 1) or the impact of modern civilization (chapter 5) as imperial, or even global, problems that the Pastorians were well-positioned to solve, precisely because of the scope of their network.

Imperial infrastructure and political priorities supported Pastorian scale- making projects. Other imaginaries constrained them. The most important were emerging international scientific institutions and the countervailing networks of colonial subjects who became increasingly adept at mobilizing biomedical language to their own ends. In the early 1900s, and during the interwar years in particular, organizations aimed at facilitating information exchange, establishing common standards, and setting ethical guidelines led to new debates in which Pastorians had to defend their vaccines, containment programs, and research agendas. Vietnamese journalists, activists, and doctors and African representatives, activists, and soldiers all traveled, acquired allies in France and elsewhere, and pushed back against Pastorian reforms, often using the language of social hygiene and microbiology. Sometimes, their action shifted Pastorian agendas. In other cases, Pastorians adapted. The game of scales was rigged for the Pastorians, who defined the terms of engagement and moved more easily between international, imperial, colonial, and microbial dimensions. But they were still only players; others, if they had good strategies, good allies, or good luck, could also play to win.

Bacteriology between National, Imperial, and International Visions of Health

The Pasteur Institute was born into a transforming world. In the fin de siècle, scientists across Europe, the United States, and Asia, were challenging, if not fully transforming, dogmas of medical science and public health. Louis Pasteur stirred French science through his work on the microbial causes of anthrax in France. In England, Ronald Ross demonstrated the importance of the mosquito vector in malaria, and Joseph Lister introduced sterilization to surgery.[21] Robert Koch's work on tuberculosis made him the German candidate for the title of "father of bacteriology," and the work of Japanese bacteriologists Kitasato Shibasaburō and Hideyo Noguchi led to Nobel Prize nominations in the early 1900s.[22] Advances in science accompanied military advances: in the 1880s and 1890s, French and British empires expanded to cover most of Africa and consolidated their grip on Asian colonies; the French formally colonized northern Vietnam, Cambodia, and Laos, and all European powers chipped away at Chinese sovereignty.[23] Finally, Pasteur's empire emerged at a time of dense, though uneven, global connectivity, which included the rise of various international bodies, from sanitary conferences to professional societies, dedicated to scientific exchange.[24] In charting how Pastorians navigated these new conditions, *Pasteur's Empire* connects, complements, and challenges their respective historiographies as well: the history of bacteriology, the history of imperial governance, and the history of medical globalization.

The nineteenth century was the century of hygiene. In response to industrialization and urbanization, and in conjunction with the emergence of statistical sciences, intellectuals and reformers developed disciplines of public health. They investigated how social, environmental, and moral conditions influenced the health of communities and national populations. Elite concerns over contagious epidemics, and the need for healthy laborers and soldiers drove research, as they often do. Influential studies catalyzed action. Edwin Chadwick's reports on the health of English workers (1842 and 1843), Louis-Réne Villermé's tableau of the moral and physical condition of French workers (1840), and Rudolph Virchow's articles in the journal *Medical Reform* all framed health as essentially a social and moral issue, interchangeable with other social ills, such as crime, poverty, and licentiousness. Countries established public health boards, constructed sewage systems, and put in place building codes, turning personal cleanliness and the elimination of filth into a responsibility toward the nation.[25] From the 1850s onward, the tension between early nineteenth-century statist contagionists and liberal anticontagionists gave way to a broad consensus, where the state assumed responsibility for hygiene, clean citizens became markers of a strong nation, and the moral and physical health of the individual body became a proxy for the health of the social body.[26] In the United States, the case of Mary Mallon—better known as "Typhoid Mary"—showed how the New York City Health Department was willing to use a hygienic state of exception to curtail basic freedoms in the name of the public's health.[27] In Germany, Virchow became one of the prominent cheerleaders of Otto von Bismarck's social reforms.[28] Hygiene became a marker of civilizational progress and was taken up by non-Western powers as well, most notably in Japan, China, and the Ottoman Empire.[29]

France was central to both the rise of modern public health and bacteriological science. The French Revolution declared health a right of a democratic citizenry, established the first Institute of Hygiene in 1794, and sponsored statistical studies of populations around the country. France led the way intellectually; in politics, it embodied the central tension in nineteenth-century social reform: between a belief in the ameliorative power of reason and commitment to laissez-faire liberalism. Though the Paris Board of Health was established already in 1802, and the provinces followed suit by 1822, effective regulation remained haphazard for some time. From the 1850s onward, however, the state—or, more likely, municipal authorities—began to construct sewers and monitor residential salubrity.[30] Nowhere but France did hygiene gather such obsessive levels of public attention, guiding discussions of sexuality, criminality, mental health, urban planning, morality, and physical health alike.[31] And nowhere but France did bacteriology attain an almost religious level of reverence, and Louis Pasteur, the godfather of bacteriology, the status of a national saint.[32]

Third Republic France, born out of a crushing military defeat against Prussia in 1870, had a uniquely low birth rate in the Western world. Experts, critics, and legislators alike came to see both hygiene and bacteriology as potential solutions to the variety of social and moral conflicts generated by tensions between republicanism, urbanization, and industrialization. David Barnes has termed this mixture of hygienic principles linking health to society, morality, and the environment with bacteriological ideas of the microbial causation of disease the "Sanitary-Bacteriological Synthesis."[33] Setting the genesis of the Pasteur Institute in the context of nineteenth-century hygiene explains the ambitions of Pastorians and the level of attention accorded to them by metropolitan statesmen and journalists as they were moving their operations into the colonies.

This standard chronology, however, also poses problems by folding bacteriology into the history of Western hygienic modernity writ large. Indeed, even though many historians have highlighted the role of colonial networks in the making of Pasteurian science, from Alexandre Yersin's discovery of the plague microbe to Charles Nicolle's Nobel Prize–winning research on typhus, they have often reinforced the intellectual flexibility of bacteriology and its cohesion with developments in the metropole.[34] Kim Pelis sees Nicolle's identity as an "imperial missionary" to follow from Pasteur's dictum to "go forth and educate the nations of the world."[35] Anne-Marie Moulin describes the "elastic ideology" of overseas Pastorians as having interacted with colonialism with "relative autonomy."[36] Bruno Latour, too, in his magisterial study *The Pasteurization of France*, shows bacteriology as a force enrolling the empire to advocate on its behalf but assumes that bacteriology itself remained unchanged in this process.[37] The point, however, is neither to show bacteriology as essentially flexible and part of a larger project of hygienic modernity nor to claim for it a specificity and rigidity that establish it as a revolutionary science. The point is precisely that Pastorians were flexible or rigid *strategically*. In the metropole, the language of bacteriology melded with social hygiene, while Pastorians in the colonies increasingly saw the two modes of intervention as in opposition. In the interwar years, as enthusiasm for social medicine grew internationally, Pastorians used their colonial resources to convince France and the world of the viability of their "magic bullets."

A central problem in the historiography of colonialism, in health as in many other domains, is the tension between the ideology of a "civilizing mission" and its limited impact on the ground. Scholars have argued that colonial public health produced "biomedical citizenship," "medicalization," or "hygienic modernity."[38] This ideology justified vast expansions of state power and intensified imperial control over the bodies of colonial subjects, while always keeping them at arm's length from the colonizers. Hygiene, in this view, was part of a broader array of Western scientific discourses— ethnography, studies of sexuality, and others—through which distinctions between European colonizers and the indigenous peoples of Africa and Asia were articulated and reproduced.[39] In the French empire, this "civilizing mission" provided colonial officials with a justification for radical reforms, which included the abolition of precolonial institutions—slavery, customary law, chieftainships, and local languages—and the development of modern infrastructure, industry, education, and health institutions, all designed to inculcate subjects with the habits of proper (i.e., French) civilization.[40]

Yet these projects never amounted to all that much on the ground. The constraints of running an empire on the cheap reined in administrators. Colonial power in the pre–World War II French empire (with the exception of Algeria) was, in reality, thin. Administrators, numbering fewer than in a middling French province, ran territories much larger than France itself, largely with the help of local intermediaries. Colonies had to balance their budgets, since Paris was unwilling to invest money in their development. Officials had to mediate conflicts with missionaries, businessmen, and foreign agents, all of whom carried significant political clout.[41] Accordingly, studies of hygienic modernity have been complemented by work showing the limits of Western medical practices, the thinness of its power, and the degrees to which Western medical expertise mixed with local knowledge and sometimes even worked against the interests of the colonizers.[42]

Pasteur's Empire argues that bacteriology offered an ideology and a set of tools, which allowed politicians in Paris and administrators in the colonies to resolve this conflict between boundless ambition and tightly bound reality. Vietnamese and African activists turned out to be quite adept at using the language of social health to demand improved housing, education, and labor rights, as well as the abolition of coercive and racist policies of quarantine and forced segregation. Discourses of Pastorian progress functioned precisely to *contain* the expansion of public health promises. Bacteriologists in the colonies came to see their role as that of limited technical experts, not as philosopher-kings.

The Pastorian age, with its focus on spectacle, universalizing promises, and increasingly profit-oriented ambitions, on the one hand, and its consciously limited scope, technical focus, and suspicion of social determinants of health, on the other, resembles more the current era of global health than cautiously optimistic histories of early twentieth-century international institutions would allow.[43] Scholars working on the League of Nations Health Organization (LNHO), as well as a variety of humanitarian catastrophes, such as the Congo-Ocean railway, emphasize how international bodies created forums, where issues of health, nutrition, and labor could be raised and debated, if not addressed.[44] In the domain of health, Deborah Neill has argued, the shared "epistemic community" of tropical doctors reinforced international connections and solidarities.[45] Paul Weindling, Iris Borowy, and others have seen the LNHO as a significant, if limited, force countervailing the dominant currents of nationalism and isolation that characterized the interwar years.[46] By contrast, scholars of twenty-first-century global health are more likely to highlight "the persistence of the colonial past in the biomedical present," revealing how the work of humanitarian organizations in the Global South is predicated on unequal relationships forged in the age of empire.[47]

In examining the movement of bacteriologists between France, colonies, and international institutions, *Pasteur's Empire* argues that organizations such as the LNHO, the Office International d'Hygiène Publique, and the International Health Division (IHD) of the Rockefeller Foundation brought interimperial competition into stark relief. New arenas for international debate incentivized the Great Powers to rely more, rather than less, on their colonial resources. The LNHO developed new, uniform epidemiological and experimental standards. In meeting those standards, however, Pastorians turned to what is known today as "regulatory arbitrage." In other words, they took advantage of lax oversight in the colonies in comparison to the metropole. Similarly, competition with the self-consciously internationalist Rockefeller Foundation's IHD generated distrust among French and British researchers, who all sought American funding for their yellow fever projects in Dakar and Lagos. Increased global connections only heightened the importance of long-established imperial networks.

Continuities between the "heroic" Pastorian age and the current global health era of spectacular, yet insufficient, interventionism are largely effaced by the outsize reputation of the Pastorians in France and the postcolonial world alike. It is no accident that the only French street names left in Ho Chi Minh City are named after Louis Pasteur, Albert Calmette, and Alexandre Yersin. As Noémi Tousignant, P. Wenzel Geissler, and others have documented, the dire state of African health infrastructure today rests on the ruins of post–World War II developmental colonialism and the brief period of *coopération* after political independence, when the French state invested in postcolonial research institutions and helped usher in a generation of local experts who took custody of them.[48] From the vantage point offered by this book, however, the current era looks much like a postcolonial return to Pasteur's empire, not simply a retreat from postwar developmentalism.

The chapters of this book trace the construction of Pasteur's empire, with an equal focus on its microbial and global building blocks. Each chapter follows a particular scientific and political project, from its initial articulation through development, contestation, and praxis, highlighting different aspects of Pastorian technopolitics. Together, these chapters trace the history of the Pastorians' colonial network, its rise, expansion, and contestation, and also develop a series of conceptual interventions required to help explain this historical change. Chapter 1 centers on the role of interimperial and international networks in the emergence of a specifically Pastorian disease ecology; it shows how Alexandre Yersin's movement between British, Chinese, and French empires and up the ranks of the colonial hierarchy shaped his epistemological commitments. Chapter 2 turns to local technopolitics and shows how engineering decisions surrounding the production of intoxicants shaped industrial policy in French Indochina. Subsequent chapters investigate the Pastorian expansion across colonies and their relationship with international organizations, focusing on the Pastorians' heroic masculinity (chapter 3), the construction of a pan-imperial Pastorian epidemiology (chapter 4), and the role of the empire in the deployment of BCG (chapter 5). Finally, the case of yellow fever in West Africa shows how biological agents—viruses and mosquitoes—could shift racial politics (chapter 6) and foregrounds the interplay between microbial and global politics in the construction of the yellow fever vaccine (chapter 7). Punctured by a brief period of developmentalist colonialism and cooperation in the postwar era, the legacy of pastorization continues to shape policy in the postcolonial world. The apparent success of Pastorian projects generates new enthusiasm for magic bullets; experience with "hygienic" intoxicant monopolies in Indochina or deadly vaccinations in West Africa has catalyzed opposition to Western promises of Pastorian modernity. Pasteur's ghost seems to be everywhere in the postcolonial world; it is given life by a diverse set of alliances that were hard to forge and that remained always unreliable. This book is about the politics of those alliances.

1

The Invention of Pastorization

The coalition between Pastorians and colonial administrators has a history. It began in French Indochina in the late nineteenth century. In 1891, Albert Calmette established the first bacteriological laboratory in Saigon but found little support from colonial administrators. Like the Pasteur Institute in Paris, the Saigon laboratory offered primarily vaccinations against rabies. This mattered little in Indochina, where the disease was rare. Colonial officials were more concerned with pacifying newly conquered territories than sponsoring research without immediate practical benefits. In 1893, another bacteriologist, Alexandre Yersin volunteered to study plague outbreaks in the Chinese province of Yunnan, just north of French Tonkin. The governor-general of Indochina, Jean-Marie de Lanessan (a doctor by training), remained uncooperative, stating: "There has never been plague in Yunnan, and if it was to appear, I should deny it; the burden of poor Tonkin is heavy enough without laying the plague on its back as well."[1]

This chapter charts the emergence of the Pastorian alignment with French officials in colonial Indochina. It shows how "pastorization," the public health model that won the support of the colonial state, developed in international debates over political stability, commerce, and Great Power cooperation. Its emergence is set in the context of the great plague pandemic, which spread on cargo ships and passenger boats from China to Hong Kong, then to British India, and then across the world. In 1894, on a mission to Hong Kong, Alexandre Yersin discovered the causative agent of the plague—the microbe *Yersinia pestis*. A few years later, another Pastorian, Paul-Louis Simond, identified rats as the primary agent of transmission.[2] Scientists and historians have highlighted the seminal importance of this moment in the history of bacteriology. Andrew Cunningham has argued that the discovery of the plague cemented the laboratory as the site of defining disease identity. Bruno Latour showed how Yersin's description of the plague microbe linked laboratory science to the broader concerns of social hygiene.[3] But in terms of state responses to epidemics, scholars argue, the bacteriological revolution changed little, whether in the colonies or in European metropoles. Indeed,

Pasteur's Empire. Aro Velmet, Oxford University Press (2020). © Oxford University Press.
DOI: 10.1093/oso/9780190072827.001.0001

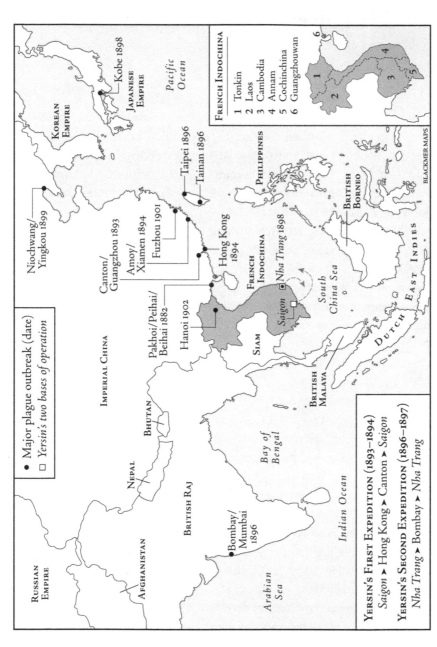

Map 2 Alexandre Yersin's plague expeditions.

many scholars credit the success of germ theories of disease *precisely* to the fact that they "did not require colonial officials to change any of the routines they had used to control disease in the past."[4]

In French Indochina, however, Pastorian bacteriology itself changed, and it changed state thinking about epidemics in turn. In the plague years, growing international attention, changing political needs, and new bacteriological tools allowed Pastorians and colonial administrators to work out their relationship and reconfigure the political boundaries of plague containment measures, leading to the emergence of "pastorization"—the technopolitical strategy that would become the backbone of the cooperation between Pastorians and imperial rulers. This chapter charts the shift in Pastorian responses to the plague. It surveys Yersin's initial reporting from British Hong Kong, which critiqued coercive containment policies and recommended cooperation with indigenous authorities. It ends with the set of measures that emerged under Pastorian guidance at the International Sanitary Conferences in the early 1900s, focusing on technical interventions, namely, claytonized disinfection, vaccination, and the destruction of microbe-carrying rats. These measures were technical fixes, which the Pastorians portrayed as "civilized," cheap, effective, uncoercive, and conservative (in the sense that they did not imply radical changes to the colonial situation). This narrow approach extended the geographical reach of the Pastorians. Once bacteriologists imagined the local sociopolitical and environmental context as essentially passive, Pastorians could import containment measures from places as far as away as Copenhagen was from Dakar.

The new, "pastorized" strategies were rarely very effective, as they overlooked various ecological, political, and infrastructural problems in specific colonial locales. Indeed, prefects and public health boards in Indochina—and even Yersin himself—quickly fell back on older strategies, such as the incineration of infected houses or the establishment of sanitary cordons, using them in conjunction with Pastorian methods. Yet Pastorian containment measures were politically useful in other ways. They projected competence and hygienic modernity to both colonial subjects and France's imperial competitors.[5] Officials in Indochina and elsewhere could reassure trading partners and international bodies, on the one hand, and Vietnamese and Cambodian elites, on the other. Pastorian methods communicated that the French had cutting-edge tools to prevent the spread of the disease. Their means were *civilized*, and officials could claim they resorted to coercive methods only in the last instance. Failures of

Pastorian policies were blamed not on the limits of Western expertise but on the inability of local populations to properly cooperate.

The Genesis of the Pasteur Institute's Imperial Mission

The overseas Pasteur Institutes were born in the middle of the bacteriological revolution. This new discipline had a particularly powerful impact in France, through the work of Louis Pasteur. The scientist rose to national fame through a series of public experiments. He showed how microorganisms caused fermentation, arguing that the seemingly spontaneous generation of life in hermetic flasks was actually the product of microbial activity and that anthrax vaccination could prevent livestock from dying. Pasteur linked his spectacular experiments to explosive political and cultural issues of the day. His experiments disproving spontaneous generation became central to debates between evolutionists and Catholics. The former argued, following Jean-Baptiste Lamarck, Étienne Geoffroy Saint-Hilaire, and, of course, Charles Darwin, that the spontaneous generation of living matter proved the veracity of a materialist worldview, while the latter used Pasteur's work to argue that in biological processes, life could only be transformed and not generated.[6] Pasteur's research had equally many practical uses. The development of pasteurization—the heating of liquids to a temperature of between sixty and one hundred degrees Celsius, killing bacteria and molds within them—made beer and milk safer and extended their shelf life. Pasteur's work on fermentation prolonged the lifespan of wines. His vaccines brought tangible benefits to farmers struggling with anthrax and, most famously, provided a method for preventing rabies, a relatively rare but tortuous and fatal disease.

By the 1880s, Pasteur's ideas had been widely accepted by social hygienists, who dominated expert discourse. The bourgeoisie and the popular classes, who talked increasingly of sanitation and the preventing the spread of germs, embraced Pasteur's thought as well.[7] Public health boards routinely prescribed measures such as disinfection and isolation for halting epidemics, ordered laboratory studies of potable water, and put in place hygiene guidelines in schools. Still, Pasteur's ideas faced stiff resistance, particularly by the "medical mandarins" of the Academy of Medicine, who accused the scientist of overreach or even incompetence.[8] The death of a vaccinated child in 1886 created particular controversy. Opponents of Pasteur blamed the vaccine, and popular journals reminded readers of Pasteur's "bonapartism," suggesting that he was claiming credit for medical advances that properly belonged to social hygienists.[9] Pasteur remained frustrated with the unwillingness of the medical establishment to accept his vaccines. The foundation of the Pasteur Institute and its expansion into Indochina therefore have to be seen in the context of Pasteur's ongoing struggle for legitimation, the expansion of the French empire, and the creation of the Colonial Health Service (Service de Santé [SdS]).

The Pasteur Institute became a way for the scientist to distance himself both from the state, which—mistakenly, in Pasteur's view—resisted making vaccination compulsory in deference to the liberal values of the republic, and from the medico-scientific establishment, where his most staunch opponents resided.[10] It was a self-consciously international means for capitalizing on the rabies vaccine, distributing it to patients "not just in France, but in Europe, Russia and even North America."[11] Finally, the new center would become a hub of bacteriological research, where a new generation of scholars from all over the world would be able to research and publish new bacteriological discoveries. To that end, Pasteur proposed establishing a house journal for the institute—*Annales de l'Institut Pasteur*—"a more intimate and less solemn [publication] than the proceedings of the Academy of Sciences," as well as prizes and honors to inspire bacteriological research elsewhere.[12] Opened to great fanfare in 1888, the Pasteur Institute was supported by an international fund drive, which raised nearly 3 million francs and included donors ranging from Nicholas II, the Russian tsar, to Peter II, the emperor of Brazil.[13]

The laboratory was a success. By the 1890s, the microbiology course taught by Émile Roux, Pasteur's closest collaborator, had become a legendary feature in the Parisian medical landscape, attracting, among others, two young medical men: an aspiring Swiss physician called Alexandre Yersin, and a naval doctor named Albert Calmette. Both men excelled at Roux's bacteriology course but felt out of place in the Parisian scientific world. They pined for the colonies, and soon enough, changes in imperial administration would provide them with an opportunity to leave.

In the 1880s and early 1890s, France began to consolidate its conquests in North Africa, West Africa, and Indochina, conducting extensive missions of "pacification" in some regions and replacing military officials with civilian administrators in others. Politicians in Paris sought to streamline colonial administrations and regularize their governance, leading to the creation of an independent Ministry of the Colonies in 1894. Questions of development—*mise-en-valeur*—became salient again; after all, the very purpose of colonization was the economic empowerment of France. Naval medicine already had accumulated its own schools, institutions, and career tracks. Policymakers in Paris imagined that these could now become the basis for a Colonial Health Service, providing a steady career for the would-be explorers, with promises of long leaves in France and more stability than a traditional naval career.[14] The Health Service was finally created in 1890 and tasked with both the safeguarding of the health of the colonizers and—for the first time—improving the sanitary state of the *indigènes*. In the words of its head, Georges Treille, the SdS would "limit [colonial health institutions] not just parsimoniously to the defense of hygiene, . . . but making it the basis of our entire civilizing mission."[15] According to this vision, the doctor would become the representative of "the administration even in the remotest district," demonstrating the moral and technological superiority of the French and lifting the prosperity of the colonies almost as if by osmosis.[16]

The organizers of France's new medical mission adopted an eclectic, often contradictory, set of views. Their plans contained the geographical determinism of naval doctors, the principles of social hygiene dominating France, as well as the vaccine- and serum-oriented bacteriology of the Pasteur Institute. Treille himself was committed to a climatic view of disease. He believed that certain illnesses were specific to certain locales and environmental conditions, and that the health of different races was ultimately a function of their natural geographical habitat. He argued even that under "normal" circumstances, "white races" in the colonies would never be able to maintain population levels without immigration.[17] At the same time, he believed that hygiene, when combined with medical geography, could improve the health of the colonizers in the short term and accelerate the conquest of the colonies.[18] This could mean a moral and hygienic re-education of *indigènes*, "who were, until now, abandoned to the mortal fatalism of their traditional customs and social practices"; it could mean urban renewal and the construction of sewage systems, but it could also mean vaccination and bacteriological research focused principally on fighting specific epidemics.[19] In his writings, Treille outlined an ambitious agenda for the new Health Service, drawing on all traditions of hygiene in circulation in France at the time.

Critically, the founders of the new SdS imagined operating on the scale of the entire empire, not just within individual colonies. One of the purposes of the Health Service was to establish an independent, civilian pan-imperial authority on matters of hygiene and sanitation. Military doctors, Treille argued, would inevitably find themselves torn between loyalties to the military command and the civil authority.[20] Instead, Treille imagined the Health Service as the first step toward a "central bureau of colonial hygiene in Paris," which would allow sanitary officers to overcome "local influences, which are often in conflict with the general interest and can paralyze [health experts'] actions."[21] The centralized, pan-imperial institution could then be complemented by a corps of locally trained colonial health officials, prepared to treat ailments specific to the specific region.

The Pasteur Institute shared many of Treille's medical and organizational goals. Research in microbiology offered new methods for studying and treating tropical diseases. Calmette prided himself in being one of the "first subscribers to the *Annales de l'Institut Pasteur*," after having witnessed the limitations of naval doctors' expertise in treating diseases such as typhoid fever and malaria during a trip to the Congo and Gabon.[22] The Pastorians' international ambition fit the bill for Treille's vision of a network of standardized but locally embedded research institutions.[23] Treille and Émile Roux, the acting director of the institute, quickly joined forces and lobbied the ministry to attach a bacteriological laboratory to the Health Service in Indochina. On 9 October 1890, Calmette received word that Eugène Étienne, the undersecretary of the colonies, had appointed him to begin work in Saigon. The Pastorian left immediately.

In Saigon, Calmette oversaw the construction of the new laboratory, with its adjacent buildings, stables, and warehouses. Initially, he focused on getting the rabies service off the ground and on networking with local French elites. On 27 February 1891, Calmette met Yersin, who was passing through Indochina as the doctor on a postal ship, the *Volga*, having left the institute in Paris for colonial adventures.[24] Yersin needed little convincing: in 1892, he joined Calmette in Saigon.[25] There, the situation was precisely as Treille feared. Officials in Indochina had many conflicting concerns and treated the new bacteriological laboratory with indifference at best and a degree of hostility at worst.

French colonizers aspired to access the silk, tea, and textile markets of Chinese Yunnan. Tonkin, Vietnam's northernmost province that shared a border with Yunnan, had been the object of French imperialist ambitions since Francis Garnier's siege of Hanoi in 1873. The province became a protectorate of France in 1884, but this only served as a clarion call for a protracted period of guerrilla warfare. Pockets of resistance to French rule

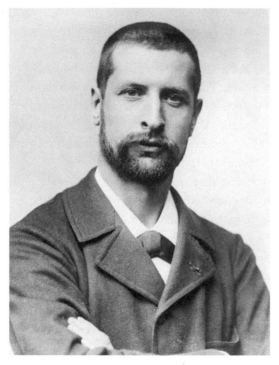

Figure 1.1 Portrait of Alexandre Yersin at age thirty in 1893. Photo by Pierre Petit. © Institut Pasteur/Musée Pasteur.

known as Cần Vương (Help the King) fought French colonizers in support of the exiled king Hàm Nghi for several years. Chinese warlords effectively occupied northern Tonkin, overseeing trade in opium, weapons, and slaves. Densely forested mountain ranges in the west proved excellent hiding places. Local mandarins provided leadership for the resistance movements, whose members were easy to recruit given the harsh policies of "pacification" enacted by French generals such as Henri Frey.[26] Governor-General de Lanessan was appointed to deal with the colonizing of Indochina at a moment when it seemed to have completely stalled. By 1894, the French had decreased their military presence in Tonkin to fewer than five thousand, and Vietnamese mandarins remained intransigent in their opposition to French rule. De Lanessan's main priorities were reducing the burden of taxation and labor placed on the village populations and using the breathing space to mount a strong counterinsurgency in particularly troublesome highland regions.[27]

In this context, the nascent Pasteur Institute of Saigon had little to offer de Lanessan. In the first two years of its existence, Calmette's work on snake venoms had won him some public recognition in France but had done little to convince colonial interests that the laboratory was worth the yearly subvention by the Cochinchinese government.[28] Calmette described his interaction with the governor-general's office as one of profound indifference (it took him nearly half a year to secure an audience from the governor in 1893), which intensified to "some disagreements" with an "arrogant and not at all intelligent" lieutenant governor during budgeting time.[29] When Yersin proposed to study reports of plague outbreaks in Yunnan in 1894, de Lanessan saw this as another expense the colony could not afford. "Who is going to pay for it?" he asked Yersin. "You believe [it will be the colony]. Well, you are wrong."[30]

The governor his reasons for minimizing the plague threat. A serious response to plague outbreaks by the Indochinese border would disrupt trade and affect the already precarious fiscal situation of the colony. Some steps were still taken: responding to outbreaks in Hong Kong and Yunnan, Charles Grall, the chief medical officer in Annam-Tonkin, instituted mandatory sanitary checks and disinfection on all ships coming "directly or indirectly" from Hong Kong and mandatory ten-day quarantine on incoming Chinese ships in May 1894.[31] Yet Chambers of Commerce in Saigon and Haiphong opposed similar measures, arguing that quarantine would stifle trade and prove impossible to enforce in larger ports.[32] When Grall proposed a broad decree mandating that medical officers board and examine *all* ships arriving in *all* Indochinese ports, and to give them the power to condemn suspicious ships into quarantine for up to fifteen days, de Lanessan returned it with the brief note that read: "I oppose this project, which I find useless. The plague is currently in Hong Kong and we have taken sufficient provisional precautions. As far as I'm concerned, there is no need to go any further."[33] It was only because of a personal intervention by the newly appointed minister of the colonies, Théophile Delcassé (a personal friend of Émile Roux), that on 9 June 1894, Yersin received a telegram ordering him to study the plague, which had, by that point, spread to the British-held port city of Hong Kong.[34] The Pastorians may have had the rhetorical and institutional support in the Health Service and in the ministry in Paris, but in Indochina, officials had other concerns on their mind. As representatives of the civilizing mission in the abstract, Pastorians were hugely valuable to the visionaries in France; as practical agents of empire in Saigon, they were yet to demonstrate their worth.

Bacteriological Critiques of the Colonial Situation in Hong Kong

Yersin's expedition to Hong Kong, his discovery of the plague microbe, and his publication of the expedition results in the *Annales de l'Institut Pasteur* have now become legendary moments in the history of bacteriology.[35] Yet focusing on Yersin's scientific publications obscures the fact that, in Hong Kong, he was first and foremost an agent of the Indochinese government. The Pastorian was studying the plague in order to advise his skeptical superiors on how to prevent and contain an outbreak in Tonkin or Cochinchina. Well before publishing his article in the *Annales*, Yersin sent a series of reports to the governor-general, Albert Calmette, and the Ministry of the Colonies in France, relaying the lessons learned from the British experience.

In these reports, a different picture of Yersin's disposition emerges. Rather than emphasizing laboratory identification of the plague microbe and focusing on vaccination as the primary solution, his early reports highlighted how British policies, from careless experimentation to coercive policing of the streets, made even the few good containment measures at their disposal useless, underscoring the close connection between disease and politics. Yersin's social position as an outsider both in the Indochinese administration and in British Hong Kong shaped his reports to the Government-General and helps explain why, in this early stage of his career, the Pastorian could adopt what would later become a very un-Pastorian view of disease and politics.

Other scholars have termed his approach "ethnographic" or "flânerie," emphasizing Yersin's ongoing negotiation with British and Chinese authorities, as well as with native agents, and his need to go outside the laboratory, form alliances, and explore in order to construct knowledge about the plague.[36] Microbiological debates about the precise form of the plague microbe mattered, but identifying the plague microbe using laboratory tools did not become the final arbiter of biomedical truth in those years; rather, it was dependent on epidemiological knowledge Yersin gathered ethnographically. As important as Yersin's ethnographic disposition was in determining his actions in Hong Kong, the following discussion emphasizes his relationship to the British and Chinese as essentially a foreign agent. Yersin was in Hong Kong to evaluate and criticize the practices of the British (who already had their own bacteriological expertise in the form of a Japanese team) and report back to officials in French Indochina. With the antagonistic relationship with the British, Yersin had no other choice than to seek allies elsewhere. In French Indochina a few years later, he would not be so eager.

Hong Kong in the time of Yersin's mission was the largest port in Southeast Asia, shipping twenty-two million tons of goods annually. The city was notoriously insalubrious, having grown explosively after the Second Opium War (1857–1860). Roughly two hundred thousand mostly male Chinese laborers worked the docks and helped sustain the trade that brought the twenty-four thousand European and Chinese businessmen their wealth. The city had established a sanitary board in 1883, but it lacked a chief medical officer. Hong Kong housed six hospitals: two established by the British government, two run by the army, one by the London Missionary Society, and one hospice run by the Chinese charity Donghua.[37] As the plague spread, the government quickly established a new makeshift hospital on the ship *Hygaea* and converted several buildings in the western part of the city, Kennedy Town, into hospitals for the Chinese. It was there that the British government allowed Yersin to set up his laboratory.[38]

Yersin's critiques of the British containment policies focused on three issues. First, he argued that conditions in British hospitals "lacked humanity," a fact that British officials "did not see as the least bit important."[39] The facilities at the hospitals were insufficient for the needs of the population, demoralizing both doctors and the sick. The British Sanitary Board, led by Dr. James Lowson, had made isolation of the sick mandatory months before Yersin's arrival in Hong Kong.[40] Yersin saw that hospitalization did nothing to halt the spread of the disease. The terrible conditions within the hospital, however, created fear in the hearts of Chinese patients. "The first and the last feeling in these horrible halls is one of absolute discouragement, experienced both by the doctors who no longer even attempt to cure their patients, and by the sick themselves. . . . It seems that neither are under any illusion about what awaits them—this discouragement is easily explained if one reflects on the fact that not one of the Chinese that has entered the hospital has ever come out since the beginning of the epidemic."[41] Yersin also wrote, without commentary, that European patients were shipped to the *Hygaea*, where, he confirmed, "they received excellent care."[42]

Second, Yersin argued that British urban containment measures were coercive and violent, and ultimately helped to spread the plague instead of preventing it. Two of Yersin's reports described the "severe sanitary discipline" of the British: every day, three hundred British soldiers marched through the Chinese districts of Hong Kong, forcibly transporting the diseased to the hospital and destroying housing deemed "too insalubrious."[43] The British evacuated entire neighborhoods and either disinfected the housing stock with a mixture of chloride and sulfuric acid or burned dwellings to the ground, if the quality of construction did not permit such disinfection. The British in Hong Kong focused on the living conditions of the urban poor—which in this case meant the Chinese—and did not hesitate in applying extreme force to address what they saw as the chief causes of the disease: "The poison . . . developed from atmospheric conditions underneath houses in certain districts . . . is caused simply by poverty and dirt."[44]

Yersin believed these measures to be counterproductive. The fear of British authorities, the destruction of property, and forced internment caused mass emigration of the Chinese to the province of Canton, spreading the disease

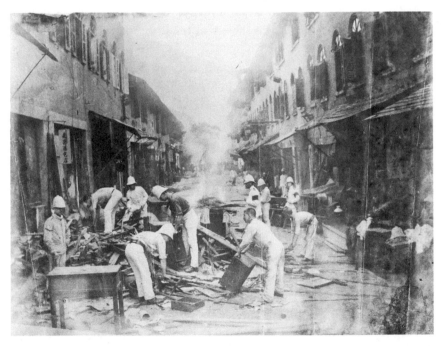

Figure 1.2 Staffordshire Regiment cleaning plague houses, Hong Kong. CC4.0 Wellcome Library, London, United Kingdom.

farther to the countryside. Rather than maintaining political stability and combating disease, the British were spreading fear and unrest through the city. For several weeks, violent mobs prevented the isolation of patients, and British doctors had to carry weapons in order to assert their authority in some regions of the city.[45]

Yersin's reports highlighted a number of lessons the Government-General could draw from the British experience. Of course, as a Pastorian, he highlighted the potential of vaccination and serotherapy. Implicitly, all of his reports focused on the importance of trust and cooperation between authorities and indigenous populations in containing the plague. Explicitly, the Pastorian outlined a number of infrastructural and political problems in the urban environment, which helped spread the disease. For one, he argued, Hong Kong had built up a "bad system of sewage," where the narrowness of sewers, particularly in indigenous parts of the city made it impossible to "disinfect the sewers or hunt down [the rats]" responsible for spreading the plague. The Pastorian also criticized quarantine, which limited Chinese access to hospitals and forced them to bury their dead in places where the disease could easily spread back into the city. He noted that mortality rates among Europeans were much lower than among the Chinese. Yersin ascribed this difference to the better sanitary conditions of European homes, the quality of European hospitals, and the persistent overcrowding of Chinese houses. "Here is," he concluded, "an example for us not to follow."[46] If Yersin's publication in the Annales, as Bruno Latour has argued, aimed to direct the attention of legislators and social hygienists to the bacteriological laboratory, then his letters to the governor-general were more equivocal. He did indeed highlight the potential of bacteriology but also connected the spread of the plague to the specific deficiencies of Hong Kong urban planning, the inefficiency of quarantine, the disparity between European and Chinese standards of habitation, and questions of trust and cooperation. In this rendering, containing the epidemic required political change and urban renewal, as well as biomedical innovations.

Why did Yersin choose this broad frame to critique British containment policies and recommend such demanding alternatives for Indochina? For one, his approach cohered with the sanitary-bacteriological synthesis as it was being practiced in France. While French naval doctors at the time focused on the importance of place—the geographical, climatic, and cultural specificity of an epidemic location—and many British hygienists continued to believe in a miasmatic theory of disease generation, Yersin's approach resembled more the bacteriologically informed yet broadly enviro-social methods used by sanitarians during the 1880 "Great Stink of Paris."[47] Like Parisian health councilors then, who recommended "complete stud[ies] of the air, the housing, the ground, and the underground" in order to stave off epidemics, Yersin too considered diverse aspects of the Hong Kong urban environment, from the soil and the built environment, to the social relations between the British and Chinese.[48]

Second, Yersin was an outsider in the British hierarchy, which forced him to improvise in securing cadavers for study and to collaborate with Chinese doctors, French, and other actors on the margins of the plague epidemic. When Yersin arrived in Hong Kong, a Japanese mission, led by the Robert Koch–trained bacteriologist Shibasaburō Kitasato, was already working with British health officials on isolating the plague microbe.[49] Kitasato claimed he had already discovered the disease agent, while Yersin's lack of English skills and his reluctance to socialize with British bigwigs made it difficult for him to lobby for laboratory space and official endorsement.[50] Yersin ended up working in a makeshift laboratory in the Chinese hospital of Hong Kong, and he paid workers at the docks tasked with transporting the deceased to deliver them to him instead for study.[51] Against the recommendations of both British and French authorities, Yersin traveled to nearby provinces and toured hospitals run by Chinese doctors, judging them to be generally in much better condition than the indigenous facilities organized by the British. Yersin saw the British as panicked, careless, and too eager to experiment with new treatments, while "in Canton, more prudent Chinese doctors rely on their old experience, and I do believe that mortality there is much lower than in Hong Kong."[52] Yersin even cooperated with some Chinese doctors in treating patients in the surrounding regions. One doctor, Lei, from Xiamen sent Yersin a letter, thanking him for sharing his expertise and administering treatment to patients.[53] Most likely, Yersin's position outside the British administration allowed him to perceive and study alternatives to the drastic British measures.

Finally, Yersin had to secure his own position in Indochina. Highlighting the threat a plague epidemic represented to political stability, and a language of "riots," "unrest," "mass emigration," and a loss of political control reframed the severity of the threat for French administrators. His rhetorical work justified his antagonistic relationship with British health officials on scientific grounds—a more flattering argument than the lack of personal rapport emphasized by the French consul. In Hong Kong, Yersin adopted an approach to plague containment that focused on the importance of political relations in the colonial situation and took indigenous actors seriously as rational agents. In the following years, as the epidemic spread, this approach would change dramatically.

International Crisis and the Pastorization of Plague Containment

As trade vessels carried the plague from Hong Kong to India, Australia, Egypt, Hawaii, San Francisco, Buenos Aires, and Cape Town in just a little under a decade, epidemic control moved from being a colonial issue, resolved by local health boards, administrators, and councilors, to a global problem, which imperial powers and top experts discussed on the international diplomatic stage.[54] The Great Powers quickly repurposed the International Sanitary Conference, a forum established for the standardization of quarantine measures in the wake of cholera outbreaks in 1851, to address questions of plague containment. Diplomats struggled with balancing the safety of as-yet-uninfected ports with the needs of international trade, which uncoordinated periods of quarantine disrupted. The Pastorians, too, changed their approach. As Yersin's discoveries helped him secure funding for his own laboratory in Nha Trang, and as Émile Roux and Albert Calmette became involved with French diplomatic efforts at the Sanitary Conferences, the Pastorians' recommendations shifted from broad political and social hygienic reforms to emphasizing specific technical interventions.

This new vision of bacteriology—pastorization—had its own political consequences. It considerably narrowed the field of intervention for Pastorians and the colonial state but empowered them in other ways. The following discussion will situate the emergence of the Pastorians' three technological solutions—vaccination, steam disinfection, and deratization—in the global politics of the plague pandemic. Pastorians developed a uniform, aspirational language of "progressive" containment measures, which acknowledged the violence of earlier interventions such as sanitary cordons and the destruction of property. These new measures were portable, limited technical fixes, promising states a reduction of quarantine times and the prevention of the spread of the plague to neighboring ports while simultaneously minimizing risks to political stability.

A critical component in the development of Pastorian containment measures was the discovery of the rat vector. In 1898, Paul-Louis Simond, a Pastorian, traveled to India on Roux's recommendation and began to study the role of vectors in propagating the disease, paralleling the work of Robert Koch, Ronald Ross, and Alphonse Laveran, who had recently started investigating the role of mosquitoes in the transmission of malaria.[55] Like Yersin, Simond contrasted the potential of bacteriology to the fruitless, although drastic and extensive, containment efforts of the British. He wrote: "We owe the Indian government the justice of admitting that they spared no expense in getting the plague under control; the results sadly did not correspond at all to the expenses and the effort."[56] Unlike Yersin, Simond assumed that calling for the alteration of India's political and urban conditions was beyond his remit, and he focused instead on the physical destruction of rats as the single most effective way of halting the disease.[57]

Not everyone agreed that identifying rats as disease carriers pointed inevitably to vector control as the best solution. In a response article to Simond published in the Pastorian *Annales*, Ernest Hankin, a British microbiologist, drew more fatalistic conclusions:

> The role of rats in the propagation of the disease in a big city leads to the conclusions that it is impossible to halt the plague once it has been declared. First, because it is impossible to completely evacuate a large city, and secondly because nobody knows how to completely and on location destroy a whole population of rats.[58]

Hankin's perspective was not entirely without hope: he had more faith in precautionary measures, including wholesale urban renewal. "The best measure of defense," the British scientist wrote, "is the construction of such housing, which rats cannot enter."[59] Ultimately, Hankin saw no magic bullet solution that emerged from the discovery of the rat vector, concluding instead, in the words of Daniel Defoe, "The best remedy against the plague is to flee."[60]

Some public health authorities rejected the idea of rats as plague carriers; others did not agree that vector control was the most promising response. The controversy was wide open. Yet the international situation worked in the Pastorians' favor. The plague continued to spread, finally reaching Europe in 1899, with an outbreak in Porto. Epidemics in Rio de Janeiro, Honolulu, Buenos Aires, and San Francisco in 1900 were relatively mild but raised the specter of civil unrest. Most of all, these outbreaks highlighted the speed at which modern commerce could spread illness. Different countries experimented with different containment measures. In Brazil, South Africa, and British India, medical elites blamed poverty, overcrowdedness, and lack of civilization among populations considered racially inferior. In other places, like Sydney, health officials embraced bacteriology, distributed vaccines, and attempted rat control. In San Francisco, Porto, and elsewhere, officials pragmatically mixed both approaches.[61]

The variety of approaches and lack of coordination between countries caused suspicion and led to harsh unilateral action against travelers from known plague ports. Maritime commerce slowed down, as ships arriving from India, Hong Kong, or other locations of known outbreaks often found themselves moored for weeks, unable to land passengers, and sometimes unable to sell their wares (such as rawhides and skins from Bengal), which were suspected of being capable of transmitting the plague.[62]

For decades, International Sanitary Conferences had provided a forum where (mostly European) Great Powers could solve precisely these kinds of coordination problems. These were ad hoc meetings, originally conceived for the purposes of standardizing quarantine laws during a period of cholera epidemics. Quarantine, for a long time, had been used for political purposes to police borders and impede trade by rival powers. The period following the Congress of Vienna, however, decreased the political need for quarantines. New, liberal regimes in Britain and France desired freer trade, leading to the first conference in Paris in 1851.[63] These meetings consciously combined politics and science. Each country sent a medical expert and a diplomat to ensure that both political and medical considerations were taken into account.[64]

The central problem delegates at the conferences faced was the following: how to ensure the continuity of ever-faster commerce, while preventing ever-faster spread of disease. Existing rules of quarantine seemed to accomplish neither. One way to solve this dilemma was to coordinate sanitary responses between states, making sure that there was no doubling of sanitary precautions. If ships were disinfected in departing ports, for example, there would be no need to redo the procedure in ports of arrival. More important, however, European states, which dominated the conference, increasingly differentiated between kinds of mobility. European troopships were not subjected to the same kinds of rules of quarantine and inspection as commercial ships. Asian and Middle Eastern travelers were looked at with suspicion. Compared with orderly and easily surveilable European border crossers, European powers described oriental travelers as uncivilized itinerants who "only subject themselves to material force and do not have the least respect for the law, be it sanitary or civil."[65] Muslim pilgrims traveling to Mecca became the subjects of particular concern and stringent surveillance. Increasingly, European delegates came to agree that the most reliable way of avoiding disruptions to trade would be to cut off the disease at its source, which inevitably put the focus of intervention on the "Orient."[66]

At the Venice conference of 1897, the delegates began to discuss the plague. The French proposed modeling antiplague measures on anticholera measures, which the Great Powers had adopted five years earlier.[67] The resulting agreement required thorough inspections of outbound ships and the disinfection of contaminated goods but also mandated surveillance and isolation of infected vessels for up to ten days in ports of arrival. It simultaneously permitted receiving countries to ban the import of certain goods that were thought to carry the plague.[68] Delegates specifically excluded European colonies from the agreement and underscored that it would not proscribe public health measures *within* contaminated territories—these would be left to the best judgment of local authorities. When the plague continued to spread to European and American ports, states had to reevaluate their options. The chapter on plague containment was reopened in Paris in 1903.

Most delegates expressed deep dissatisfaction with the results of the 1897 conference. Adopting the cholera prevention framework had done little to stop disease, but it hurt global commerce. Neither Greece nor the Ottoman Empire had joined the 1897 convention, meaning that ships originating from their ports were still subjected to older quarantine regimes. This damaged countries like Italy, which relied on Mediterranean trade.[69] Italian and Russian delegates argued that disinfection and surveillance requirements imposed high costs on receiving states, without actually limiting the spread of the plague. "Thus, the Convention regime did not save neither Oporto, nor Glasgow, Liverpool or Naples; it did not prevent the plague from arriving in Australia, in any case, any more than quarantine regimes did not free Beyrouth, Smyrna, Constantinople etc," concluded the Italian delegate Santoliquido.[70] Instead, the Paris conference took a different approach, seeking to "determine whether experience and progress of the prophylactical sciences in the past six years would allow us to modify the rules in a liberalizing direction."[71] Faced with continuously high costs to trade, the French organizers proposed bacteriology as the solution.

The delegates harbored several assumptions, which nudged their views closer to those of the Pastorians. For one, observing the costs of policing maritime commerce, delegates concluded that the best course of action was to "determine the source of the infection, concentrate on the contaminated point with all the means that science provides us in order to surround and smother this initial outbreak as fast as possible."[72] This meant that the brunt of the containment operation would be borne by oriental states, cohering with the conviction of European powers that the Orient was less civilized, and therefore harsh measures would be more acceptable there. The imperative of catching the outbreak quickly also raised the importance of first-order and preventive measures, drawing attention to Pastorian vaccination and serotherapy. Second, delegates were particularly frustrated with embargoes on tradable goods, which were often impounded, destroyed, or devalued in the process of disinfection.[73] Simond's discovery of the rat vector promised to draw the focus of containment measures away from humans and goods, and onto a rodent population with no economic value whatsoever.

Pastorians, too, had already begun to frame their work in terms of its impact on commerce. Yersin suggested that a system of sanitary passports could exempt properly vaccinated travelers from quarantine measures.[74] Calmette promised in a speech that Pastorian measures would "henceforth obviate the need for quarantine" and reduce the time for sanitary control from ten days to "hardly twenty-four hours, and implying only a minimum of discomfort for commercial transactions."[75] No wonder, then, that French hosts of the conference listed vaccination as the first among several interventions that would allow governments to review the length of quarantine measures and facilitate trade.[76] The technical committee at the conference, tasked with bringing plague containment in line with the latest bacteriological insights, was expanded to include two new French delegates: Albert Calmette and Émile Roux.[77]

Though Pastorians praised the potential of vaccination and serotherapy in public, privately they acknowledged that these technologies were far from perfect. Yersin's first attempt at treating select patients during an outbreak in Amoy, China, had resulted in seemingly spectacular success: out of twenty-four treated patients, twenty-two were cured, and only two died.[78] These initial results earned Yersin quite a bit of attention in the medical and popular press.[79] Yet he could not replicate this success. In Bombay in 1897, Yersin's serum gave mixed results: one batch, shipped from Paris, appeared to work. The second batch, from Yersin's own laboratory in Nha Trang, failed—thirteen out of nineteen patients treated died, a 73 percent mortality rate. The third batch, again from Paris, showed improvement with a 38 percent mortality rate—but still nowhere near the promising results seen in Canton.[80] A different vaccine, developed by the Russian Pastorian Waldemar Haffkine, was equally controversial. It conveyed only temporary immunity, ranging from fifteen to twenty-five days.[81]

Without a reliable vaccine, Calmette and Roux emphasized disinfection not just of infected ships but also of entire port towns that had been exposed to the disease. Here, other members of the committee expressed caution, noting that the technical committee should limit itself to discussing cross-border traffic only, and not impinge on the rights of governments to decide on their own public health policies. Delegates were careful not to prescribe specific methods of rat destruction. Instead, they provided an overview of different options that could be used on ships, largely based on gaseous pesticides containing sulfuric acid or carbonic acid.[82] Still, the final agreement, best known for calling for the establishment of an international body for the exchange of health data (what would later become the Office of International Public Hygiene), brought rat control and disinfection into the international limelight, replacing the previous focus on isolating infected goods and people.[83] This expertise propagated quickly, even among colonial authorities, who were not necessarily bound by the convention.[84] As for *how* authorities were to control the rat population in port towns—the Pastorians once again came to the rescue.

The Pastorian solution had Danish origins. From 1900 to 1904 the Danish sanitary reformer Emil Zuschlag embarked on an international campaign to gather support for "the rational destruction of migratory rats."[85] Drawing attention to the immense agricultural cost caused by the carnivorous rats eating small birds, chicks, and other vulnerable livestock, as well as their role in spreading disease, Zuschlag proposed a system of bounties, whereby municipalities would pay teams of volunteer rat-catchers for the capture and killing of rats. The tails of the rats would serve as proof, and local municipalities would pay bounties of ten øre per rat. This method, Zuschlag remarked, would prove more reliable in urban settings where steam disinfection with Clayton machines was not practical, since rats could always escape to the streets or adjacent housing.[86] The plan was all the better, given that it would draw the attention of "the poor and their children," and prove cheaper than frequently ineffective rat traps. Zuschlag's plan doubled as a form of social assistance and a potential source of fiscal savings.[87] It was, Zuschlag remarked, a truly "rational method" for sanitary reform.[88]

Zuschlag's plan fit neatly into an ongoing struggle in Danish public policy. The increasingly evident costs of urbanization and the emergence of a pro-letarian underclass motivated social reformers to lobby for wide-ranging, state-run sanitation schemes that married a concern over the danger posed by the economically and morally "deficient" with an imperative to overcome the drastic changes of an urbanizing society.[89] While popular with landlords and farmers eager to put the responsibility for public health on the shoulders of the state rather than on themselves, Zuschlag's plan still faced an uphill struggle.[90] He attempted to convince the Danish Folketing to turn his rational rat-catching project into national policy, but the legislation stalled as state leaders feared the excessive costs such a project would impose on the gov-ernment.[91] Hoping to win international support and credibility for his pro-ject, which had thus far been tested only in Copenhagen and Frederiksberg, Zuschlag embarked on a four-year international tour in search for allies.

He did not have to look for long. Other Scandinavian countries embraced the system—rat-catching bounties were soon in place in various Swedish cities, from Malmö to Helsingfors. Zuschlag made connections in the European diplomatic and scientific communities through conferences, such as the International Maritime Congress, and at various international expositions. It was through this process of internationalization that Zuschlag realized the relevance of his method for plague control. Zuschlag's orig-inal letters to the Danish Folketing only referenced the general threat to agriculture and public hygiene, without singling out a specific disease. By contrast, his 1904 French publication focuses squarely on the plague, spe-cifically the importance of battling the rat vector and preventing the disease from reaching Europe.[92] Pastorians such as Calmette purchased Zuschlag's pamphlets and attended his conferences, seeing in his work a potential policy output for their scientific work. This was a mutually useful cross-pollination: the bacteriological interest in the rat vector lent additional force for Zuschlag's battle back home in Copenhagen, while his "rational" system provided a specific technological fix for Pastorians, who were under pressure to deliver concrete policies at Sanitary Conferences and other imperial and international meetings.

The path from Simond's discovery of the rat vector to the acceptance of Pastorian measures of vector control was never preordained; it was forged through many alliances. International interest in alternatives to quarantine shifted the attention of Pastorians to measures that did not impact the move-ment or value of goods and humans. Networks with other hygienists helped to secure a method—Zuschlag's rational destruction of rats. Pastorian proposals for plague control were then quickly disseminated in French ad-ministrative discourse through policy papers authored by, for example, Calmette and Alexandre Kermorgant, the senior councilor for health at the Ministry of the Colonies. In these writings, Pastorian authority became the foundation of progressive plague containment: "Insisted by Dr. Roux, in his high authority," "our colleague Yersin, who found himself struggling against the plague, . . . advocates for the following general measures," "wherever in the world a pestilential epidemic ravages, . . . other 'pastorians' are always there to combat it."[93] This model, which played up Pastorian heroics, simultaneously abstracted away the importance of local sociopolitical context, which Yersin had emphasized in his critiques of the British. Instead, Pastorians offered technical fixes—vaccination, disinfection, and deratization—which they portrayed as universal features following logically from the discovery of the rat vector. In reality, these measures responded to an environment that priv-ileged trade, liberalization of quarantine, and the safety of European ports.

The Practice and Performance of Pastorian Plague Containment

In subsequent years, plague outbreaks in Nha Trang, Hanoi, and elsewhere showed the difficulties of actually implementing deratization, disinfection, and vaccination methods. Yersin himself had to come to terms with the gap between his vision of mass vaccination and the messy reality of producing and administering the vaccine in provincial Indochina. In 1897, the plague broke out in Nha Trang, the village that housed Yersin's new laboratory. The outbreak provided Yersin, the highest medical official in the region, with an opportunity to demonstrate proper measures of plague control and to apply his knowledge of vaccination, consider the importance of rats as disease vectors, and properly cooperate with the villagers.

Initially, Yersin did indeed seek the help of Vietnamese elders, who were supposed to report cases directly to him. He responded sympatheti-cally to local concerns, reassigning an unpopular subprefect, whom the villagers blamed for causing the epidemic by upsetting the village spirit with his behavior.[94] He ordered all patients isolated in a makeshift lazaret, families and neighbors vaccinated, and infected houses destroyed by fire (Nha Trang lacked the technology for steam disinfection).[95] However, his plans for treating the infected with his new serum proved more complicated. Quarantine measures imposed on Nha Trang made it difficult for him to obtain the serum, which had to be shipped in from Paris. Yersin also feared that if the plague spread to adjacent villages—Ninh Hòa and Phan Rang—he would effectively have to coordinate medical responses in three different places, prompting him to request that the Government-General send over more doctors from Saigon. The government rejected his request.[96]

As the plague returned in 1897 and 1898, Yersin considered more radical measures. Realizing that not all cases were reported and that he could not maintain proper isolation in lazarets, he decided to take protective action. He ordered the evacuation and quarantine of entire populations and ultimately decided to burn two infected villages, Phường Cầu and Văn Thanh, to the ground.[97] French authorities moved village populations several miles away to virgin territory, where Yersin ordered the construction of new housing, in hopes that the plague had been defeated in the fire.

Particularly revealing here is how differently Yersin chose to explain these events to his colleagues and to his superiors in Hanoi. In a letter to Émile Roux, Yersin admitted that the plague may have originated from his own labs, from the cultures he had brought back from his various trips to China and the British colonies. Yersin hypothesized that rodents attracted to the food in the holding pens of his lab might have carried highly virulent strains of the disease from infected monkeys into the nearby village. He noted that the plague had also killed several of his mongoose, even though the animals were kept far away from his plague labs.[98] The scientist ultimately admitted that in the process of developing new ways of protecting French Indochina from the plague, he may have inadvertently introduced the disease to the land.

In his official report to Alexandre Kermorgant, Yersin made no mention of this hypothesis. Instead, he suggested that Chinese pork merchants from Canton and Hainam, who had visited the nearby island of Bay Mien, were responsible for transmitting the plague.[99] His claim rested on the fact that the disease had broken out in the neighboring village of Cu Lao (which did business with the Chinese merchants) around the same time as it appeared in Nha Trang. In his report to the governor-general, Yersin outlined a third option: In one of the infected houses Yersin's team had found a cage allegedly stolen from the laboratory in which test mice were being held. The villagers used the cage for storing nuts, and Yersin speculated that the scourge might have escaped the laboratory. As for the aggressive containment measures, Yersin spread responsibility for his strategy between poor resources and native ignorance: "Had [the original] instructions been followed to the letter, it is likely that the epidemic would already be extinct. This, sadly, is impossible owing to the ignorance of the villagers and the limited means at our disposal."[100]

Reporting to his superiors, Yersin faced a dilemma other medical officers would encounter repeatedly: Pastorian bacteriology had been sold as a magic bullet to solve the terrible epidemic. Yet the reality turned out to be far more complicated. At stake was nothing less than the credibility of Pastorians. "This is bad news," as one Pastorian wrote regarding the Nha Trang epidemic. "This sad accident may have an influence on him, and perhaps on all of us."[101] The solution, for many health officials, was to place blame on outsiders: ignorant natives or Chinese migrants.

In the following years, as plague outbreaks multiplied, it became apparent that both colonial infrastructure and politics obstructed Pastorian plague control. On numerous occasions, decision makers in Hanoi and Paris attempted to push local health officials to embrace Pastorian measures, low-level officials kept reminding their superiors in angry letters that the lack of funds, machinery, labor, and political stability could not be overcome by technological genius alone.

The most comprehensive reforms took place after the Hanoi epidemic of 1903–1904, as part of a broader attempt to overhaul the Indochinese health system. Some years earlier, Governor-General Paul Doumer had brought the four French domains in Indochina (Cochinchina, Annam-Tonkin, Laos, and Cambodia) together under the Indochinese Union. He initiated a series of administrative reforms intended to unify governance across the colonies, including the establishment of a "director of health" in each colony, drawn from the ranks of the navy.[102] Real reforms took off under Paul Beau, who established a number of institutions for curing both the colonizers and the colonized in 1905, the most important of which was the Indigenous Medical Assistance (AMI), comprising navy doctors and local auxiliaries trained at the newly formed Hanoi Medical School (established by Alexandre Yersin).[103]

The ambitions of the reformers were broader still. As Dr. Maurice Clavel argued, curative medicine could do little without preventive hygiene.[104] He outlined an ambitious plan of sanitary reform, ranging from the construction of sewers to vulgarization programs intended to increase popular knowledge about Western hygiene. Yet these plans went nowhere, as they demanded resources and a commitment to deepening governance that the state simply did not have. Instead, administrators in Hanoi and Paris focused more narrowly on epidemic control and prevention. The governor-general ordered prefects and residents-general to purchase Clayton apparatuses required for steam disinfection and implement preventive measures in a series of circulars and decrees from 1903 to 1906.[105] A series of reports from local prefects, filed in 1904, brings into focus the chasm between the aspirations of Pastorian reformers and the reality of colonial governance.

These reports reveal how budgetary constraints and priorities of local administrators limited the spread of nondestructive disinfection. In response to a circular ordering local prefects to purchase state-of-the-art mobile steam machines, many prefects returned a laundry list of budget deficits, concerns over reimbursements, and ballooning health costs. One inspector noted that he was hesitant to take on more expenses, given that he had already constructed a makeshift lazaret under orders from the Government-General and had not yet been reimbursed for the 6,400-piaster project.[106] Another stated that he did not see a purpose in spending several thousand piasters on a machine for a job that "had little value, where complete destruction by fire could be practiced in appropriate cases."[107] Largely, provincial leaders shifted the responsibility back to the resident-superior, demanding advances or at least assurances of budget allocations so that the prefects would not be left paying for the steamers from discretionary budgets.

As a result, administrators distributed Clayton steamers very unevenly. Port towns—Hanoi, Saigon, Haiphong, Tourane, and a few others—had both more funds and more motivation to purchase the machines. Customs officials were required to disinfect goods coming in from known plague ports, making the existence of Clayton machines almost a given in these urban centers. Sometimes municipal authorities simply replaced outdated steamers with newer, mobile models that could be used in harbors and driven out to the city or adjacent provinces when needed. In the countryside and by the Chinese border, Clayton machines remained an exception rather than the rule.[108] Even in Hanoi, disinfection was not always an option. During the 1903 outbreak, city officials destroyed 130 houses in three districts, noting later that "clearly, if the city had a steamer it would have been possible to disinfect [the houses] completely and thereby avoid destruction by fire. Sadly, we do not possess a steamer: therefore we were obliged to destroy by fire all contaminated objects where ordinary disinfection was impossible."[109]

Deratization faced less resistance from officials. It was still almost impossible to implement. The plan was to have Vietnamese volunteers capture and kill rats, in exchange for a bounty of one to three piasters for every one hundred rats. The measure, which had worked well in Scandinavian urban centers with few rats and many people, turned out to be less practical in low-population-density regions of Annam-Tonkin. The prefect of Van Bu declared the plan "useless," noting that in his region "population is sparse, with often considerable distances between villages. The forests, which cover most of the province, are infested with rats, and paying a bounty for their destruction would be ineffective."[110] Another prefect noted the difficulty of administering the system in regions with a low-level French presence, fearing that without strict oversight the funds would be embezzled: "Administrative oversight in other communities is not as strong as in the capital, and bounties allocated in these conditions run the risk of not being completely used for their intended purpose."[111] Others noted the impossibility of capturing all the rats in the region, particularly during the periods right before and after the rainy season, when the critters were particularly abundant and plague outbreaks particularly likely.[112]

More problems surfaced in implementation.[113] In Hanoi, deratization seemed initially successful beyond expectations. On the best days, rat-catchers claimed upwards of ten thousand kills per day (they were only required to deliver the tails of rats as proof).[114] The payment for killed rats proved lucrative enough to encourage complicated ways of gaming the system, as Michael Vann has documented. Over time, municipal authorities started noticing that tails brought in for collection were in various states of decay. Reports from neighboring provinces indicated that instead of heading to the sewers of Hanoi, catchers were heading out into the surrounding forests to catch rats, leading to high collections rates but no effect on the hygiene of the city.[115] In Hanoi itself, people started noticing rats running around without tails, leading authorities to conclude that catchers were simply collecting the tails, leaving the rats to breed and keep business going. Indeed, some of the more entrepreneurial Vietnamese were reported to be raising rats themselves.[116] It is unclear how widespread these practices were, and to what degree they reflected the municipal rumor mill, where racist assumptions about the Vietnamese were surely heightened during a disease outbreak. Still, it is hard to dispute that in the French administrative mind and on the street level, deratization failed to dent the epidemic, which claimed 110 lives according to official statistics in 1903, and a further

263 (mostly Vietnamese) lives a few years later.[117] Although deratization remained a priority in official documents, officials during later epidemics—in Phnom Penh in 1910 or Hanoi in the 1920s—thought of deratization as a nice idea in theory but did little to actually implement it.[118]

Quarantines, forced isolation, and the destruction of infected houses and sometimes entire neighborhoods remained in the French playbook across the empire, even in the age of bacteriology.[119] Indeed, the most controversial example of French public health intervention comes from 1914, almost two decades after the isolation of the *Yersinia pestis* microbe, when colonial authorities in Dakar, in West Africa, destroyed almost the entire African medina to contain a plague outbreak.[120] Although Pastorian recommendations proliferated in medical literature and in high-level policy texts, officials on the ground continued to complain about the lack of consistent legislation, noting that the procedures for combating epidemics were scattered and often contradictory.[121] Bacteriologists had learned to think like an empire, developing mobile technologies that could be implemented across great distances and that enacted politics that mattered in Paris—reducing quarantine, improving trade, and maintaining fiscal probity. On the local level, these methods proved utterly useless.

Yet, the pastorization of plague control served a number of other functions. It legitimized bacteriology as a critical imperial science. Even though the effectiveness of Pastorian measures could rarely be demonstrated, Pastorians explained their failures largely as problems of "indigenous ignorance," while the promise of their technologies helped colonial governments demonstrate their competence in the face of epidemic crises. In 1905, the Indochinese Government-General signed agreements with the Pasteur Institute in Paris, which institutionalized governmental subventions to the Pasteur Institutes in Saigon and Nha Trang, citing in particular their role in combating the plague.[122] This agreement obliged Pastorians to conduct research "with useful applications for French Indochina"; deliver vaccines, sera, and other public health services to the government; and undertake special expeditions and missions for the benefit of the colony.[123] In a 1907 circular, the Indochinese governor-general outlined this policy for improving public health measures:

> To avoid trial and error, and to achieve the highest returns, one condition is indispensable: a constant collaboration between the administrative and technical elements. No public health measure should be mandated without prior study and without consulting the sanitary authorities; all

bacteriological, chemical and other potentially necessary studies should be completed, and only then, with certain and truly scientific data, can we accomplish the vast project of sanitary reform.[124]

Second, Pastorian innovations, particularly plague sera and vaccines, became useful means of performing French technoscientific prowess on both local and international stages. French administrators and diplomats became greatly concerned with the symbolic gesture of delivering plague vaccines, even when they themselves were aware that the quantities involved were clearly too small to make a practical difference. The Pasteur Institute regularly received demands for small quantities of the Haffkine vaccine or the antiplague serum, when the scourge broke out in surrounding regions: Bangkok, Manila, Singapore, Macau, Quang-Tchéou-Wan, the Chinese province of Canton, and various locations in Japan.[125] Because of the small quantities involved, these deliveries clearly functioned primarily as diplomatic gestures rather than serious attempts to limit the spread of the disease.

Similarly, vaccination became a symbol of an effective state response for those local notables who maintained cordial relations with the French. During the Hanoi outbreak, French administrators received complaints, both individual and collective, protesting—as Yersin had predicted—the destruction of housing and the inability to follow burial rituals, as all bodies were required to be handed over to French sanitary authorities. In particular, the complaints emphasized their preference for vaccination as an alternative to these practices, highlighting them alongside other modernization efforts of "incontestable utility," such as the construction of roads and sewers. "When the doctor comes to visit [the patient], and has him transported to the lazaret to be inoculated and to prevent the spread of the disease, we welcome this good measure."[126] Whether this tells us anything of the disposition of the Vietnamese toward vaccination as a practice is debatable, but it certainly shows that the citizens of Hanoi, too, had understood the symbolic connection between vaccination and progress, in contrast to "disinfection by fire."

French administrators also felt the power of this symbol. When the plague broke out in Phnom Penh, the governor-general sent out a memo cautioning health officers from using the antiplague serum as a substitute for the Haffkine vaccine. Although the serum allegedly conferred short-term immunity, it was much harder to produce, requiring large amounts of livestock, and in the early 1900s was manufactured only in the Paris institute, which also supplied the rest of the world. In 1907, the institute had to reduce its deliveries to Indochina because of increased demand in Rio de Janeiro.[127] In response, local officials sent a series of strongly worded complaints, demanding permission to use the serum in lieu of the vaccine, in order to avoid undermining hard-won credibility with local notables:

> If we consider the persistent efforts that we had to deploy to overcome the instinctive, and still imperfectly won, resistance of the indigenous population, if we consider the importance that this may have to first of all, hygiene, and for securing our moral influence through the repeated proof of acquired immunity . . . it seems clear that the local Health Service could not have received more frustrating orders.[128]

What administrators were concerned with was maintaining a symbolic economy in which the distribution of vaccines in the Phnom Penh region would be accepted as a marker of French hygienic modernity. What was at stake with vaccination was more than simply health—it was the very authority of French civilizing mission that vaccination could affirm or call into question.

Conclusion

In 1905, Albert Calmette authored an article in *La Revue Scientifique*, in which he laid out general principles for "the role of medical sciences for colonisation." Imagine, he began, a colonial city, somewhere on the coast of West Africa or "in any colony, where governors and administrators have the wisdom to use the expertise of doctors and scientific laboratories."[129] This city would have no sanitation, no proper sewage, no regulation of marketplaces, no disinfection service, not even a code of hygiene, since "the local authorities have up to now respected local customs."[130] How, then, could the colony be protected against epidemic disease, be it cholera, yellow fever, or the plague? Calmette offered a three-point plan, focusing on "isolating the sick," "suppressing the vehicles of the disease," and "protecting the healthy."[131] While the particular technologies for achieving these goals varied from disease to disease, Calmette ultimately returned to the three methods the Pastorians had developed during the plague epidemic: disinfection, vector control, and vaccination.

Whether discussing the destruction of mosquitoes to prevent malaria, or deratization to prevent the plague, Calmette cited examples from other parts of the world, where such methods had proved effective, and focused on technologies that either destroyed the microbe or prevented it from entering the human body. When it came to disease ecology, Calmette was interested only in using a bacteriological method to disrupt the microbe-vector-human linkage. There was no discussion of general sanitation, of urban renewal, of construction of larger housing, or of education in the rules of hygiene. Calmette simply asked his readers to assume that respect for local customs—or "superstitions and prejudices" of colonial subjects—stood in the way of large-scale public hygiene projects.[132]

Calmette showed no interest, too, in the complexity of local political relations or the tenuous issues of trust between administrators, doctors, subalterns, and entrepreneurs of various sorts. Instead, the Pastorian asked his readers to assume unlimited authority for the Health Council. The only political issue Calmette discussed was how, under his proposed regime, "ships would no longer be subjected to quarantine, unless they came from an infected port and were accused of having plague victims on board."[133] He concluded his story of progressive epidemic containment with an anecdote of a Chinese response to Yersin's first experiments with antiplague injections, which, he claimed involved nothing less than calling Yersin a "god of healing, descended on the earth."[134] Would this example not prove, Calmette concluded, that the "penetration" of "European influence" into the "abdomens and chests" of *indigènes* would surely and peacefully replace the piercing force of "destructive projectiles"?[135]

This article succinctly summarized the main principles of the Pastorian method of intervention. Calmette's ecology contained only the microbe, the vector, and the human body. His politics assumed unlimited authority for the health administrator, and his priorities were imperial, rather than colonial or local. He thought in terms of machines and mobility: vaccines and Clayton machines could easily be transported from Rio de Janeiro or Copenhagen, and the specific location of his hypothetical colonial city did not matter. At the same time, his technologies delivered much more than just vaccines. The syringe became a metaphor for European influence, as powerful as the gun, a symbol of the awesome technological superiority of the French. The sanitary-bacteriological synthesis, which continued to reign in France, and which shaped Yersin's approach to studying the epidemic in Hong Kong, had, in Calmette's vision, all but disappeared.

Of course, colonial officials also talked about education, social hygiene, and curative medicine. The medical reforms of Paul Beau, Albert Sarraut, and others were supposed to deliver education, infrastructures for training indigenous medical corps, urban sanitary codes, and much else. The language of colonial medicine was capacious. Yet, as Laurence Monnais and others have noted, these reforms remained largely on paper, particularly outside major metropolitan centers.[136] When choosing between competing alternatives, as we will see, colonial officials regularly went with the Pastorian option. During the plague pandemic, Pastorian technologies became measures of progress, a model for administrators to follow when planning new interventions. A rhetorical commitment to the destruction of germs, whether through vaccination, disinfection, or vector control, provided aspirational proof of administrators' progressive credentials, even when, in practice, drastic, coercive epidemic control measures remained in the colonial arsenal. As one health officer wrote in the 1920s: " Deratization, antiplague vaccination are doubtless destined to represent the entirety of antiplague defense in some more or less distant future. For now . . . we have to remind here the diversity of measures that are still found in the prophylactic battle of today."[137]

The invention of pastorization in Indochina opened up new political strategies for the colonial state. The following chapter explores how pastorization was put into practice outside the sphere of public health, in the service of industrial and fiscal interests. In this case, as in the case of plague containment, once political decisions were relegated to the level of technological choices, then technological logics themselves began to influence politics.

2

Pastorization and Its Discontents

From the 1910s onward, readers of colonial newspapers were likely to come across page-length advertisements for the Société Française des Distilleries de l'Indo-Chine (SFDI), the corporation holding monopoly rights to the production of Vietnamese rice wine in Tonkin, northern Annam, and Cochinchina. Illustrated with aerial photos of large factories, these ads impressed on their readers a vision of rationalized, hygienic, and efficient modern alcohol production. This new process had replaced indigenous methods, with their "repulsive filthiness and very irregular methods of fermentation."[1] At the heart of the factory's success was a Pastorian: Albert Calmette. The corporation, so the texts claimed, owed "its creation and rapid development . . . to the adoption of scientific methods perfected by the research of doctor Calmette."[2] Longer exposés were even more specific: the key to the SFDI's success was a particular fermentation technique called "the Amyloprocess, a product of the learned studies of Albert Calmette, director of the Pasteur Institute of Saigon, on certain microorganisms of the Far East."[3]

On the ground, the SFDI's success appeared fleeting. Since the administration brought alcohol production and sales in northern Vietnam under monopoly rule in 1902, consumers had protested against the new regime. The SFDI portrayed its rượu (rice wine) as a modern, rationalized, and hygienic product, but Vietnamese aficionados experienced it as tasteless and unhealthy—"an affront to taste and to custom," in the words of one Vietnamese councilor.[4] Protests against the alcohol monopoly made it into petitions, popular plays and often led to street fighting. In a letter to the minister of the colonies written in 1912, Governor-General Albert Sarraut called the alcohol protests "a serious question" that "risked costing us all that is left of our prestige among the indigenous populations."[5] The Pastorian Amyloprocess, which the SFDI praised as the hallmark of modernity, created strife and resistance among Vietnamese consumers.

A parallel, but ultimately divergent, story unfolded within the other big Indochinese state industry: the opium monopoly. There, too, factory

Pasteur's Empire. Aro Velmet, Oxford University Press (2020). © Oxford University Press.
DOI: 10.1093/oso/9780190072827.001.0001

owners called upon Calmette's expertise in order to rationalize their fermentation process using Pastorian bacteriology. Alas, the Pastorians' attempts to eliminate unnecessary biological agents from the mixture and to cut down fermentation time culminated in a fiasco; the final product was deemed unusable, the procedure was abandoned, and Chinese experts were brought in to run the monopoly instead.[6] The opium monopoly never became a hallmark of French modernity. Lacking that rhetorical cover, the state, when challenged, openly admitted its true purpose in taking this industry under monopoly control: selling opium was an "ideal form of an indirect tax" in a colony where balancing the budget was a perennial problem.[7] As Calmette himself noted, "If the government brought [these industries] under state control, [they] would supply French industrialists with robust and considerable profits."[8] In both cases, Calmette positioned himself as the central expert on defining the parameters of "modern" production, focusing on the identification and manipulation of what he deemed the central microbiological agent in both alcohol and opium fermentation. In other words, he sought to pastorize the intoxicant industries.

In comparing the attempts to pastorize the opium and alcohol monopolies, and the consequences this had for colonial politics, this chapter highlights the bacteriological technopolitics of colonial industry. Other studies of colonial intoxicants have analyzed the political and economic purposes of drug monopolies, as well as their effects on controlling a colonial proletariat or creating new criminal underclasses.[9] In these cases, the political logic of intoxicant monopolization and the technical logic of intoxicant production have remained largely in separate spheres.[10] This chapter argues that this separation is untenable. The technical success of pastorization and the political success of monopolization were inextricably linked. Scientific and technical questions, such as the shape of a "pure" or "hygienic" fermentation process, carried with them political consequences. Many different actors could leverage Pastorian expertise to achieve their own political ends. Using Pastorian arguments, administrators and their clients could override political commitments to free trade, which guided the Ministry of the Colonies and competing French entrepreneurs. Opium reformers used racialized arguments about the health consequences of opium smoking in orientals to underwrite the monopoly in Indochina, while committing to stamping out the drug among French consumers. Vietnamese consumers used the language of biomedicine and hygiene to contest the alcohol monopoly. In all these cases, actors channeled expertise and the logic of bioindustrial engineering as weapons in political fights.

At the same time, Pastorian engineering choices, once cast into the factory mold, produced material consequences that colonial officials did not anticipate or even desire. Factory alcohol did not suit the taste of consumers; Calmette's opium fermentation process failed and reignited a long-standing debate over the limits of state control over Indochinese industries. Ironically, it was precisely because pastorization *succeeded* in placing the alcohol monopoly outside the realm of politics and turning it into a symbol of French scientific modernity that it became particularly vulnerable to attack. The opium monopoly, which the French admitted was primarily a fiscal instrument, never became such a source of instability. In criticizing the taste of rice wine, however, Vietnamese consumers set into question the very foundation of the French civilizing mission.

The Politics of Drug Monopolies

In the 1890s, French governors in Indochina constructed a new fiscal base to reform infrastructure, finance pacification efforts in Tonkin, and protect French entrepreneurs seeking to capture new markets from metropolitan and Chinese rivals. The establishment of drug monopolies served all of these goals. In the early years of French rule, rượu and opium were taxed eclectically. In Cochinchina, alcohol policies sometimes meant creating tax farms, where a syndicate of approved distillers were required to pay the state an annual license fee. In other cases, the state used excise taxes, charged per liter of pure alcohol.[11] The Vietnamese Nguyễn dynasty in the North began taxing alcohol in 1874 in order to pay war indemnities to the French, adopting in effect the license fee system used in Cochinchina.[12] As the French consolidated their power over Indochina in the 1880s, they tended to adopt the taxation systems and middlemen already in place, such as the licensing system implemented by King Norodom in Cambodia, or contracts established by the Nguyễn emperor Tự Đức in Annam-Tonkin.[13] Opium smoking had been outlawed under the Nguyễn dynasty, but in the 1860s war concessions forced the Vietnamese regime to begin selling tenders of production or dealing directly with individual Chinese producers supplying the increasingly heterogeneous Sino-Vietnamese market.[14] French officials replicated this model in Cochinchina, signing contracts with large producers. These attempts at regulation were incomplete at best; contraband retained a huge market share, and Vietnamese producers working from small home distilleries continued to evade the state.

The French initially resisted radical reforms within the alcohol industry because of its centrality to Vietnamese everyday life. When Résident-Supérieur Paul Bert considered monopolizing alcohol production in 1886, he mused: "It would have to be acceptable to the population; alcohol consumption is common, it even plays a ritual role in many annamite celebrations, and any restrictions would appear as insults."[15] This was true: rượu was a daily beverage at Vietnamese dinner tables, consumed primarily by men, and a crucial part of many holidays, including New Year's (Tết), birthdays, weddings, and funerals. Jugs of rượu were exchanged in ritual wedding processions to the houses of the groom and the bride, offered on the altars of the newlyweds' families, and drunk by the couple themselves from the marriage cup during their wedding night. Infusions of rượu with herbs, such as ginseng, or animal products, such as snake venom or bear bile, were understood to have medicinal properties. Finally, rượu provided a frame for male socialization. The drink was (and remains) so common in Vietnamese society that signaling the end of a satisfying meal in Vietnamese literally means saying "rice and rượu—full and drunk."[16]

Opium smoking was largely the domain of Chinese immigrants, though it spread also among Vietnamese and Cambodian upper classes. By the 1890s, the French were purchasing raw materials in the form of roughly dutch cheese-sized boules from the Benares region of British India, where poppies were grown in large fields and harvested in late April. Contraband from the Chinese province of Yunnan made up for shortfalls.[17] One giant Chinese factory in Saigon and smaller factories in Langson, Haiphong, and Luang Prabang in Laos processed the imported raw material. These Chinese refineries were crucial to delivering quality product, and their owners were powerful local businessmen. Since French officials collected substantial revenue from farming out production rights to these factories, they initially were in no rush to reform.

Opium consumption took two forms: as chandoo smoked in opium dens by the wealthy, and as dross, chandoo residue scraped from used pipes, which still contained small quantities of the intoxicant and could be smoked or mixed with wine.[18] Smoking dens run by Chinese proprietors often contained little more than the minimum amount of furniture, a few statues of deities, and sofas for the smokers. Statistics on consumption are unreliable, but the

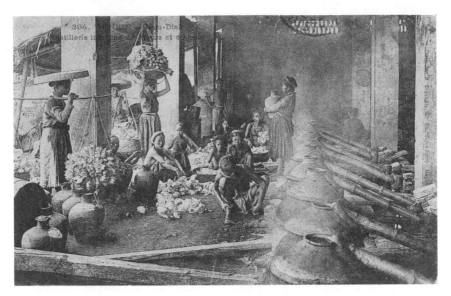

Figure 2.1 Postcard of an indigenous distillery of flowers and alcohol.
Collection of the author.

most regularly cited figures reported around 20 to 50 percent of the Chinese
population and 10 percent of the Vietnamese were regular smokers.[19] On
average, the French estimated, some eighty-five thousand regular smokers
in Indochina consumed between approximately three hundred grams (in the
case of Vietnamese consumers) and two kilograms of opium (in the case of
Chinese) per capita. Most opium was consumed in Cochinchina and in the
cities of Saigon and Cholon, homes to the wealthiest Chinese communities.[20]

In the 1890s, administrators started to consider drug monopolies as part
of broader fiscal reforms. The efforts began under de Lanessan's pacification
program but took off properly under Paul Doumer. First, officials needed
more tax revenue. From 1882 to 1891, the Tonkin province cost metropolitan France nearly half a billion francs.[21] The pacification of the region was
expensive, and Paris was not willing to pay. Taxation, particularly in the
comparatively wealthier colony of Cochinchina had to make up the shortfall. Direct taxes, such as the land tax or the corvée, were collected by village chiefs (the lý trưởng) and covered only a fraction of the population.
Cadastral registers, such as they were, had not been updated since the time of
the Nguyễn dynasty. The French had no accurate information on population
numbers.[22] Rationalizing and broadening direct taxation could therefore

not solve the French fiscal problem. Second, the reliance of the Vietnamese economy on rice (which accounted for 90 percent of trade) created fears that the Chinese market would not be able to absorb the agricultural surplus, given rising yields. This would lead to depressed prices and less tax revenue.[23] Finally, French industrialists wanted Doumer to invest in infrastructure. The governor-general sought a loan of 80 million francs to finance a series of ambitious public works projects. These developments included the construction of a railway from Phủ Lạng Thương near Hanoi to Lạng Sơn by the Chinese border, potable water purification projects in Hanoi and Haiphong, and a number of other smaller ventures. Expenses swelled, and ultimately the colony borrowed a considerable 200 million francs to finance its public works in 1898.[24] No wonder that Doumer was willing to consider forms of taxation that his predecessors had dismissed.

Drug monopolies presented an attractive alternative with precedents in both Europe and Asia. In France, Jean-Baptiste Colbert had established a tax farm monopoly on tobacco already in 1674. By the eighteenth century, similar monopolies existed in Spain, Portugal, and the Hapsburg Empire and in German and Italian states.[25] Completely state-run monopolies, however, were rare, as most early modern states preferred to build up patronage systems and not rely on centralized tax collection. In the nineteenth century, European states, motivated by higher revenue needs and concerns over the equity of taxation, moved increasingly toward direct collection and away from monopolies. At the same time, in Asia, British and Dutch colonial states still established centralized monopolies, which could extract more revenue by appropriating profits that previously went to license holders and by eliminating common forms of tax evasion.[26] Meanwhile politicians in Paris, who saw monopolies as anathema to republican principles of free trade, and businessmen in Indochina, who realized that most of them would inevitably remain excluded from profits made by a *state* monopoly, remained skeptical about such schemes.[27]

In 1893, de Lanessan instituted taxes on a wide variety of goods: petrol, candles, tobacco, salt, and finally alcohol.[28] The new alcohol tax, which applied to commodities as well as to alembics and other distillation equipment, did not substantially increase revenues.[29] Defenders of free trade, the so-called ultraliberals suggested that revenue might be increased by a better-equipped and better-staffed Douanes et Régies department, but this reform required substantial investment. Pro-monopoly "ultrafiscalists" argued that self-sustaining finances were preconditions for the moral growth of the indigenous population, teaching them the restraint and economics necessary for eventual self-government. Such moral education ultimately superseded concerns over free trade.[30] The Doumer administration decided to bring alcohol production under the control of the state and cut out middlemen altogether.[31]

Former Douanes officials used this moment to leverage their connections and gain privileged access to the profits promised by drug monopolies. Two brothers, Lucien and Auguste Fontaine, raised capital from small French landholders in Indochina and founded the SFDI, which lobbied for monopoly contracts in regions where the French regulated alcohol production.[32] Another former Douanes agent, René de Saint-Mathurin, formed the Société Fermiere in 1887 and pursued opium contracts colonial administrators had traditionally signed with the Chinese. By 1890, Saint-Mathurin had acquired control of opium production in Tonkin-Annam and set his sights on Cochinchina and Cambodia.[33] Both Chinese and French competitors, however, cautioned against favoritism, noting that existing producers had more expertise and more efficient production methods than either the Fontaines or Saint-Mathurin.

Meanwhile, Calmette in the Saigon microbiological laboratory keenly felt the need to impress the importance of the colonial government funding his research. Expertise in agrobusiness and fermentation had been central to Pastorian science since Louis Pasteur. In a groundbreaking paper, "Study on Lactic Fermentation," Pasteur argued that anaerobic microorganisms—yeasts—and their biological activity caused the fermentation process that transforms sugar into lactic acid in substances such as wine or sour milk.[34] This paper shot Pasteur to the forefront of French science and contained "the central theoretical and methodological features of all of Pasteur's work on fermentation."[35] The scientist himself highlighted the potential advantage France would acquire if it could improve its beer industry, which lagged behind that of Germany, playing to the Franco-German rivalry that consumed France after 1870.[36] According to a legend, Pasteur's work on lactic acid fermentation was inspired by his encounter with a viticulturist named Bigo (sometimes rendered "Bigot"), who was having trouble producing beetroot alcohol, which often had a sour taste. In this telling, Pasteur's entire oeuvre became a symbol of the fertile encounter between industry and science. Although there is no evidence this encounter ever took place, the persistence of this legend among bacteriologists demonstrates the extent to which industrial development had become a key part of Pastorian self-identification.[37] It is hardly surprising, then, that Calmette focused on industrial agriculture. French monopoly makers faced many obstacles. In the metropole, officials saw drug monopolies as distinctly antimodern and anti–free trade. Both Saint-Mathurin and the Fontaines had inferior technologies, which existing producers did not hesitate to point out. Calmette's expertise proved crucial in resolving all of these tensions.

Pastorizing the Alcohol Monopoly

After arriving in Saigon in 1891, Calmette quickly made contact with the director of the Douanes et Régies and pitched him the potential of Pastorian expertise for the alcohol and opium industries.[38] The bacteriologist was planning to reverse-engineer Vietnamese methods of distillation and modernize them according to Pastorian principles. Ultimately, he developed a new method of fermenting rượu. He called it the "Amyloprocess," named after what he believed was the critical yeast in the Vietnamese-Chinese process, the *Amolymyces rouxii*. This method became the centerpiece of the SFDI's business model and the basis for the company's claims to purity and hygienic and scientific rationality.

A closer look at how Calmette conceptualized and developed the Amyloprocess reveals how technopolitical concerns guided his study from the beginning. There were no obvious answers to some of the conceptual questions facing Calmette. How much could he alter the fermentation process while still being able to claim it was identical to the traditional Vietnamese product? What was it that made rượu rượu? Was it the taste of the drink? The grounding of Calmette's research in Vietnamese tradition? The chemical composition of the wine? And if so, which biological processes were critical to maintaining the identity of the drink and which could be discarded in the interests of cutting fermentation time or reducing costs? What constituted "pure" wine, and what made the drink "contaminated"? Technical knowledge alone could not answer these questions; Calmette's answers were animated largely by politics.

Calmette began with reverse-engineering local practices. He drew on an ethnography of the Saigon distillery published in the *Journal Indochinois* in 1887, as well as visits to the Thủ Thiêm distillery outside Saigon, where he obtained a recipe used in the fermentation process.[39] The recipe, which the Pastorian translated into both French and Latin, contained "the complete list" of forty-six plants used to grow the mysterious "Chinese leaven."[40] Calmette noted that the plants only added aroma to the product, and that the recipe omitted the active agent itself—the yeast. Having secured a sample of the leaven from the distillery, he could grow an active culture in a Petri dish and discover which of the many yeasts was responsible for the saccharification of the rice starch. He named the critical microorganism in honor of his teacher Émile Roux: *Amolymyces rouxii*.

Distinguishing between the "active ingredient" and plants of secondary importance was crucial for Calmette's framing of the process as scientific and rationalized. He argued that it was only through Pastorian science that the process of wine fermentation could accurately be explained, and therefore modernized, while the Chinese recipe arrived at its results only by accident. He argued that rather than being introduced to the rice mixture through a forty-six-plant mixture—as the Chinese recipe seemed to imply—the critical yeast attached itself to the outer shells of unhusked rice. This explained why Chinese distillers had to "insert moist rice husks in the still-soft loaf [of leaven]."[41] Calmette then noted that this process bore a curious resemblance to the fermentation of wine as described by Pasteur, where the crucial yeast was found on the skins of grapes, implying that it was Pasteur's insight that helped him arrive at the correct explanation.[42] In Calmette's telling, the Chinese had focused on secondary aspects of the fermentation process, while he, building on the genius of Pasteur, could now focus on the one transformation that mattered.

Calmette then proposed several alterations to the fermentation process, which "improved" on the Chinese recipe. First, by optimizing temperature, limiting oxygen flow, and adding small quantities of antiseptics, Calmette promised to double the yield of alcohol and significantly reduce fermentation time in laboratory conditions. Second, the Chinese process involved many colonies of different yeasts, some which aided the fermentation process, while others impeded it and could even prove toxic. Calmette's "improved" method only preserved the "alcoholic ferments" in the recipe, while the Chinese process also preserved "the ferments of disease."[43] Calmette assumed that efficiency in production time clearly indicated progress, outlining how Chinese "imperfections" reduced yields and increased fermentation time. He made only passing mention of the fact that the particular combination of yeasts in the Chinese process also gave the rice alcohol its distinctive, smoky ("empyreumatic") taste. His "perfected" method, which Calmette named the Amyloprocess, held the promise of handing the

French a monopoly on rice alcohol production in Indochina.[44] Here, again, Calmette assumed that processes that did not directly relate to the production of alcohol were impediments or toxic and should be excised in order to speed up fermentation time. The rhetoric of "purity" and "disease" hid the degree to which these distinctions were arbitrary and reflected the concerns of the administration, rather than a specifically Pastorian method.

The SFDI quickly obtained rights to Calmette's Amyloprocess and gave the Pastorian a seat on the company board. The advantages conferred by the Amyloprocess, combined with clever legislative reforms, helped the company to secure control of virtually all wine production in Tonkin and northern Annam, as well as to become the largest producers alongside Chinese industrialists in Cochinchina. The monopoly-building, which took place gradually from 1897 to 1902, was a difficult process, and its success owed much to the creative interfacing between technology and legislation.

When Governor-General Doumer decided to make alcohol taxation one of the "beasts of burden" of the colonial budget, he ran into serious opposition from the Ministry of the Colonies. Officials in Paris, in true republican fashion, were concerned about protectionism and other impediments to free trade.[45] While in the metropole, the 1890s marked a resurgence of protectionism, with the introduction of measures such as the Méline tariff on agricultural products, the Ministry of the Colonies remained committed to equal opportunity. Ministry officials had already scolded the Indochinese administration for its existing tax regime, which differentiated between alcohol manufactured with local raw materials and imported raw materials, as well as between locally produced and imported alcohol. Ministry officials called such distinctions protectionism and noted that "the illegality of this sort of taxation is incontestable."[46] In this climate of heightened metropolitan attention, handing over *all* rice wine production to a French company by administrative fiat was inconceivable. Instead, the administration passed a number of decrees that, combined with the economic advantage provided by the Amyloprocess, enabled the SFDI to simply corner the market.

On 1 June 1897, Governor-General Doumer decreed that all distillers in northern Vietnam had to apply for a license from the Douanes et Régies. To get licensed, distillers had to produce liquor with a minimum 35 percent alcohol content and sell the product to retailers at prices set by contracts negotiated by the administration.[47] Thirty-five percent alcohol content was a relative rarity for Vietnamese rice wine, with the most common strength ranging just below, at the 26 to 35 percent range. The Amyloprocess, however, delivered higher alcohol content. The ability of the French to set wholesale prices meant that producers had to deliver relatively high yields in order to turn a profit—again, something that few Vietnamese distillers could achieve. The Amyloprocess, by contrast, had been explicitly designed to raise yields. Finally, the SFDI further increased its competitive edge through economies of scale by using French capital to construct huge new factories in Hanoi and Nam Định.

Later legislation stacked the deck even further toward the SFDI: a decree from 9 March 1900 required all distilleries to have tiled roofs and walls made of either brick or clay, ostensibly to "perfectly close" the distillation area and to establish fixed entry and exit points. This would facilitate surveillance by Régie agents and prevent contraband from getting out of factories.[48] In reality, the capital costs for these improvements were so high that only French distillers could afford them.[49] The final nails in the coffin were the decrees of 20 and 22 December, 1902, which gave the administration the right to refuse to issue new licenses if the region in question was already "adequately" served by existing distillers, to set caps on the quantity of alcohol suppliers were allowed to buy from any one distiller, and, in cases of unexpectedly high demand, to assign increased production quotas to factories delivering the lowest prices.[50] By the time these decrees were passed, the SFDI already enjoyed a near-monopoly status in many regions, and since the decrees effectively made it impossible for new distilleries to be established, the 1902 decrees ensured the Fontaines' Amylo-aided dominance of the northern Vietnamese market for decades to come.[51]

The emergence of the SFDI monopoly depended, ultimately, on the mutual interaction of legal and technical changes, on administrative action, and on Pastorian innovation. Calmette's Amyloprocess delivered a higher concentration of alcohol at a higher yield. The reduced variety of yeasts and aromatics made the process easily scalable. Once the administration made efficiency in production, high yields, and high alcohol content the metrics of licensing, the SFDI suddenly found itself at a competitive advantage. True, not everywhere. In Cochinchina, Chinese distillers had access to large factories and capital, so they could meet French regulations even using older methods that delivered lower yields. In central Annam and Cambodia, inadequate infrastructure worked against centralization and helped local distilleries remain dominant. But in northern Vietnam, the technopolitics of the Amyloprocess transformed alcohol manufacturing into a monopoly regime in the span of only a decade.

The rượu monopoly continued to leverage the language of Pastorian hygiene and the connection Calmette's research process established to traditional Chinese fermentation methods as justification of its existence. French administrators and entrepreneurs fused orientalist stereotypes about Vietnamese habits with Pastorian claims about the "purity" of their product. For the Vietnamese, alcohol was not an intoxicant, the monopoly supporters claimed, but a "necessity of the first degree," used by "men, women, children and elderly alike" for ritual and everyday purposes. "Guided by his instinct," the Vietnamese never abused alcohol, and therefore a state-run monopoly could not pose a danger to public health. On the contrary, centralized production and strict surveillance would help safeguard "the public health and interest of the country."[52]

Descriptions of the improvements achieved through the Amyloprocess often involved a slippage between economic and hygienic dimensions. The isolation of productive yeasts in the Chinese process provided primarily an economic advantage, decreasing fermentation time and increasing yield; but Calmette himself was purposefully fuzzy, describing his innovation as distinguishing the "ferments of illness" from the productive *Amolymyces rouxii* and suggesting that the Chinese process was unpredictable and could also influence the taste and quality of the alcohol.[53] In official correspondence and public propaganda, the emphasis was almost always placed on the hygienic effects of Calmette's procedure. "While the products obtained through the Amyloprocess invented by Doctor Calmette of the Pasteur Institute are more or less pure, Chinese alcohol contains impurities in great quantity. . . . Limiting ourselves only to the hygienic perspective, it is desirable that the Chinese alcohol consumed every year in Cochinchina be replaced by the French product," Governor-General Albert Sarraut wrote to the Ministry of the Colonies in 1912.[54] Another defender of the monopoly similarly slipped from a discussion of yeasts harmful to the process of alcohol formation to a discussion of "extremely harmful side products, such as various essential oils, giving the alcohol a very strong odor and flavor."[55] In the course of a few paragraphs, a technical question of production efficiency had become a question of consumer taste. Vietnamese commentators, too, acknowledged these claims to purity: "Yes, I know, one can demonstrate with A plus B, in learned formulas, that the alcohol of the Societe des Distilleries is perfect, that it is exquisite, that it is not in the least toxic. . . . Chemistry possesses a certain beauty that it is not for us mortals to dispute," admitted Pham Quynh, a conservative Vietnamese nationalist in 1931.[56] Finally, SFDI routinely highlighted the hygienic and scientific aspects of the Amyloprocess, constantly emphasizing the Calmette connection in promotional materials. References to the "learned studies of Doctor Calmette" were complemented by aerial photographs of large-scale factories, where rice from the most "modern paddy fields" was processed in distilleries containing the "most careful antiseptics" overseen by chemists "permanently monitoring every phase of production."[57]

At the same time, supporters of the Amyloprocess pointed out that factory alcohol, although purified and "perfected," was still "in principle the same as that [produced] by Asian distilleries."[58] "The [European] operations, which are identical to those employed by the Chinese, . . . take place in conditions of absolute asepsis," noted another report, again emphasizing the similarity of the SFDI's procedure to the Chinese, while highlighting the hygienic improvements.[59] The connection between local tradition and Pastorian

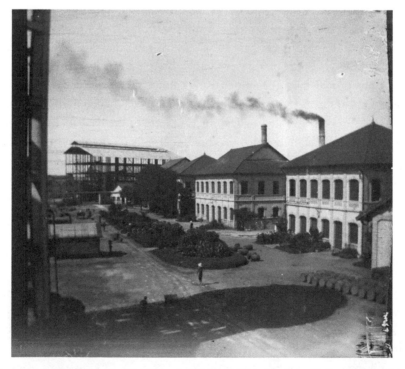

Figure 2.2 The factory of the French Society of Distilleries of Indochina, 1921. Pierre Bonnet (1888–1965). Paris, Musée Guimet—Musée national des Arts asiatiques. © RMN-Grand Palais / Art Resource, NY.

expertise, physically forged through the purchase, study, and modification of leaven from the Thủ Thiêm distillery, proved critical to the French defense of the monopoly.

How tangible was this connection, though? In many ways, SFDI alcohol was clearly *not* identical to Vietnamese rượu. The composition of rượu and the variety of herbs used to flavor it differed greatly across regions—the beverage had no single identity to begin with. The secondary yeasts, which Calmette called "ferments of illness," were responsible for giving rượu its smoky flavor. Eliminating these organisms reduced fermentation time but also altered the taste. Finally, the alcohol produced with the Amyloprocess was stronger than traditional rượu, 40 percent alcohol rather than 25 to 35 percent. As Gerard Sasges has convincingly argued, this, too, was a feature, not a bug, since alcohol content became a way of distinguishing factory alcohol from contraband. Still, the taste and quality of the drink were noticeably different. The processes were identical only by Calmette's definition, which allowed all modifications for the sake of efficiency and boiled the measure of "identity" down to the use of the single alcohol-producing yeast, the *Amolymyces rouxii*.

The final irony was that from the early 1900s onwards, the SFDI no longer used this yeast in its production process. Upon returning to France in 1894, Calmette continued to work on his method. The *Amolymyces rouxii* appeared to do the work of both malt (saccharification) and leaven (fermentation into alcohol), thereby promising significant efficiencies in industrial distilling in France as well. Hoping to innovate French distilling, Calmette's students in Lille, Boidin, and Rolants, collaborating with a French distiller named Collette, refined the study of the *Amolymyces*, increasing potential yields even further.[60] The group took out a patent on the yeast, which, by 1898, was used in more than a dozen distilleries in France and many more in Belgium. Calmette transferred his share to the Société Amylo, controlled by Collette, for 250,000 francs. This allowed Collette and Boidin to continue independent work on the Amyloprocess, developing other yeasts that did the same work as the *rouxii*, surviving on temperatures above thirty-eight degrees Celsius and performing both saccharification and alcohol production. They ultimately opted for the use of the *Rhizopus delemar*.[61] It was this method that the SFDI used in its factories. The "Chinese method" had undergone several transformations: technological, in the form of Calmette's efficiency-oriented "improvements"; biological, in the form of the yeast substitutions; as well as discursive, in the translation from Chinese tradition to Pastorian science.

The last transformation—juridical—in the form of patents, which were then used to change ownership, divest Calmette from the product, and deliver the SFDI the rights to exploit the method in Indochina, black-boxed all the other transformations and cemented the Amyloprocess as a Pastorian-improved method rooted in Indochinese local custom.

The development of the rice alcohol monopoly posed both political and technological problems. Pastorization provided answers to both. It provided the SFDI with technology to actually produce rượu on a competitive basis, as well as the conditions of possibility for legal changes that privileged French factory alcohol over local products. The logic of pastorization embedded in the choice to focus on one yeast culture as the defining characteristic of the Amyloprocess provided both a rhetoric of "purity" and "science" to justify the monopoly to critics opposing it on the grounds of free trade and a rhetoric of "identity" enabling the SFDI to claim that its alcohol respected tradition.

Pastorizing the Opium Industry

The fate of the opium industry provides an illuminating contrast to the successful transformation of the alcohol monopoly. With opium, Calmette and the Douanes et Régies attempted a similar approach, studying ways of improving Chinese methods of fermentation using Pastorian science and deploying arguments about hygiene and efficiency to justify centralizing the industry in the hands of René de Saint-Mathurin's Société Fermiere. Their plans, however, faltered. Here, the fusion of technology and politics became an obstacle. When Calmette's initial attempts at improving opium manufacturing failed, Saint-Mathurin's many enemies in the business circles of Saigon and critics outside the colonial administration quickly laid blame at the feet of the Pastorian. French entrepreneurs used Calmette's failure as a proxy to talk about the overreach of the state in business. Technological failure became the vehicle of a different kind of technopolitics, one that Calmette and the administration could not predict. Opium manufacturers ultimately made more modest reforms, and administrators continued to emphasize the essential Chineseness of opium, arguing that it was an "oriental vice," which the French were regulating for purely fiscal purposes.

Initially, administrators and Pastorians argued that opium was a potentially progressive product, if submitted to proper bacteriological and state control. De Lanessan once suggested instituting an opium monopoly based on the British example, noting that opium "is, in reality, a habit neither better nor worse than smoking or drinking; it just has the disadvantage of being less easy to satisfy."[62] Administrators defending the opium regime regularly noted that the percentage of "opiomanes" in Indochina was hardly larger than the percentage of alcoholics in France. They argued that in the tropical climate, opium produced "more advantages than obstacles," helping users manage the hot and humid weather, and that opium, unlike alcohol, tended to render intoxicated consumers calm and quiet, rather than aggressive and loud.[63] Some even called opium "an intellectual stimulant," no doubt recalling its importance for writers such as Charles Baudelaire.[64] Many analysts feared that if opium use were suppressed, consumers would switch to liquor and develop "alcoholism, the effects of which are far more deplorable than those of opiomania."[65] All these qualities, administrators claimed, made opium far more amenable for state regulation than other vices, such as gambling. Once the potential virtues of opium were established, Calmette and others could claim that bacteriological expertise could render opium processing more regular, the results more uniformly consistent, and the taste more accurately reflective of consumer preference.[66]

Calmette decided to study opium after meeting the French industrialist René de Saint-Mathurin during his first voyage to Saigon in 1891. At the time, Saint-Mathurin was in the process of consolidating his hold on Tonkin-Annam, and pressuring French administrators to award him more contracts.[67] In the following years, French administrators experimented with different ways of seizing control over opium production, in some cases handing out public tenders to Chinese concessionaries, in other cases giving production rights to Saint-Mathurin, and in some cases purchasing the production plants directly. Usually, this meant that a few large factories in Cochinchina, Tonkin, and Laos changed ownership, while on the shop floor, Chinese managers and workers continued toiling away at their everyday jobs. The success of the French-run opium monopoly depended not so much on competition with local small businesses (as was the case with alcohol distillation) as with offering a product competitive with rampant contraband and extracting enough revenue to support the colony's tax base.

Calmette's research on opium drew heavily on a paper published by a French colonial pharmacist, Lalande, in the *Archives de Médecine Navale et Coloniale*. Unlike rice alcohol, which the French had struggled to understand, opium processing could be easily observed in the Saigon factory. The plant had been brought under French control in 1882 and operated under the supervision of a naturalized French-Chinese manager, Tang Thai, and the "wise and intelligent" Monsieur Piétri, who provided Lalande with details of chandoo production.[68] In the factory, opium was brewed with water in a series of vats until it acquired a homogeneous consistency. It was then flash-heated, washed and filtered, turned into cakes (*crêpes*), and then, finally, left to ferment. This last process gave chandoo the smell of burned plaster and the acrid taste that Indochinese consumers expected.[69] After an initial month-long fermentation, the chandoo was packaged and left to ferment for another period of up to a year. Lalande described the "Chinese" or "Cantonese" method but did not propose any improvements to the process, nor did he identify the leaven responsible for the long fermentation.

Calmette had help from the director of the Douanes et Régies, who had unlimited access to raw opium (it was, after all, purchased from India by the colonial state). Studying Lalande's description of the "Cantonese method," Calmette soon discovered that a species of the fungus *Aspergillus* was responsible for consuming excess glucose and dextrin in the product and transforming tannin into gallic acid, creating the distinctive taste of quality chandoo. The Pastorian knew that *Aspergillus* fungi grew particularly well in a mixture of water, candied sugar, ammonium nitrate, tartaric acid, and a variety of sulfates, known as Raulin's medium. By cultivating these fungi and seeding them in fermenting opium, Calmette was able to cut fermentation time from a year to a month. To convince the administration, he then conducted a blind test with a Frenchman, a Chinese aficionado, and the director of the Douanes et Régies. Calmette proudly reported that none could tell the difference between Chinese opium and his own.[70]

Alas, taking the research from the laboratory to the factory proved more complicated than Calmette had believed. The first large-scale batch of opium produced with the Calmette process failed miserably for mysterious reasons, leaving the Douanes et Régies with nearly five thousand kilograms of subpar product and a net loss of 3,000 piasters.[71] Later attempts did not fare any better. The fast-fermented product lacked the distinctive smell and taste of chandoo, sold poorly, and even prompted a series of vituperative op-eds in the *Courrier de Saigon*, where a representative accusation read: "You are urinating in the fermentation vats to poison us."[72]

The failure of Calmette's experiments quickly became a talking point in an ongoing conflict between the colonial administration and business interests. A special commission of the Colonial Council, the advisory body made up of French entrepreneurs and some Vietnamese notables, evaluated the promises the Douanes et Régies had made on the basis of Calmette's new method and concluded that "regretfully, [the commission] is obliged to contradict the Administration in almost all of its assertions."[73] "The empirical ways in which experiments were conducted," the commission concluded, led to an inconsistent and subpar product, which caused French opium sales to plummet, and in itself caused significant damage to the finances of the factory. The administration had proceeded too ambitiously, scaling up an essentially untested method, without accounting for potential downsides. This sort of meddling in the affairs of the factory, several councilors noted, was inevitable, given that the state was appointing managers who had no real knowledge of the industry. Instead of large-scale reforms, the administration should finance piecemeal experiments and leave business decisions to the factory owners, the commission stated. One councilor, Bérenguier, accused the administration of placing too much faith in Calmette, who in his opinion had mistaken a secondary fermentation agent for a primary one, and in his attempts to streamline the process eliminated a crucial yeast.[74] Even years later, analyses of opium processing still referred to "Calmette's elementary error" that had spoiled the batches of 1894–1895.[75] These arguments at the Colonial Council were largely attempts by French economic interests to discourage the administration from large-scale experimentation and claw back fiscal and managerial freedom from the increasingly interventionist Douanes et Régies.

At the same time, Douanes officials and some councilors defended Calmette and blamed factory owners instead. Some commentators believed that greedy managers had deviated from Calmette's instructions and, in their attempts to raise yields and deliver a more profitable product, had diluted the brew beyond its limits.[76] The director of the Douanes et Régies pointed out that the problem might lie with the quality of the raw materials imported from India, since the defects disappeared with the following batch of boules.[77] Finally, Calmette himself accused the rigid business cycle of the opium trade, which depended on yearly harvests in India. The limited supply window of raw opium meant that the Régie often had to ship unfermented chandoo out to retailers in order to meet demand, making fast fermentation (which required sophisticated tools and a controlled environment) impossible.[78] The material failure of Calmette's modernization efforts became a tool in political contests between French entrepreneurs and the Douanes et Régies. Even though the various parties ultimately agreed that Calmette's fault could not be conclusively established, Calmette's reforms became too toxic to revisit. The pastorization of the opium monopoly failed.

Improvements to the Saigon factory did happen over time, but they were initiated by factory managers, not administrators. In the decade after Calmette's fiasco, engineers and biologists working at the factory tinkered with all aspects of the process. A dedicated laboratory was attached to the factory, tasked with quality assurance. Factory owners replaced manual threshing with machinery, replaced gas heating with charcoal, refined the brewing process, introduced the sterilization of opium cakes, and ultimately increased yields from 50 percent to 60 to 70 percent, while decreasing water use.[79] Owners reduced staff and hired more European middle managers. Opium barons even employed the help of visiting researchers from the Pasteur Institute.[80] Opium production was made more efficient, but it never acquired the symbolic heft of a Pastorian modernization process.

Factory alcohol became a symbol of local tradition improved by Pastorian (and therefore French) science. In the case of opium, manufacturers and administrators emphasized the essential Chineseness of their product, playing down the alterations the French had made to the process, which ranged from bacteriological improvements to changes borrowed largely from Dutch factories in Java. Yet commentators consistently referred to the procedure as "the perfected Cantonese method" and highlighted the importance of Chinese labor.[81]

Technological failure, like technological success, was embedded in politics. Calmette's problems in translating his fast fermentation from the laboratory to the factory setting hurt his reputation and made him an easy target to blame for underwhelming sales. At the same time, blaming Calmette's method became a tool for French economic interests frustrated with the Douanes et Régies interference in management, even though it was entirely possible that the failure of opium modernization could have been caused by many other factors. The opium batches' failure to ferment halted Calmette's rise to the top ranks of opium experts, empowered factory managers' resistance to the state, and dissolved the discourse of scientific modernity around opium reforms. Here, again, technology was critical to shaping the politics of opium monopolies, though in a very different way.

One might ask if the differences between the rượu monopoly and the opium monopoly were, at the end of the day, that great. Even though the former was driven largely by administrators, and the latter more by factory owners who operated state contracts, and even though the former was imbued with a rhetoric of progress and Pastorian hygiene, while the latter was not, both industries were successfully seized by the French, and contributed massively to the Indochinese tax base. Did the French state not achieve its goals? Yet differences in the ideological justification and the material structure of these two industries ultimately mattered substantially when Vietnamese, French, and international critics began to challenge these monopolies in the early 1900s.

Challenging the Alcohol Monopoly

Despite its seeming initial success, maintaining the alcohol monopoly required enormous effort. Wine sales failed to deliver the expected tax revenue, leading to violent police action in attempts to contain contraband. This, in turn, contributed to broad opposition and resistance to factory alcohol. In opposing the regime, Vietnamese, Chinese, and French actors all drew on the very rhetoric that had allowed the French to consolidate rượu production—that of Pastorian hygienic modernity. The conflict came to a head in 1911–1913, when Albert Sarraut attempted to reform the system but quickly discovered that the very success of the Amyloprocess regime vastly limited his options for reform. In the following discussion, I draw substantially on previous research by Erica Peters and Gerard Sasges, who have looked at alcohol protests through the lens of everyday consumption and the politics of policing, respectively. Here, however, our interest is on the role of the rhetoric and technology of pastorization during the decades of protest.

Monopolies were supposed to be the "beasts of burden" of the Government-General's budget. Their revenues formed the fiscal basis for loan repayments, infrastructure projects, and other expenses, which encompassed the entire Indochinese Union.[82] On paper, the alcohol monopoly appeared to serve these purposes well. Governor-General Doumer reported that in 1901 almost half of the general budget's revenue came from the three monopolies—alcohol, opium, and salt—with alcohol accounting for 13.6 percent of total revenue, and opium accounting for 26.4 percent.[83] Yet, as Sasges has argued, these figures were wildly optimistic, based on projected sales, exclusive of administrative expenses and the fluctuating rates of purchasing prices. They were effectively magic asterisks, helping to demonstrate the soundness of the general budget and establishing the creditworthiness of the union to lenders. More realistic figures, provided by two missions of inspection (audits ordered by the Ministry of the Colonies) in 1912 and 1930, suggested that the alcohol monopoly netted between 2 and 4 percent of the general budget's revenue, less than one-third of Doumer's estimate.[84] While creative accounting did provide additional leverage for the state, actual fiscal benefits were deeply underwhelming.

Pressured by the SFDI to maintain price levels, the Government-General ordered local prefects and the Douanes et Régies to crack down on contraband.[85] Some provincial administrators, incentivized by the promise of increased budget allocations for every liter of alcohol sold over a certain minimum, reportedly established village quotas.[86] For example, Trinh-ca Giang, the the lý trưởng of Ha Xa, filed a complaint in 1910 noting that the local French resident required villagers to purchase five large bottles of factory alcohol for permission to slaughter a pig. The "tax" for killing a cow was twelve bottles, and a bison cost twenty-four bottles. He even attached a letter requesting permission to kill three pigs for a funerary festival in exchange for fifteen bottles of alcohol.[87] Similar incidents were reported across the Tonkin province.[88]

The Douanes et Régies also became increasingly coercive in its attempts to curb contraband. By 1908, it was the single largest department in the Indochinese Union, with 1,290 European officers in the Vietnamese colonies– a tenfold increase over ten years—and an additional two thousand indigenous employees.[89] Douanes agents were allowed to search Vietnamese homes between 5:00 a.m. and 6:30 p.m. and conduct body searches and exterior searches at any time and for any reason—while searches of Europeans required due cause.[90] Any attempts to resist the douaniers were classified as "rebellion" and brutally suppressed. The Vietnamese could file complaints, but these were processed by Douanes officers themselves, leaving little hope for fairness.[91] Lenience in policing was, in the words of the Douanes director Jules Morel, "a case of truly misplaced humanism."[92]

Efforts to curb contraband culminated in 1902 with the infamous "Article 96," which imposed collective responsibility for failing to report contraband. The law allowed the Douanes et Régies to impose collective fines on villages if douaniers discovered illegal distilleries without information from local notables. Even though Article 96 was legally ambiguous (it failed to specify which village notables should be held responsible and how the fine was going to be paid), as well as simply illegal under the Napoleonic Code (as many legal experts at the time noted), it remained on the books until 1908.[93]

Article 96 had severe unintended consequences for political stability. Administrators noted that it became a vehicle for resolving intravillage strife: villagers looking to rid themselves of an unpopular mandarin could simply put up a secret distillery, tip off the Douanes et Régies, and wait for the other shoe to drop.[94] The law eroded trust between village notables and French administrators and made municipal posts unpopular among the Vietnamese. In 1904, in the village of Hoi-an, douaniers caught the family of Nguyen Van Buong illegally distilling rượu and, following Article 96, put the village mayor on trial facing a fine of 1,000 francs. The mayor, knowing he would be convicted, stepped down from his post days before the trial. Predictably, all proposed replacements declined the nomination. Finally, Monsieur Doceul, the local prefect, had to nominate Nguyen Van An, a civil servant, for the post—who promptly fled the village and hid in the nearby forest for a day. Doceul finally managed to convince Van An to accept the post but only after extensive handwringing.[95] Incidents such as these caused much bad blood between French administrators and the Douanes et Régies, the former accusing the douaniers of eroding their authority and making their job harder.[96] It was under this sort of pressure that Article 96 was finally repealed.

Contraband policing, Article 96, and coercive sales intruded deeply in Vietnamese lives and probably were the main causes of resistance to the monopoly.[97] However, Vietnamese critics found it difficult to verbalize this dissatisfaction, since the legal system left them with few options for proving Douanes abuses. Douaniers could counter complaints by pointing toward high levels of contraband and arguing that being tough on crime was a crucial part of their mandate.[98]

Instead, Vietnamese consumers attacked the monopoly itself, rejecting the Pastorian claims to purity, efficiency, and quality through letter-writing campaigns, opinion pieces, theatrical plays, pamphlets, and arguments advanced at sessions of the Colonial Council. Most common complaints had to do with the strength and taste of SFDI rượu. Vietnamese critics claimed it was too strong—40 percent alcohol instead of 25 to 35 percent, as was common in locally distilled products. It also lacked the characteristic smoky taste, a byproduct of the variety of herbs and secondary ferments used in local distilling, that the Amyloprocess had excluded as ferments of illness. Factory alcohol was also reported to cause "nausea and unbearable headaches."[99]

The Vietnamese did not simply complain about taste; they consciously contrasted problems with flavor to Pastorian promises of scientifically assured purity and hygiene. When French residents reminded the Vietnamese that factory alcohol, while less flavorful, "had an enormous advantage by being more pure and less detrimental to health," the Vietnamese responded that nausea, headaches, and stomachaches were not exactly signs of fitness.[100] Some even claimed that drinking factory alcohol endangered not only the drinker but also his offspring.[101] Others suspected that the efficiencies of factory production came at a cost to the consumer: at village meetings, Vietnamese peasants accused the SFDI of replacing quality *nep* rice with lower-quality rice or even with potatoes.[102] Rather than outright challenging the French monopoly, or focusing on the repressive practices of the Douanes et Régies, Vietnamese consumers accused the French of not living up to their promise of hygienic, Pastorian modernity.

A second line of attack focused on the question of consumer choice. The SFDI claimed that its alcohol was simply a pastorized, modern version of Vietnamese wine. Yet lacking the necessary taste, Vietnamese consumers countered, it could not be used for ritual purposes. "A Vietnamese maxim says: 'without alcohol, worship is impossible.' But the Fontaine alcohol, which has neither the taste nor the title of traditional alcohol, cannot be used for worship," one councilor asserted.[103] The French, some critics argued, would not be expected to replace fine Burgundy wine with a factory-made product simply because of economic efficiency. This argument clearly resonated, as it made its way to several official reports.[104] What the Vietnamese wanted was the "taste of the land"—*le goût du terroir*—something with which the French were all too familiar.[105] The French had promised a modern product faithful to Vietnamese tradition, but they could deliver neither.

Vietnamese consumers found unlikely allies among French entrepreneurs upset with the Fontaines' dominance of a lucrative industry, as well with those staunch French republicans who opposed everything that prevented free trade. One chemist and student of Calmette, Sanguinetti, joined forces with two French entrepreneurs in Indochina, Bédat and Ajalbert. He intended, with the help of Chinese distillers and a method derived from the Amyloprocess, to provide competition to the SFDI while still meeting the requirements set by the administration. Their case rested on consumer choice and a disdain for monopolies: partnering with Chinese producers would enable them to retain the smoky taste and ritual qualities customers sought, while the use of a variant of the Amyloprocess would provide the modernizing edge the French promised. Finally, their venture could break the SFDI monopoly, which in turn would lead to further innovation: "In my eyes all monopolies are an industrial shame, contrary to free innovation and the development of new technologies—nobody has the right to declare that they've reached industrial perfection."[106] Privately, Calmette warned Sanguinetti against using a method so close to his Amyloprocess, and the application was rejected by the Government-General, on the grounds that demand in Cochinchina was already being met by existing distillers, that distillers were prohibited from engaging in retail sales, and that it was "unsuitable to the needs of the consumers."[107] Still, entrepreneurs repeated these critiques often in the years to come, both in newspaper articles and at the sessions of the Colonial Council.[108]

When Albert Sarraut arrived as the governor-general of Indochina in 1903, just as the ten-year contract signed with the SFDI was coming up for renewal, the situation escalated further. The alcohol monopoly had become a rallying cry for a variety of anti-French movements. One year into Sarraut's tenure, a bomb exploded in a cafe in Hanoi, killing two French officers and a Vietnamese man and injuring dozens. Phan Bội Châu, the Vietnamese revolutionary inspired by the ongoing Chinese revolution who organized the bombing, accused the French of poisoning the country with factory alcohol.[109] The political stability of the colony was at stake. Sarraut, a former Radical deputy, agreed firmly with the Ministry of the Colonies in opposing the alcohol monopoly because it violated principles of free trade. Residents-superior of Annam and Tonkin, troubled by the recent rebellions and the vocal Vietnamese opposition to the monopoly, stood with the governor-general. So, Sarraut set out to change the regime.

First, Sarraut ordered local prefects to collect opinions from Vietnamese consumers and village elders, both collecting complaints about the current regime and charting potential alternatives.[110] The responses, collected by local prefects and mandarins at village meetings and delivered to local French administrators, were predictable: few took outright issue with methods of policing contraband. Most repeated criticisms about the unhealthy effects of factory alcohol, its prohibitively high price, and its unsuitability for ritual purposes. Almost all unequivocally endorsed ending the monopoly and suggested a variety of alternative tax revenues, ranging from returning to a tax on alembics to a personal income tax.[111] Based on these recommendations, analyses solicited from the Douanes et Régies, and expert opinions from the Ministry of the Colonies, the Government-General came up with three options for an alternative system. The first involved returning to a system of free commerce. Second, Sarraut considered an "ameliorated monopoly," which would force the SFDI to lower prices, change the production methods to improve taste, and ease the contraband regime. The third option was a "mixed system," which would allocate indigenous distilleries a quota of thirty thousand hectoliters of pure alcohol per year (leaving monopoly producers seventy thousand hectoliters), and tax it at rates favorable to the indigenous producers.[112] Sarraut's own preference was free trade, noting that previous administrators had effectively promised the end of the monopoly to the Vietnamese.

Reforms, however, proved difficult to accomplish. Sarraut's advisers feared that the Fontaines, who controlled production in Tonkin-Annam and two-thirds of production in Cochinchina, might halt production once he learned that the administration was not going to renew the contract with SFDI. No one, not even Chinese industrialists, would be able to triple their production overnight, leaving a several-month lull in alcohol supply, creating disorder, and putting pressure on the administration to cave. Under a free trade regime, Fontaine might use his position as market leader to buy up Chinese distilleries in Cochinchina, leading to an expansion of his empire rather than increased competition.[113] Even without market dominance, European distillers had the advantage of nearly two decades of research into the Amyloprocess and various industrial improvements to the distillation procedure, which provided higher yields and more flexibility against volatile rice prices. Indigenous distillers would remain at a disadvantage.[114] Finally, a system of free commerce would have required a new taxation regime to replace the lost revenue. All the options on offer came with significant drawbacks, ranging from enforcement issues to augmenting the power of local mandarins.[115]

Ultimately, the administration reached a compromise with the SFDI. Contracts with the company were renewed for another decade on 12 April 1913 but with significant changes. The SFDI pledged to lower the price of factory alcohol by 7.5 piasters per hectoliter of pure alcohol, making it cheaper than contraband. The new contract put stricter requirements on the quality of rice used in the distillation process and mandated that SFDI alcohol exhibit the smoky flavor of proper rượu.[116] Finally, Sarraut relaxed the contraband regime, reducing the number of alcohol raids from 350 to fewer than 50 per month.[117] The monopoly regime remained in place, but the Vietnamese complaints were heard: the taste of the alcohol was changed, and the contraband regime relaxed.

Technology and ideology operated together as resources for various parties struggling to enact their own vision of an Indochinese industrial empire.

Vietnamese opposition to the repressive regime was grounded in turning French promises of purity and scientific efficiency against them, but this argument only worked because Fontaine factory alcohol had demonstrably different taste from locally distilled rượu. Vietnamese rhetoric was made possible by the combination of Pastorian language used in alcohol reform and the physical properties of factory alcohol, which resulted from the specific engineering decisions made in the development of the Amyloprocess. Similarly, Albert Sarraut's plan to return to free trade was constrained not simply by the complexities of tax collection and the lobbying power of the Fontaines but also by the very material limits of the sociotechnical system Calmette, the SFDI, and previous governors-general had set up. Armed with the Amyloprocess, a system of high-volume factories with two decades' worth of improvements, and the history of a favorable legal system, the SFDI was likely to dominate the market even under a system of free exchange.[118] Technology set limits to the political choices that both the French state and Vietnamese critics could pursue.

The construction of the alcohol monopoly as a Pastorian modernization project turned out to be a double-edged sword. The language of pastorization provided a rhetorical cover that justified monopolization to free-trade critics, but Pastorian engineering decisions also created material consequences that offered fodder to Vietnamese and French critics of the monopoly. The material form of the monopoly, at the same time, constrained the French in their attempts to reform the system and return to a more liberal sales model. The monopoly survived until 1934, but it was the product of compromise, made in conflict between colonial administrators, Pastorian scientists, SFDI monopolists, and their Vietnamese and French critics, and structured by the technopolitical logic of the Pastorian Amyloprocess.

Challenging the Opium Monopoly

At an initial glance, the opium monopoly closely resembled the alcohol monopoly. The opium industry too was run by a large, centralized French company, the Société Fermiere, which had its largest factory in Saigon. Like the SFDI, the Société Fermiere was led by a larger-than-life businessman, René de Saint-Mathurin, who had big ambitions and close connections to the colonial state. Like rượu, chandoo taxes were supposed to become the backbone of the general budget: Governor-General Doumer estimated that a quarter of the state's revenues came from opium sales in 1904.[119] Contraband was a problem with opium as well, particularly in northern Vietnam, which, with its weak border controls and proximity to China, became a hotspot for smugglers. Repressive state interventions gradually multiplied not simply because of concerns over contraband but also because reports of "opiomania" among French soldiers, middle-level administrators, and Vietnamese go-betweens unsettled officials. Yet despite these similarities to the alcohol monopoly, the French opium industry never became a controversy that "threatened to tear the colony apart." Instead of being challenged from within the Vietnamese society, the opium monopoly was threatened by changing international norms around prohibition. The French, however, managed to deflect critics on pragmatic grounds, and the Société Fermiere's monopoly survived mostly unchanged until World War II.

As with rượu, contraband chandoo became a major issue for the colonial state. A 1899 decree mandated fines from 500 to 2,000 francs for selling contraband, along with imprisonment from fifteen days to three years.[120] The politics of contraband opium, however, differed from prohibition of local moonshine. Rượu distillation was integrated into Vietnamese village life in a number of ways: it was a way of storing surplus rice, its byproducts were used as pig feed, and distillation was an important activity for women.[121] Declaring locally distilled wine illegal disrupted all of these social and economic relations, creating deep dissatisfaction in Vietnamese villages. In contrast, contraband opium was almost exclusively imported to the French colony from China, across borders in northern Tonkin and Laos, since poppies did not grow in most of Indochina. Some regions in Laos and Tonkin had temperate enough weather to support poppy cultivation, and French ethnologists indeed noted that some villages did indeed grow the plant, but the practice was clearly limited.[122] Changes to the opium regime involved fewer changes to local social relations and upset fewer people, who depended on the opium economy for livelihoods.

Nor did factory opium provide opponents with such an easy rallying point as French rượu, which, with its altered, unpleasant taste, became a proxy for concerns the Vietnamese could not openly voice. The Société Fermiere essentially took over the Chinese factory in Saigon and continued production with old staff, using well-honed methods while avoiding changes that would drastically alter the taste of the product. Factory managers were aware of how sensitive customers could be to changes in taste. During the Calmette incident in 1894 and a few years later, when British bans on opium trade forced the French to buy poppies from Yunnan, questions of quality were discussed at the level of the Colonial Council, and production processes were altered accordingly.[123] They did not become political flashpoints.

Instead, challenges to the opium regime came from outside Indochina. In the early 1900s, international opinion turned decisively against opium. Britain, which had fought two wars with China over the right to export Indian opium to the Celestial Empire, changed its mind. It was now seeking to crack down on the trade, as moral reformers and a Liberal government in London put pressure on imperialists and traders. The Chinese government too, under nationalist pressure after the 1900 Boxer Rebellion, had begun to see opium as an impediment to modernization, which dragged the country backward and allowed foreign powers to influence the empire. The United States, which had just acquired the Philippines, faced a robust opium economy in the colony, as well as increasing numbers of smokers in West Coast cities. Supported by temperance movements at home and seeking to reduce British influence in the Far East, President Theodore Roosevelt pushed for an international conference to regulate the opium trade. This conference was held in 1909 in Shanghai.[124] In this polite company, the French budgetary backbone looked increasingly embarrassing.

Representatives of all the major empires, including China and Japan, met for four weeks at the Shanghai conference in 1909 and delivered a strongly worded report encouraging participating governments to limit nonmedicinal opium use to "prohibition or careful regulation."[125] The recommendations, however, were not binding, and soon after the end of the conference, the United States and China began to lobby for another meeting that would deliver real commitments. This meeting took place in 1911–1912 in the Hague and delivered a promise to phase out both opium cultivation and opium trade.[126] Administrators in Indochina were unphased by the requirements of the convention, since the colony did not actually grow any poppies, and diplomats felt confident that China would fail to implement its reforms, thereby remaining a reliable trading partner for Indochina. The only active measures they would have to take in response to the convention were the regulation of cocaine and morphine, both used as medical anesthetics.[127]

Still, international pressure combined with increasingly vocal critics in the metropole accusing colonial officers of bringing an oriental habit to France. Newspapers in the metropole published articles with headlines that referred to "a national threat," "a scandalous monopoly," and "a poison for victors and defeated alike."[128] "Did we acquire colonies so that they would poison us?," asked one French deputy concerned with the newly acquired habits of young French soldiers.[129] Recruits, after all, might forget themselves in drug-induced daydreams when they were supposed to be ever-vigilant.[130] This moral panic drew metropolitan attention to the monopoly in Indochina and increased the pressure for reform.

The administration's response was twofold. First, it sought to deflect criticism by arguing that the monopoly was a pragmatic necessity and not dangerous for social order. Because opium was not fused to a broad modernizing vision, French administrators could tell it like it was: opium sales brought in tax revenue, which remained a priority for the colonial state. In 1907, the Hardouin Commission studied the possibility of suppressing opium sales in Indochina, providing the most complete survey of official attitudes toward the regime and outlining arguments that would be marshaled for decades. After the commission had filed its report, the governor-general delivered the following conclusions to the minister of the colonies: Indochina was not an opium producer, addiction was an exaggerated problem, and opium was "the ideal form of an indirect tax" as it was a nonessential luxury good, thereby weighing more heavily on the rich who voluntarily made the choice to smoke. Finally, the governor-general concluded, opium was consumed mostly by the Chinese, who were not French subjects and toward whom the government held no civilizing responsibility.[131] Administrators argued that only China itself could take responsibility for halting the opium trade and securing the health of its citizens. Moreover, officials recalled, foreign residents of Indochina were exempt from many burdens, such as the corvée, that weighed on the subject population and could therefore bear the burden of the tax.[132] The fiscal argument and the argument that the French were not responsible for civilizing the Chinese became cornerstones for supporters of the monopoly, circulating from newspaper articles to official inquiries at the National Assembly and the quai d'Orsay.[133]

Defenders of the monopoly still had to respond to the moral panic over recreational opium use in port towns.[134] These arguments relied on old-fashioned orientalism. While, previously, colonial officials had touted opium as a less noxious alternative to alcohol in universal terms, they now claimed that opium was an "oriental vice," to which the Chinese were particularly accustomed. "The Chinese have enjoyed the drug for many years, and the race has not degenerated," wrote one analyst. "Centuries of experience" have taught the Chinese to moderate their use, wrote another.[135] While limiting opium consumption for Europeans was a solid public health measure, officials reasoned, for "people that have used opium since time immemorial ... such measures would be both ineffective and bad politics."[136]

Thus, the Government-General passed a series of half measures designed primarily to curb European opium use. Opium was banned for all European civil servants, the opening of new dens was severely restricted, and retail prices were raised in 1907 and again in 1908.[137] However, no existing dens were closed, and the majority of opium, which was consumed privately, was left unregulated. Administrators themselves had mixed feelings about price rises, which they felt encouraged contraband.[138] The state remained intransigent in the face of international pressure to reduce consumption and to reform or eliminate the monopoly system, without bearing heavy costs. When high-level officials discussed "the monopoly problem" in Indochina, they always meant the alcohol, not the opium, monopoly.[139] With the rượu monopoly, the administration had restructured the manufacturing process and turned it into a symbol of pastorian modernization. Once this vision had been implemented, the colonial state had to stand by it, and due to the unforeseen consequences of Calmette's Amyloprocess, it turned out to be all too open to attack. With the opium monopoly, the old manufacturing process remained intact, and officials declared opium an oriental oddity, which, from the point of view of the state, was nothing more than a source of tax revenue. Having made no grand promises, the administration could not be accused of either hypocrisy or failure.

Conclusion

Pastorians gladly offered the benefits of their research to both colonial and imperial rulers. While Yersin's research on the plague impressed diplomats and politicians in the Ministry of the Colonies, Calmette appealed to the immediate concerns of local administrators, promising that pastorization represented "a great undertaking ... with immense practical consequences for our colonies."[140] Calmette's reforms fused technology and ideology. In the case of the alcohol monopoly, Calmette's Amyloprocess offered a language of hygiene, progress, and scientific management, which countered accusations of favoritism, illiberalism, and interventionism. This language was enacted through a method that focused on modifying the growth of a single, fermenting microbe, enabled centralization and economies of scale, distinguished French rice wine from contraband, and helped the SFDI to meet regulations that were designed to exclude alcohol made using conventional methods. The Amyloprocess machinery and the resulting factory alcohol turned ideological claims of hygienic modernity into physical reality, sometimes quite literally, such as when the SFDI countered criticisms of its products by offering tours of its clean and scientifically run factories. The methods, technologies, and products enabled by Calmette's research enacted the political objectives of the reforms by helping centralize alcohol production in French hands and thereby simplifying tax collection.

The technopolitics of alcohol and opium monopolies could also shift ideologies, empower critics, catalyze new forms of conflict, and constrain French officials. The consequences of the Amyloprocess, most notably the poor taste of factory alcohol, provided a vehicle for Vietnamese critics to express a much broader range of complaints, including attacks on the contraband regime and the coercive Douanes et Régies. At the same time, the method enabled the SFDI to drive other medium- and large-scale producers out of business, limiting the Government-General's options for reform. The struggles over the alcohol monopoly and the eventual compromise were all structured by the technical and ideological form of Calmette's Amyloprocess.

Setting alcohol and opium reforms in the same frame reveals the fragility and contingency of Pastorian technopolitics, as well as the consequences that followed from it. In the case of the opium monopoly, the *failure* of Calmette's attempts in pastorizing opium fermentation took on a political quality. For French business interests who opposed the Government-General's interventions in factory management, Calmette's experiments were prima facie evidence of the damage that overeager officials could do. It was not clear that failure of the 1894 vintage was Calmette's fault, but it provided a powerful argument in an ongoing debate between the douaniers and French businessmen. As a result, the opium monopoly never became a symbol of Pastorian progress. Officials defended the opium regime against attack from international critics with arguments founded in fiscal expedience, and did so with remarkable success.

In reality, then, Pastorian technopolitics had highly variable outcomes. Microbial transformations and macroeconomic reforms were highly unpredictable and created unintended consequences that profoundly altered the balance of colonial power. All actors—colonial officials, Pastorians, Vietnamese middlemen, critics and entrepreneurs, Chinese traders, French businessmen, and metropolitan journalists—learned how to operate in this novel playing field and could leverage microbial successes and failures to their advantage. Neither the Government-General nor the Pastorians commanded this arena as well as they desired. Yet, Calmette was undoubtedly successful in leveraging this process to the advantage of himself and his institute. The money made from selling his stake in the Amyloprocess patent enabled him to start his own Pasteur Institute in Lille, where he dedicated the rest of his life to the study of tuberculosis—to which I shall return in chapter 4. Alcohol reforms and the potential industrial benefits of Pastorian fermentation caused at least as much buzz in official circles as its work on public health and led to the establishment of Pasteur Institutes in Morocco and Tunisia by the Departments of Agriculture of both protectorates.[141] Forced to operate on an economic and political landscape they did not fully control, colonial officials gladly accepted the help of the Pastorians, setting off their expansion from Indochina to the rest of the French empire.

3

Monks and Warriors, Bureaucrats and Businessmen

A key episode in Céline's classic novel on interwar France, *Journey to the End of the Night*, takes place at a prestigious research laboratory, a clear proxy for the Pasteur Institute, where Céline himself had studied. The Pasteur Institute was familiar to the public, both in France and abroad, as the place where "intrepid" and "heroic" students of Louis Pasteur—"microbe hunters," as Paul de Kruif's popular book called them—developed vaccines, sera, and antitoxins that promised to eradicate dangerous diseases ranging from rabies to diphtheria.[1] Céline, however, portrays the institute as a "a decomposing space" packed with "gutted bodies of small animals, cigarette butts, chipped gas jets, cases and jars with mice suffocating inside them." It is populated by "small, unshaven, whispering" scientists, hardly microbe hunters, but at best second-rate cooks in "microbe kitchens," made frail by "old age" and only interested in "problems of heating and hemorrhoids."[2] Far from being "full of passion, of purpose" in a "million-franc Institute," Céline sees the microbiologists as "listless" and "riveted by starvation wages."[3] The director of the institute, named Parapine in the novel, is "an old Bachelor" with perverse desires. He spends hours sitting on rue de Vaugirard, stalking underage Lycée girls in the afternoon, commenting that he knows their "legs by heart."[4] All the bacteriologists, Céline concludes, found "the habit of filling one's stomach" through poorly remunerated and largely useless science easier than "courage."[5] Bardamu, the novel's protagonist, comes to the institute searching for help for a working-class boy who has fallen ill, but he does not succeed; the boy dies some days later of typhoid fever. This literary depiction of Pastorians is cynical and pessimistic, but exactly like the hagiographic story of Paul de Kruif, it links the virility of scientists to the economic vitality of their institutions.

This chapter contextualizes the interwar crisis of the Pasteur Institute in gendered anxieties over degeneration and imperial conquest, changing economic fortunes, and a rethinking of the institute's business model in the wake

Pasteur's Empire. Aro Velmet, Oxford University Press (2020). © Oxford University Press.
DOI: 10.1093/oso/9780190072827.001.0001

of the Great War. I argue, following the language of Céline and de Kruif, that understanding the transformation of the Pastorians' scientific ethos requires analyzing gendered fears of failure and experiences of institutional economic success together in the same frame. A vibrant scientific laboratory did not simply enable cutting-edge research but also helped its staff to provide for their families and allowed them self-fulfillment as men. There were very few women employed at the Pasteur Institute before 1940, and they held relatively low positions. One of the most remarkable female scientists, Germaine Benoit, worked as an assistant in chemical therapeutics from 1923 onward and became head of the laboratory in 1943, ten years after winning the Prix Louis from the Academy of Medicine. Aside from the few cases, when the leadership of the institute discussed specific cases of women seeking work at the institute, Roux, Yersin, and others always assumed that the research staff were, without exception, specifically *men* of science. By the dawn of the Great War, however, what it meant to be a man of science had changed considerably from metropole to colony.

Colonial researchers like Albert Calmette, Alexandre Yersin, and Charles Nicolle came to think of themselves not as ascetic, charitable, and secluded monks but as profit-oriented, worldly, and ambitious conquerors. Completing this transformation required both a rethinking of what it meant to be a masculine scientist and the institutional-economic success of the institute's colonial offshoots in comparison to the Parisian *maison-mère*. Overseas Pastorians socialized in the world of explorers, administrators, and other "heroes of empire," for whom maintaining prestige meant upholding military valor and whose exploits and conquests the reading public saw as counterweights to degeneration in the metropole.[6] The war experience delegitimized ascetic science, which became associated with the horrors of mechanized, industrial warfare and the slaughter it caused on the battlefield. In Céline's words, "In the trenches of the Great Debacle, a Doctorate of Medicine is as good as a Prix de Rome"—put differently, worth nothing at all.[7] Colonial Pastorians advocated for a different model of scientific conduct, based on military courage, individual heroism, engagement with the state, and most critically, a different attitude toward profit and institutional expansion.

Literature on scientific masculinities has highlighted how the production of authoritative knowledge depended on shared masculine cultures— joint sporting ventures, all-male schooling, even dueling.[8] Being perceived as unmanly could undermine the scientist's credibility. Like Heather Ellis's work on Britain, this chapter highlights the anxieties of ascetic, and potentially effeminate, scientists in an age of "degeneration."[9] Historians have recently begun to chart the varieties of masculine cultures that have structured scientific activity; work on how these cultures changed is still rare.[10] Understanding how interwar Pastorians resolved their masculine anxieties requires attending to both the ideological and the experiential role of their colonial laboratories: how work in the empire offered "regeneration," instantiated through the experience of entrepreneurial success.

Second, this chapter shows how French debates over the relationship of degeneration and colonialism created tensions within a scientific culture. From the 1870s onward, commentators in France feared that the nation was "in decline," "decadent," and "degenerating" both morally and physically. Everything from poor diet, venereal disease, alcoholism, and lack of physical exercise to the feminist movement, indulging in luxury commodities, and an overly sedentary lifestyle could render French men effeminate, incapable of defending the nation, and potentially dangerous for the future of the republic.[11] Recent scholarship has shown how many French experts believed colonial ventures could regenerate French men through geographical and carnal conquests—exploration and métissage.[12] Given how enlightenment through science was central to the mission civilisatrice and, indeed, as we will see, to Louis Pasteur's conception of science, there was obvious potential in colonialism for re-establishing the Pastorians' male prowess.[13] This chapter, however, argues that while on the surface the Pastorian colonial mission may have appeared as a unified outgrowth of the civilizing mission, it generated a number of new tensions within the Pastorian community.

Finally, this chapter extends the importance of public image-making beyond the figure of Louis Pasteur himself, looking at how Pastorians repurposed his memory for new ends. Gerald Geison has studied the ways in which the success of Pasteur's research and his reputation as a national hero were the product of careful rhetorical crafting. Others have analyzed the self-portrayals of his disciples. Here, I am concerned with how Pasteur became a "scientific persona" and how his biography became a model of conduct that was constantly reframed and reinterpreted. What aspects of Pasteur's life his disciples remembered and celebrated depended on how these followers envisioned a proper scientific life. Roux, Calmette, Yersin, Nicolle, and Pasteur's grandson, Pasteur Vallery-Radot all sought to show that the strategies they envisioned for the institute and for their own conduct were directly inspired by the legacy of its founder. In this analysis, events like Pasteur's centenary or the institute's fiftieth anniversary were not just commemorations but moments for constructing a model for truly Pastorian behavior.[14]

The Paris Pasteur Institute and the Monastic Ideal

When Pastorians expanded their operations overseas in 1890, they joined two different professional communities, both with their own, occasionally overlapping and often conflicting cultures. Colonial bacteriologists were the students of Pasteur, members of a research community defined most often through graduation from Émile Roux's bacteriology course at the Paris institute and membership in professional societies. The norms of these institutions impressed on Pastorians the importance of indifferent, dispassionate observation, the pursuit of knowledge as a communal effort, and proper science as abstracted from individual subjectivity, national belonging, or economic interest. As Robert Nye has argued, scientific credibility and the ability to speak truthfully in this period depended on the speaker's possession of noble honor, expressed through intense loyalty toward one's peers and a constant affirmation of the scientists' proper qualities through peer affirmation.[15]

Overseas Pastorians found they had to navigate two different moral economies, both of which demanded the expression of specific, often conflicting, values in order to gain access to resources and achieve professional success.[16] To prove their worth to colonial bigwigs, Yersin and others had to impress peers whose background was largely in the military. Pastorians had to become explorers, intrepid geographers, and conquerors, demonstrating independence, economic and political ambition, and dominance. Tales of exploration and conquest published in geographical journals helped demonstrate his initiative to colonial councilors doubting his abilities at budget meetings in Indochina. Yet these same qualities undermined his credibility with bacteriologists in Paris, who saw his colonial adventures and empire-building ambitions as reflecting his "egotism" and lack of commitment to research, demonstrating he was unfit for promotion. Pastorians in the metropole and in the colonies spilled much ink in personal correspondence and in publications to convince each other of the worth of their particular version of scientific masculinity.

Pasteur's own efforts at turning himself into a figure of legend have drawn considerable scholarly attention. Bruno Latour, David Barnes, and Gerald

Geison have all shown how Pasteur's career was contradictory, a "mixture of audacity and traditionalism," full of confidence in public and plagued by self-doubt in private.[17] Pasteur dedicated himself simultaneously to helping the French wine and beer industries, and to the self-proclaimed charitable improvement of all humanity. He famously stated that "science has no fatherland," only to add that "science has to be the highest personification of the fatherland."[18] Pasteur carefully managed his public face, emphasizing the virtues of patriotism and confidence while simultaneously asserting that those qualities were underpinned by a scientific ethos focused on following a strict method, a disinterested approach free of a priori convictions or personal stakes. His was a "superficially antirhetorical language [that was] itself but another rhetorical resource."[19]

Pasteur knew how to put on a public spectacle, but he espoused, particularly later in life, what Lorraine Daston and Peter Galison have called an ethos of "aperspectival objectivity," which rested on denying individual genius in favor of discipline and peer collaboration. Scientists were supposed to render the natural world in a way that was free from individual idiosyncrasies, providing the scholar with "a view from nowhere."[20] This principle stood in contrast to earlier understandings of empirical observation, for example, those of eighteenth-century botanists and physicians, whose authority derived from *individual* experience and skill, and their rhetorical and artistic ability to render the qualities of plants and organs in a *subjective* manner. Scientific atlases in the early nineteenth century routinely exaggerated and modified images of plants or skeletons, attempting to achieve not accuracy but a "truth-to-life."[21] During the Romantic period, philosophers began to distinguish between the human self as a source of individual subjectivity and nature as the locus of "objective" phenomena.[22] In this view, objectivity in science was required precisely *because* the self could only have a subjective, impassioned perspective on the world; it was only through the suppression of individual subjectivity through discipline, mechanical action, and peer review that true knowledge could be acquired.[23]

In France, the physician Claude Bernard defined this ethos most forcefully. In his major work on method, *An Introduction to the Study of Experimental Medicine*, the scientist laid out the central tenets of "objective" experimentation and described the character of the person best suited to carry out these tasks. Bernard argued that it was only through the exercise of self-control, "by means of reasoning and facts," that men could overcome the primacies of feeling and ideation and gather "objective" truths from the natural world.[24]

Several safeguards ensured that scientists did not remain on the level of feeling but moved on to reason and experiment. The most important of these safeguards were facts, acquired with the help of mechanical appliances and disinterested observation. However, Bernard also emphasized the importance of community (since not all scientists were naturally skilled in both observation and experiment) and doubt, the "absolute freedom of mind."[25] For Bernard, the search for truth, fueled by constant doubt, was fundamentally opposed to "personal vanity or the diverse passions of man."[26] Emotional restraint and discipline of the body were key elements of Bernard's ideal scientist. It was not by accident that these qualities mirrored the codes of honor of nineteenth-century male bourgeoisie.[27]

Bernard's principles became accepted wisdom in France, to the degree that Pasteur used his own words against him in 1878, when a series of posthumously discovered notebooks revealed Bernard's hostile feelings toward the microbiologist, who, Bernard believed, wanted "to direct nature . . . and to submit the facts to his ideas."[28] Pasteur responded by referencing Bernard's own seminal text and accusing him of being wedded to the "tyranny of preconceived ideas," and presenting himself as a follower of the "inductive scientific method, working outside theories."[29]

In its public presentation, the Pasteur Institute carried the same values of asceticism, restraint, and isolated community. Journalists recognized these virtues in the very structure of the laboratory. As usual, patriotism and pomp worked together with scientific restraint. At the institute's inauguration in 1888, observers noted that, although all the adjacent streets were decorated "as if for a national holiday," the building of the institute itself "was simple, without ornamentation or sculpture."[30] Some authors drew parallels with the "small house, on an obscure street of Dôle," where Pasteur had been born.[31] Constructed in simple neoclassical style, the building had "no luxury neither on the exterior, nor the interior," with only the busts of principal donors: Baron Rothschild, Mme Boucicaut, the Russian tsar, and the Brazilian emperor decorating the central gallery.[32]

Though in popular parlance the Pasteur Institute was named "the palace of rabies," journalists reported that "nothing could be further from the truth. This is, if anything, a scientific factory, but an admirably stocked factory, perfectly designed for the task at hand, spacious (11,000 m^2), well-ventilated, where everything is at one's fingertips, and everything has its proper place."[33] The industrial qualities of the institute were further emphasized by the state-of-the-art heating systems, which maintained accurate temperatures

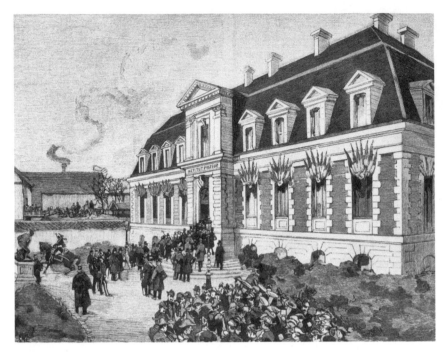

Figure 3.1 The inauguration of the Pasteur Institute in 1888. L. Tinayre, *Le Monde Illustré*, 15 November 1888.

in laboratories and made the principal building resemble a factory more than a hospital.[34] Journalists interpreted the simplicity of the architecture, combined with the institute's technical prowess, as essential to productive scientific work.

The institute also appeared as a space for male collaboration. The structure of the compound itself was designed to accommodate the everyday needs of scholars across generations, while establishing a patriarchal hierarchy between teachers and students. Beyond the main building, the grounds contained many annexes, buildings that housed lab animals, and stables.[35] Pasteur and his preparators lived next to his private laboratory in the main building. Most staff lived on the premises, moving out only if they got married and started families. Even then, many stayed in special housing on rue Vauquelin donated to Pasteur by the local municipality.[36] The institute often employed siblings and relatives, with women and younger members in custodial and secretarial positions.[37] All the members of the institute did "considerable work for really the most modest of salaries."[38]

Descriptions of the work within the institute emphasized community as well as technical skill. Journalists writing about Roux's microbiology course highlighted the collaborative, physical aspects of training: the preparation of the bouillon for microbial cultures and the sterilization of instruments. Commentators took great care in highlighting that Pasteur himself "lived and worked alongside his collaborators" in the institute, describing how "the architect facilitated by all means available the work of teachers and students" and praising the "vast halls where students could work together."[39] Drawings of the everyday work inside the institute focused on the machines, test tubes, Petri dishes, and retorts, but equally importantly on experience of communal work. These pictures portrayed respectable men in suits rather than lab coats, together, observing each other's work, and collectively witnessing processes such as the making of bouillon. In one such image, bacteriologists hunched over Petri dishes recalled artisans in training by their workbenches; in another, the dark space of the laboratory is overwhelmed with steam coming from a bouillon machine, not unlike a factory steam engine.

Critical to the ideology of the new institute was its funding structure. Its endowment, a substantial sum of 1 million francs, produced an annual

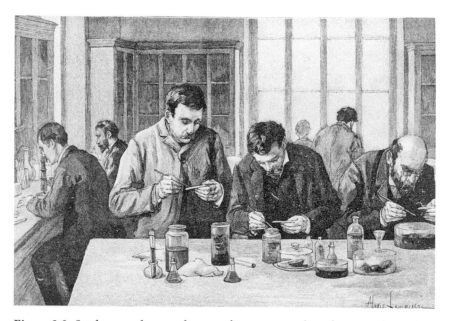

Figure 3.2 Students and researchers working on microbe colonies at the Pasteur Institute. Alexis Lemaistre. © Institut Pasteur / Musée Pasteur.

return of 30,000 to 40,000 francs, complemented by national and municipal subsidies. Commentators emphasized the international dimension of charitable giving, which lent the institute both a cosmopolitan flair, represented by the "consoling spectacle of people forgetting their conflicts and grudges" and the "spirit of charity," while also demonstrating the influence of French science on the global stage.[40] The institute's treasurer talked about its foundation as a "fairy-tale" where "the architects, M. Petit and M. Brébant, before beginning their work, declared that they would refuse all honoraria."[41] The rabies service was to be provided free of charge. In these foundational acts, Pastorians set up the institute as an idealistic counterpoint to a society oriented around profit.

Alexandre Yersin's letters to his mother from the 1880s indicate how the experience of learning by Pasteur's side inculcated the ascetic ideal in bacteriologists. The Swiss student was frustrated with the disorganized state of medical education in France. He listed ten reasons for leaving and continuing his studies in Germany, and only two for staying ("*internat* [residency], if one gets to that point, and intellectual development") but changed his mind when a supervisor introduced him to Pasteur's laboratory.[42] Pasteur's reputation loomed large in the public—a female acquaintance asked Yersin to procure an autograph from the scientist, a task he found most embarrassing. In reality, Yersin found Pasteur to be unremarkable. Upon entering his crowded laboratory for the first time, the student did not realize "the small man" telling him off for blocking the door was Pasteur himself.[43] Yersin quickly developed strong teacher-student relationships with both the elderly Pasteur and the director of the bacteriology course, Émile Roux. Simultaneously, Yersin continued to emphasize the collaborative, factory-like atmosphere at the laboratory: he always noted how many scientists from different countries came to work with Pasteur, as well as the daily circulation of literally hundreds of patients who were being vaccinated for rabies.[44]

In late 1886, Yersin was invited to work under Roux as a preparator. Soon after, the Swiss scientist moved into a room in Pasteur's compound, replacing another bacteriologist who had to move out due to marriage. By 1889, Yersin's living quarters were located on rue Dutot, on the premises of the Pasteur Institute. In his mentor, Roux, Yersin found a "true scientific spirit." He described Roux as "modest" to the degree that he let others steal the results of his work, not keen to show off his considerable knowledge, and, indeed, sometimes airheaded and forgetful. To the Swiss student, Roux appeared as a solitary man with "many enemies and few friends," but nevertheless greatly esteemed by those in his inner circle.[45]

As important to Yersin's education as the mentorship of Roux were the tools, technology, and lab animals available at the Pasteur Institute. As often as Yersin wrote about Roux, he wrote also about the sophisticated gas system that was being installed in the new institute, about electrical regulators that helped maintain precise temperatures in various ovens, and about animal pens that housed everything from guinea pigs to horses.[46] In Yersin's telling, his training took place in a highly technologically sophisticated, and self-contained environment, where men of different backgrounds studied under the eye of a mentor who, while brilliant, consciously exuded modesty and reservedness.

The community of Pastorians, like the medical community of Paris more broadly, was gendered male. Yersin remarked upon instances of "most outrageous injustice," when, for instance, a "small dandy" was selected for a residency position over an American woman with clearly superior test scores at the hospital, where Yersin, too, was a resident. Even though he recognized the injustice, he wrote of the unfairly advantaged competitor in diminutive, unmasculine terms, implying that a properly masculine challenger might have fairly beaten the "charmless woman [*guenon*]."[47] In other instances, Yersin expressed discomfort with working with female students and complained about his inability to make conversation with them.[48] For Yersin, meritocracy had its limits, and maintaining the comfortable atmosphere of a male, monastic community was a primary concern.

Louis Pasteur himself recapitulated the monastic ideal in his speech at the inauguration of the new institute. He expressed his opposition to the institute's name, "which gives a mere man the honor reserved for a doctrine."[49] In the widely circulated inaugural speech, he cautioned his students to "combine [their] enthusiasm inseparably with the most rigorous control. Do not propose anything that cannot be proven in a simple and decisive manner."[50] The search for a scientific fact, Pasteur reinforced, might take "years of combating oneself, forcing oneself to suppress one's own experience" until all other hypotheses had been exhausted.[51] The not-for-profit status of the institute and grants from internationally renowned businessmen and three different sovereigns ensured that the scientists could keep their passions cooled and "live in the serene peace of laboratories and libraries," working for the "suffering humanity."[52]

In the years after its founding, the Pasteur Institute cemented itself as a monastic, charitable organization, and as one dedicated equally to "pure" research and applied biology. It convened a regular course in bacteriology, which drew students from French medical schools as well as from abroad. It continued to develop basic research, both on the identification of microbial pathogens and on the basic interactions of microbes, the environment, and the body. After Pasteur's death in 1895, the institute garnered fame through the work of Élie Metchnikoff, whose discovery of phagocytes and theories of active immunity won him a Nobel Prize (jointly with Paul Ehrlich) in 1908.[53]

The institute also expanded its industrial activities. Its principal claim to fame when it opened was the rabies service, a wing of the institute that provided free vaccinations, with patients arriving from all over, from the French provinces to imperial Russia.[54] Over time, researchers at the institute developed new pharmaceuticals: vaccines, serotherapy, and antitoxins. The institute produced these not only for its own services but also for distribution across the country. Yet while their industrial reach expanded, Pastorians maintained their distance from commerce: Roux discouraged the use of the institute's name by doctors who offered its products or provided microbiological services developed by Pasteur. The institute refused to market its products, such as Roux's diphtheria serum, and offered many products at the price of production, completely free of charge or in exchange for reports of efficacy to any who requested them.[55] As Nathan Simon has argued, the reputation of Pastorian pharmaceuticals depended on Roux's "saintly asceticism" and on the pilgrimages conducted to the institute for the purposes of learning new microbiological techniques.[56] For some time, the Paris institute could leverage its distance from commerce and its commitment to disinterested science to build reputation and institutional power.

From Pasteur's positioning as a modest man of science in the eve of his life to Roux's policing of all associations of the Pasteur Institute with commercial activity, defenses of institutional ethos were tied up with questions of masculinity. As Robert Nye, Robert Kohler, and others have argued, the legitimacy of a producer of knowledge was predicated on the possession of honor: masculine credibility and the willingness to stand by one's words and put one's body on the line.[57] Pastorians did not duel with physical weapons, but they engaged in scathing verbal fights. In 1895, Roux published a long critique of a doctor Moizard, who blamed the death of a patient on the Pastorians' serum. Roux accused Moizard of lacking rigor and the subsequent official investigation of jumping to conclusions without consulting the literature on "thousands and thousands of cases" of successful serum injections.[58] Tellingly, one response to Roux lamented his "lack of courtesy and calm, which so befits laboratory men," and argued that instead of "losing his *sang-froid*," Roux should have let "scientific truth shine by itself, as always."[59] The critic then tied Roux's loss of character to a different form of corruption: what he considered the engagement of the Pasteur Institute in a commercial affair—the sale of the diphtheria serum. Losing one's calm (both a scientific and a gentlemanly quality) led to commerce, and that, in turn, led to irresponsibility, error, and the death of innocents.

Colonial Pastorians, the Heroic Ideal, and Conflicted Loyalties

Less than a year after the inauguration of the Paris institute, Yersin was dreaming of the sea. Reading Pierre Loti's *Island Fishermen*, the impressionistic novel of Breton cod fishers in Iceland, and hearing news of the world's fair at the champs de Mars had made the young bacteriologist dissatisfied with his career prospects.[60] His concerns blended anxieties about his personal qualities, dissatisfaction with the restrictions of the laboratory, and potential for future marriageability. In Parisian social circles, Yersin felt uncomfortable: "The theater bores me, high society scares me, and not moving around is not really a life at all."[61] In contrast to the stability, sociability, and modesty of a second-tier Parisian Pastorian, Yersin hoped the colonies would provide him with the necessary feats to finally contemplate marriage: "Marriage I do not wish to think about for some years. I would have to travel the world, to make a stir [*remouer*]."[62] At stake in Yersin's decision was then not simply his discomfort with the peacefulness, sociability, and modesty of life at the institute but his own familial fortunes.

While Calmette, Paul-Louis Simond, and many other colonial Pastorians found their way to the colonies through the military, Yersin became a doctor on a postal vessel belonging to the Messageries Maritimes. On his route from Egypt, to India, Singapore, and finally Saigon, he socialized in much the same circles composed of military men, administrators, and adventurers. In those crowds, individual courage triumphed over collective effort. Gentlemanly valor, ambition, and heroism were prized qualities. Restraint, when it was evoked, principally meant demonstrating French civilizational superiority over the supposedly barbaric natives of Africa and Asia, but a man's worth was tested through exploration and conquest. For colonial heroes, violence was an acceptable response to the cruelty of colonial peoples and the harshness of the tropical environment, particularly as French "interests" in Indochina, Madagascar, and elsewhere demanded extending territorial control in the 1890s. Jean-Baptiste Marchand and Hubert Lyautey became known for their courage under fire, the first under Fashoda, the second in Indochina, Madagascar, and Morocco.[63] Heroes of empire were ambitious, virile, and independent explorers rather than communal, restrained, and modest students.

Establishing one's credibility in the colonies meant communicating heroics to peers and the reading public. Frenchmen learned of their compatriots' colonial affairs through extensive newspaper coverage, official and unofficial biographies, book tours, homecoming receptions, and other public performances. Journalists eagerly sought out such material. In the latter half of the nineteenth century, the dominant mode of reporting shifted toward the sensationalistic, the emotional, and the scandalous—qualities best expressed in the genre of the *fait divers*. Newspapers reporting on colonial explorations saw their circulation numbers soar, the four major "penny-press" dailies—*Le Petit Journal, Le Matin, Le Petit Parisien*, and *Le Journal*—totaled 4.5 million copies a day by the early twentieth century, meaning that, extrapolating two or three readers per copy, roughly half of the French population was reading about imperial exploits.[64]

Explorers were aware of this business model and often did their best to cultivate a media-friendly image, adopting the language and tropes of the penny press even in autobiographical texts and personal correspondence. Membership in a geographical society was mandatory for the bourgeois members of the colonial class. Calmette's career in the opium and alcohol industries, after all, began with a chance meeting of a fellow of the Société de Géographie. Alexandre Yersin quickly joined not one but *two* geographical societies. Tales of exploration were a crucial component of building credibility among French colonials, and, as we will see, such adventures could be generously rewarded through career advancement and state subventions for further projects.

Yersin profited particularly well from these opportunities. He was a shy man, self-professedly antipathetic to balls, concerts, and dinners, so he had to look for other ways to make his name known within the Government-General of Indochina.[65] During his time as the ship doctor with the Messageries Maritimes, in 1890 and 1891, Yersin acquired the habit of accompanying shipowners and businessmen on expeditions inland. He wrote extensive letters about his travels to his mother, describing, for example, with hourly precision and accompanying maps a trip from Manila in the Philippines to the interior of the island, in order to deliver a steamboat to a wealthy French landowner, Monsieur Daillard.[66] In 1892, one Captain Cupet helped Yersin secure funding from two geographical societies in Paris to fund a more extensive mission to the land of the Vietnamese Montagnards in the central highlands of Annam. Yersin received official authorization and a substantial amount of funding from the Government-General, which judged the expedition "useful" for the colony.[67] Yersin was now a legitimate explorer.

Yersin took great care in shaping the public appearance of his expeditions, demonstrating to the world his transformation from a modest scientist to a heroic adventurer. He asked Roux, in Paris, to send him a camera, and had Calmette take pictures of him prior to departure "in the dress of an explorer."[68] He sent a long report of his travels to the Société de Géographie in Paris, and a summary of his travels was published in a twenty-six-part series in *Le Journal des Voyages*.[69] Like drawings of life at the *maison-mère*, illustrations in these stories too focused on groups of men interacting, but where the former pictures depicted a community of equal gentlemen, the cover of the *Journal* showed Yersin, in the garb of an explorer, towering over curious and exotic villagers offering him rice wine as a gesture of hospitality. These tales portrayed Yersin as a curious scientist, motivated by humanitarian aims. In the process, however, he found himself all too often in situations where he had to broker peace between two warring tribes, chase down "bandits" seeking to dethrone French-supported mandarins, and fight off tigers, all while studying the fermentation processes of Vietnamese rice. The role of the tropical environment was of particular importance, transforming Yersin from a modest scientist to "a strategist and a prudent and wise warrior" who displayed courage when faced with "savages who have made more than one courageous man tremble."[70] Reports of Yersin's efforts consistently emphasized his posture, strength, and energy. He appeared "very wild, the flame in his eyes illuminating his lean face," and the Chinese reportedly considered him "stronger than Hua-Tuo," the near-mythical Chinese physician.[71] Through such tales, Yersin fashioned himself as an ambitious and courageous explorer rather than a dispassionate and secluded scientist. The Pastorian abroad looked very different from a Pastorian in the Parisian laboratory.

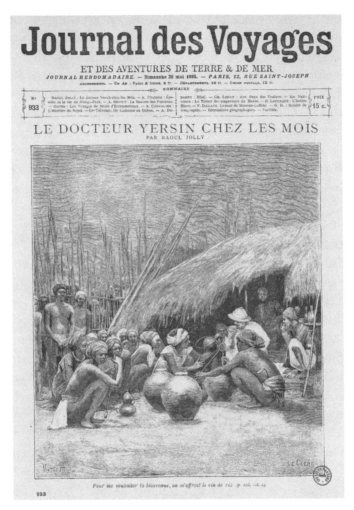

Figure 3.3 Cover of *Journal des Voyages*, 26 May 1895. "Doctor Yersin in the Land of the Mois." © Institut Pasteur / Musée Pasteur.

Yersin's reputation directly impacted his fortunes in Indochina. Journalists regularly conflated his medical missions with Hong Kong and Yunnan with his more adventurous pursuits, discussing his work on the plague and his expeditions to central Vietnam in the same breath.[72] The French consul in India invoked Yersin's "cold blood, science, dedication beyond all praise, and tremendous energy" in inviting him to study the plague in Bombay. Yersin's experience in the "land of the Mois" became a powerful argument when Governor-General Doumer chose him to scout the highlands of Annam for what would later become the hill station of Dalat.[73] Yersin leveraged his reputation to help establish his scientific presence in Indochina.

Yersin's own laboratory in Nha Trang, which became an official Pasteur Institute ten years after its founding in 1895, also diverged from the Parisian model of a secluded, modest, and monastic scientific stronghold. Here, Yersin embraced capitalism, which fit much better with the heroic image of the colonial scientists than it did with metropolitan notions of disinterested science. The Pastorian's goal was to make the Nha Trang laboratory independent from subventions from the Government-General, the predominant funding model of the Pasteur Institute in Saigon. He realized, from his own struggles, how unreliable such funds could be. Instead, Yersin became a landholder. He acquired several large plantations on the plateau of Suoi Giao and near the mountain of Lang Biang. Initially, Yersin used this land to cultivate coffee, peppers, and rice. As his operations grew, Yersin turned his eyes toward rubber. In 1898, he imported hevea seeds from Brazil into Indochina and began cultivating them on the Suoi Giao plantations, using corvée Vietnamese labor.[74] By 1911, he was harvesting enough caoutchouc that he incorporated the plantations and put the revenues toward "supporting scientific activities in the Far-East."[75] Although Yersin publicly claimed that his empire-building was all in the name of science, he himself tended to neglect the latter in favor of the former. His letters to his family spoke steadily less of his endeavors in bacteriology and more of his success with livestock farming and rubber plantations. He was now a master of his own little colony, writing excitedly about his daily drives in his new Peugeot, overseeing his lands, his laborers, and his agricultural goods.[76] This ethos, oriented toward expansion, profit, and personal mastery over the savage, exotic environment, was both an economic exigency, which responded to the difficulties of securing funding from the colonial state, and an expression of values, consistent with his new persona as a colonial hero. It was also a far cry from the monastic ideals of the *maison-mère*.

Yersin did his best to explain the economic reasoning behind his venture to his Pastorian colleagues. Construction in Nha Trang was cheaper than in Saigon, and in light of the conflicts both he and Calmette had experienced with colonial officials, ensuring the laboratory's independence was a prudent idea.[77] Still, his choices raised questions. In personal correspondence, Roux, Calmette, and others indicated that Yersin's decisions as a leader cast doubt on his personal qualities, his capacities as a scientist, and his loyalty to the mother institution. Discussions over financial decisions around the

Indochinese institutes very often turned into discussions of loyalty, fretting over public expressions of support, and accusations that one party's word could not be trusted. Remaining true to the values of Pastorian science and respecting one's colleagues were values that Parisian researchers had to police, and that Yersin had to confirm if he wanted to advance within the ranks of the institute. The moral economy within colonial high society conflicted with the moral economy of the Pasteur Institute.[78] Yersin could not simultaneously be an explorer and a laboratory scientist, a humanitarian and a capitalist empire builder. Choosing one ethos over another had very tangible costs.

In the late 1890s, negotiations over the funding of the Indochinese institutes became particularly intense. The director of the Saigon institute, Dr. Lepinay, had been mismanaging the finances of the laboratory, setting the future of the Indochinese institutes in question. As one solution, Yersin proposed fusing the Saigon laboratory with Nha Trang, bringing smallpox and rabies vaccinations over to his laboratory, and in effect turning Nha Trang into the central hub of bacteriology in Indochina.[79] Roux and Calmette strongly opposed this project. Besides citing problems of communication with Nha Trang, most of their arguments focused on Yersin's character. In letters to Paul-Louis Simond, the primary competitor for the director's post in Saigon, Calmette expressed his frustration with the "savage temperament" of Yersin and his tendency to get into "violent outbursts," which required Roux's intervention at the level of the Government-General, "without which Yersin would have succeeded in bringing [the Saigon lab] to ruin."[80] Yersin had made a number of decisions, which confirmed for Calmette that he was placing his personal pride ahead of the interests of the community. Aspiring to become the director of the Indochinese labs, Yersin ignored the primacy of seniority and training, which would have accorded the post to Simond. "I find it impossible that you would accept a position under Yersin, who does not keep up with developments, and only engages in bacteriology as an amateur," Calmette reasoned in one letter, connecting questions of personal pride with those of scientific competence.[81] In a later letter he wrote, "I explained to [Roux] that this sort of subordination would not be admissible, since you are older than Yersin, and more qualified [*plus gradé*]."[82] The problem was not simply Yersin's competence but also his character, as Calmette continued to write: "I find Yersin to be a boy [*garçon*] of merit, but I've learned that he harbors in him a good dose of egotism."[83]

The problem with egotism was that it led to disloyalty. Besides Yersin's disrespect for hierarchy, Calmette was angered by the Pastorian's attacks on his own reputation: "He told several colleagues that I was an addle-brain [*un brouillon*], and that I only got my position because of my brother in the Figaro."[84] When Yersin promised to lobby the Government-General for assistance to Simond, Calmette wrote to check if he had been "loyal" and used "his great influence with Doumer to help [Simond]."[85]

Roux and Calmette criticized Yersin for his lack of restraint and lack of loyalty, which led to unsound scientific and institutional decisions, reflecting one understanding of bourgeois masculinity, which privileged composure and esprit de corps.[86] This caused anxiety for Yersin, too. He kept writing compulsively to Roux, affirming his loyalty, but he also continued to develop his plantations in Nha Trang and style himself as an entrepreneur. Indeed, as many intellectuals discovered in the era of the Dreyfus Affair, white-collar workers and scholars could be perceived as unhealthy and prone to nervousness. Colonial masculinity could offer more "tangible proofs of manliness," and for Yersin, it certainly offered very concrete material benefits.[87] As Pastorians debated loyalty and entrepreneurship, they also debated models of masculinity.

The conflict between Yersin and metropolitan Pastorians was ultimately resolved when the Government-General appointed him the director of the first indigenous medical school in Hanoi, leaving Simond in charge of the Indochinese Pasteur Institutes.[88] But already, another conflict was brewing in Tunisia. It centered around Charles Nicolle, who became the director of the Pasteur Institute in Tunis in 1902, after Louis Pasteur's nephew Adrien Loir unexpectedly quit the post. Nicolle had just left a boring laboratory position in Rouen, and, like Yersin, he harbored imperial ambitions. In the following years, the Pastorian guided the Pasteur Institute of Tunis away from the monastic nonprofit model embraced by Roux and toward the expansive, entrepreneurial, and heroic model. Nicolle developed the agricultural exploits of the institute, embraced for-profit vaccine sales, pursued close collaboration with the colonial administration, and a used militaristic language to talk about research, all echoing Yersin's strategies in Nha Trang.[89]

The Tunis institute diverged from Roux's vision of disinterested medical research from the moment of its establishment. For many colonial administrators, the appeal of bacteriology lay in its potential to improve agricultural technologies, in the spirit of Pasteur's research on wine fermentation or Calmette's work on the Amyloprocess. In fin de siècle France, phylloxera, a pest imported from the United States, wreaked havoc in French vineyards, drastically reducing grape yields. French landholders in Tunisia hoped that this might provide them with an opportunity to jump-start a fledgling wine industry in the protectorate. To succeed, winegrowers needed the Pastorian to help protect vines against the phylloxera, improve yields, and adjust cultivation methods for the Tunisian climate.[90] In 1893, the resident-general of Tunisia discussed these issues with researchers at the Pasteur Institute in Paris and invited Adrien Loir to set up a laboratory under the Department of Agriculture. The small laboratory was officially christened the Pasteur Institute of Tunis in 1900.[91]

In part, metropolitan Pastorians hoped Nicolle's assignment would guide the Tunis institute away from Loir's narrow interests in agricultural technologies and toward medico-bacteriological research and education. Nicolle aggressively expanded the Tunis institute, integrating it with every aspect of Tunisian medical life, from public health and medical pathology to immunization and research. He established the *Archives de l'Institut Pasteur de Tunis*, a journal destined to disseminate the laboratory's research to the world, and began a personal research project with the potential for international impact: the study of typhus. The staff of the institute grew from six in 1903 to twenty-five in 1926. He also continued the agricultural and industrial experiments of his predecessor and focused heavily on the institute's fiscal stability, often running into conflicts with his metropolitan colleagues, who saw his strategies as diverging from the institute's nonprofit ethos.

The first step in Nicolle's transformation was the construction of a new home for the cramped laboratory. The new building followed the dominant model of mixing local vernacular with classical architecture, a model that Paul Rabinow has called characteristic of turn-of-the-century modern French urbanism.[92] In his public writings and personal letters, Nicolle constantly contrasted the shabbiness and the impracticality of Loir's laboratory with the well-connected and powerful new institution he was constructing. He described the old building as "a modest" and "impractical" facility "in the most precarious condition"; it was "poorly organized" and "lacking in even the most useful and familiar tools."[93] In contrast, the "walls of the new Institut Pasteur [were rising] with diligence and majesty"; it was constructed at the orders of the resident-general "resolutely" and "without hesitation" at the meeting point of the "two arteries of the city."[94] To a marginal, precarious, and struggling building, Nicolle opposed a powerful, capacious, and connected new hub.[95]

In effect, Nicolle saw his directorship as a new beginning for the Tunis institute, and to mark the moment, he organized a lavish celebration of the institute's new buildings in October 1905, with the resident-general, the French minister for public works, representatives of the Tunisian Bey, and French military and local doctors in attendance. Though Nicolle described the inauguration in a letter to his mother as a comically over-wrought affair (the director of studies fell into tears during his speech "first like a lamb, then like two, then like a fountain, then like a river and finally like the most incontinent of prostatics"), he nevertheless thought the event succeeded in convincing the attendees that the new institute would become "one of the highest places of Pastorian Science in Africa."[96] While Nicolle spent considerable time demonstrating the scientific facil-ities of the laboratory, he was equally interested in showing it as a space from which imperial power flowed; during the day of the inauguration, "outside, workers were paving roads, sanding the avenues, and painters on every corner were doing multicolor retouching."[97] Arab workers were changing the very face of the city to celebrate the new institute. Monastic research could not contain Nicolle's ambition, as he admitted in one his letters: "Though I devote almost the totality of my time outside of sleep to the laboratory and to research, I have a basic feeling that I was made for something totally different, and when I let my thoughts run free, it is in that other direction that they tend to flee."[98]

Nicolle's more active, extroverted style of leadership extended to vaccine development as well. From 1906 onward, Nicolle dedicated himself to the study of typhus, which was far from the most dangerous disease in Tunisia (malaria, cholera, and the plague had the highest death tolls) but was cen-tral for Europeans, as typhus outbreaks were common in war zones, jails, and other places that crammed together large numbers of people in unsan-itary conditions.[99] This research program led Tunisian Pastorians to a new method of vaccine production and distribution.

The most common type of vaccine at the time was produced from dead microbes and samples of immunized sera, which scientists considered safe, but which produced only short-term immunity. For the typhus vaccine, Nicolle and his collaborators discovered that microbes killed in sodium fluoride would not autolyze, but remained intact, enhancing the strength of the resulting vaccine. This discovery led Nicolle not simply to a new typhus vaccine but to higher-quality versions of many other vaccines, including those against diseases such as gonorrhea, staph infection, and cholera. Here is where his decisions differed from those of his mentor, Roux: he moved to sell these vaccines at a profit.[100]

In 1913, Nicolle, along with his head of laboratory, Ludovic Blaizot, and collaborator Alfred Conor, made an agreement with the pharmaceutical manufacturer, the Maison Poulenc, to produce and sell the typhus vaccine and other fluoridized vaccines in France.[101] The Pastorians—Nicolle, Blaizot, and Conor—as well as the Tunis institute stood to make a profit from the sales. This was in stark contrast to the attitude at the *maison-mère*, where Roux argued that the price of vaccination should only reflect the cost of its production, and not enrich the researchers themselves, as that would dilute the scientific ethos.[102]

Nicolle and his collaborators were aware of this disposition at the *maison-mère* and worked to hide their collaboration with the Maison Poulenc. In order to sell the new vaccines in France, the Maison Poulenc had to get approved by the serum commission at the Academy of Medicine, which was headed by none other than Dr. Roux himself. In lengthy correspondence, Nicolle, Blaizot, and François Billon (the manager at Maison Poulenc) discussed how best to conceal their involvement from Roux. Blaizot argued that, since Nicolle had already published his methods of vaccine production, the Maison Poulenc could be assumed to have independently developed the product based on Nicolle's publications. If the company applied for a permit without referencing Nicolle, then Roux would not be able to make the link. "All evidence of our contract has been destroyed," Blaizot wrote to Nicolle. "Nothing reveals our ties to the Maison Poulenc. Roux can, at best, simply speculate."[103] Here, economic justifications did not suffice in themselves; Nicolle and Blaizot had to contend with Roux, the metropolitan enforcer of the Pastorian ethos.

Not all colonial Pastorians had similarly tenuous relations with the Paris institute. In Algeria, Edmond and Étienne Sergent retained excellent relations with Roux and Calmette in France, while simultaneously adapting to the colonial situation. As at the institutes in Tunis and Indochina, they collaborated closely with the military and with colonial officials, running antimalarial campaigns, which they described as a "struggle," "war," and "offensive" against the mosquitoes.[104] Their highly performative attempt at eradicating (rather than containing) malaria in the "savage and killer" marsh of Ouled Mendil and their increasing construction of alliances with international health organizations outside the *maison-mère* testify to the degree to which they, too, subscribed to a colonial heroic ethos.[105] In Morocco, the

Paris institute and Algerian Pastorians pursued separate projects for nearly two decades, with people like Edmond Sergent maneuvering around the official Paris-sponsored institute in Tangier and setting up their own initiatives in colonial hospitals and in collaboration with public health boards in Rabat, and later Casablanca.[106] Generated in part by new material constraints and possibilities, in part by colonial bacteriologists' discomfort with the ascetic ethos, and in part by the social milieu of colonial geographical societies, military medicine, and belligerent administrators, the heroic ethos of colonial Pastorians alienated them in different ways from the *maison-mère*. Yersin focused on his plantation efforts in Indochina. The Sergent brothers pursued a North African strategy, trying to expand their network to Tunisia and Morocco while maintaining good relations with Paris. Nicolle was on course for a direct conflict. That conflict arrived in 1914.

Pastorians at War: Imagining the Future of the Pastorian Ideal

The Great War had dramatic impacts on both the *maison-mère* and the colonial laboratories, but ultimately, the latter suffered less. Forty-one doctors, three pharmacists, six veterinarians, and seventy-six other staff members were mobilized from Pasteur Institutes all over the world.[107] In the metropole, the Pasteur Institute's buildings were appropriated for military purposes, and the remaining staff in Paris, Lille, and Algiers "put their entire soul toward fighting for the *patrie*."[108] Metropolitan Pastorians furnished the army with vaccines against typhoid fever, typhus, tetanus, and rabies. Calmette proudly claimed that the Pasteur Institute sent more than 10 million francs' worth of sera to soldiers free of charge, totaling some 3.7 million doses. Alphonse Laveran, Émile Roux, and other notable bacteriologists traveled to the front, counseling the army on public health measures and coordinating responses to outbreaks of cholera and typhus. Wartime research yielded new understanding of diseases ranging from spirochetosis to tuberculosis.[109] Scientifically and patriotically, the Pasteur Institute came out of the war as a winner.

Still, the Pastorians had to count their losses. Twenty-six Pastorians (a fifth of those mobilized) lost their lives.[110] Many returned home wounded or maimed, and others left the scientific profession altogether. The metropolitan institutes were in ruins. Lille, under German occupation throughout most of the war, had been seriously bombed, and Albert Calmette's Pasteur Institute was effectively destroyed.[111] In 1918, German forces captured Calmette's wife and took her to a reprisal camp in Holzminden.[112] In Paris, Roux was in financial difficulty: free wartime vaccinations had eaten into the institute's budget, and inflation, which ran at 20 to 30 percent in the immediate postwar years, diminished the value of the institute's charitable donations. After four years under military command, the *maison-mère* lacked equipment and supplies. Salaries were stagnant, and the institute could not attract young researchers to replenish its staff.[113]

For colonial Pastorians, the effects of the war were more mixed. Though some of the staff in Saigon, Nha Trang, Tunis, and Dakar were mobilized, the laboratories themselves continued to function, and local directors retained control over the research agenda. Those institutes had more diverse sources of funding: Yersin sold rubber, rice, quinine, and other goods from his plantations to fund the laboratory, and most colonial institutes had long-term contracts with their respective governments for the sale of vaccines and sera. Finally, colonial Pasteur Institutes held a monopoly over laboratory analyses in their regions, securing them income from local hospitals.[114] Some colonial Pastorians expanded their research agenda during wartime. In Dakar, Alexandre Lafont and Ferdinand Heckenroth developed a plan for improving sanitation in the city; Edmond and Étienne Sergent used their research in Algiers to organize antimalaria campaigns in Macedonia and Egypt; in Tunisia, Nicolle studied the management of typhus in wartime conditions, when Serbian soldiers evacuated from Albania began arriving in the ports of Tunis in early 1916.[115]

At the same time, more overseas Pastorians felt socially marginalized. Both Yersin and Nicolle felt lonely and excluded from the common war experience shared by other men of honor in France. In 1914, Yersin repeatedly expressed to Roux his desire to return to France and serve in the war, but Roux ordered him to remain in Indochina.[116] As the war progressed, the scarcity of goods and irregular postal service with the metropole made Yersin feel increasingly isolated. "The mobilization of new classes in Indochina is going to further reduce the already meager personnel of the Pasteur Institute. Soon I will be left alone in Nha Trang," he wrote to his sister in early 1917.[117] Nicolle, too, was lonely and starving for action: he continuously pleaded with Roux to call his collaborators back from the front, and failing that, made plans to get out of Tunis himself. He briefly attempted to spearhead a campaign of typhus eradication in the Balkan peninsula, but when the project fell through, he retreated to Tunis and continued to write about his "isolation" and "solitude."[118]

Interwar public debates over the potential of disinterested medicine and the importance and character of colonial doctors added relevance to simmering conflicts over the proper ethos of a Pastorian. People in interwar France were disillusioned with the promise of scientific progress, which, as the war demonstrated, could lead to destruction as well as enlightenment. At the same time, militaristic masculinity was making a resurgence. If critics saw interwar France as weakened, unmanned, and damaged in the battlefield, then the question became how to "regenerate" the lost virility of metropolitan Frenchmen. For some, physical fitness, courage, aggression, and properly channeled passion intensified as the measures of man, leaving little room for monastic, mechanical science.[119]

In this atmosphere, medical professionals in the colonies found themselves under renewed attention, becoming symbols of France's true strength for some, and examples of pathetic, overconfident rationality for others. Responding to the many accounts of violence and abuse in events such as the construction of the Congo–Ocean Railway (1921–1934) or the Rif War (1920–1926), colonial governments produced a number of propagandistic documentaries centered on the colonial doctor in the interwar years. These documentaries, shown in schools or at the 1931 Colonial Exposition, did not deny the abjection and suffering that journalists such as André Gide had uncovered, but depicted them as products of the harsh colonial environment rather than French politics.[120] Life in the colonies was indeed nasty, brutish, and short, but not because of French intervention, forced labor, or police repressions; real responsibility lay with invisible agents, such as microbes and mosquitoes, which heroic doctors and bacteriologists could then conquer.

These films were based on a genre invented by the Rockefeller Foundation and popularized in France during the foundation's TB campaigns from 1917 onward (more on this in chapters 4 and 5). Often, they portrayed the colonial doctor as a military commander, coordinating an army of auxiliaries and patients in the African brush in the fight against invisible yet deadly diseases. Films such as *Sleeping Sickness* (Alfred Chaumel, 1930) conventionally began with a series of maps, laying out the scope of the empire and the terrains ("endemic," "epidemic," and "endoepidemic") where the battle against diseases was to be fought. Chaumel represented the mass treatment efforts of the Pastorian Eugène Jamot as military campaigns: he juxtaposed shots of nurses, auxiliaries, and doctors waiting in formation for patients with images of tribesmen emerging from the brush in the hundreds to present themselves for treatment, resembling a military parade or inspection. The camera lingered long on Jamot himself, following the bacteriologist as he oversaw the various procedures, corrected the technique of auxiliaries, and made sure statistics were properly recorded. Jamot appeared as a general overseeing the military inspection, an impression further reinforced by shots of the French tricolor at the end of the film.[121] Another film, *A Walk through French Equatorial Africa* (J. K. Raymond-Millet, 1931), recycled much of the imagery of sleeping sickness campaigns and highlighted the long journey doctors had to take to reach their research sites. Tropical doctors had to travel to Brazzaville, "far, very far from the tumultuous city [of Paris]," where they would find shelter in the local Pasteur Institute, depicted as a sort of base of operations. Their real mission was farther still, requiring long journeys on rivers, through the jungle, and across difficult terrain, all of which the film displayed in detail. Doctors, then, were not only fearless commanders fighting an invisible war but also explorers, taking the tricolor to beyond the farthest reaches of civilization, with the Pasteur Institute their only solid outpost in these foreign lands.[122]

Nicolle had grown increasingly dissatisfied with the direction Roux envisioned for the Pasteur Institute. He allied himself with Calmette and with Pasteur Vallery-Radot, Louis Pasteur's grandson, and moved to make a bid for the directorship of the Paris institute. Both Nicolle and Roux used Pasteur's centenary, widely celebrated around Greater France in 1922, as an opportunity to argue for their vision of the future of the institute by linking it to the past—specifically to the character of Louis Pasteur. In Paris, Roux organized a series of celebrations and endorsed a hagiographic film, all of which depicted Pasteur as a saintly figure, highlighted his solitary and methodical work, and connected this ethos to the successes of his Parisian colleagues. In the colonies, Edmond Sergent, Alexandre Yersin, and Charles Nicolle held celebrations of their own, portraying Pasteur as a missionary whose work promised to revitalize the colonies, and as a patriot whose scientific accomplishments complemented the use of science in warfare. The futures Roux and Nicolle imagined for the Pasteur Institute were inextricable from masculine values: virility and impotence, courage and self-restraint, and public collaboration and solitude within the scientific community, all channeled through the image of Pasteur. These were the values that guided proposals for either radically changing the direction of the institute or continuing down the well-trodden path.

Nicolle began to express his dissatisfaction with Roux's leadership privately already in the 1910s. A friend from Nicolle's university days, the medical reformer Émile Leredde, kept him abreast of the developments at the Pasteur Institute. These letters largely revolved around critiques of Roux, which jibed well with Nicolle's own experiences. "[Roux] is a man who by his disinterest . . . has gravely hurt the institute. He should have been a man who puts others in their place, who judges and stimulates people to act," Leredde wrote to Nicole in 1916.[123] In the postwar years, Nicolle commiserated with Leredde and with Étienne Burnet, another metropolitan Pastorian with interests in the tropics, over the lack of initiative Roux showed in making money off vaccinations, even though this practice—which he had pioneered with the Maison Poulenc—offered a clear way out of the budgetary quagmire that plagued the *maison-mère*.[124]

In their correspondence, Leredde and Nicolle, who held socialist sympathies, compared the state of the Pasteur Institute to the state of bourgeois Europe, fearing that the indecisiveness of stagnant leaders was leading both to ruin. Their letters moved seamlessly from one topic to another. "What unintelligence in power. What absence of decision and of clarity," Leredde complained to Nicolle, referring both to the leadership of France and to Émile Roux.[125] He believed that the institute should collaborate more closely with hospitals, training their staff in radiology and serology so that patients could benefit from the precise laboratory identification of diseases and bacteriologists would be able to develop their research agendas. "This is what needs to be said publicly," Leredde encouraged Nicolle, "a public effort to support the Pasteur Institutes, to develop pastorian research, a push by the State to create laboratories everywhere."[126] In diagnosing the causes of the stagnation, Leredde contrasted Roux's impotence ("Roux should have done it, he has been a bad member of the Pastorian brotherhood, guiding to nothingness, to negation") with Nicolle's specifically colonial potential: "You are a colonial, and a part of those colonials who have to colonize France. Those of us who left, have audacity and courage, and they know how to use both the one and the other."[127]

The financial situation in Paris also caused a crisis of vitality: the low wages offered at the Pasteur Institute prevented it from hiring young bacteriologists, further contributing to the air of stagnation. Burnet, who had been stationed in Tunis from 1921 onward, wrote to Nicolle on one of his visits to

Paris: "Everybody asks about the future of the Institut Pasteur: Where are the young? Calmette says that Roux does not care. . . . There are rumors that he has simply grown too old. The tasks of a pilot and captain are not easy."[128] The primary problems created by Roux's inertia, Nicolle concluded, remained "recruitment and remuneration."[129]

Roux had one opportunity to display the initiative that Nicolle, Calmette, and others desired. In 1919, the Greek government offered to fund a new Pasteur Institute in Athens, and Calmette was tasked with setting it up. Pastorians were offered a generous allocation of 250,000 drachmas per year for twenty years, plus an investment of 500,000 drachmas for the construction of laboratories. Still, Calmette found that staffing the new institute was more difficult than he had imagined.[130] Calmette (and Nicolle) lobbied for Georges Blanc, Nicolle's head of laboratory, as the director of the new institute. Blanc had ample experience with tropical medicine and could integrate the Athens institute into a broader system of Mediterranean laboratories, which included those of Tunis, Algiers, and Constantinople. However, Roux disagreed, insisting instead on the appointment of Georges Abt, a minor scientist at the Paris institute. Calmette was furious at this decision, writing to Nicolle that Roux continued to resist letting him take the initiative: "You know how much he fears innovations that he believes would trouble his tranquility."[131] Quiet, methodical work, focused on the laboratory itself, had become anathema to scientists trained in colonial institutes, where influence-building was the backbone of a successful bacteriological career.

Pastorians elaborated competing visions of leadership through commemorations of Pasteur at the founding father's centenary in 1922. In Paris, Émile Roux organized an elaborate celebration at the Pasteur Institute. The ceremony began with speeches by the president of the republic and prominent Pastorians, followed by a feature film dramatizing Pasteur's life and a variety of other tributes, including poems and songs composed in the bacteriologist's honor. Festivities were also held in the French provinces as well as in the colonies, where schoolchildren received special volumes on the life of Pasteur, and governments unveiled busts and statues with pomp and circumstance. The character of Pasteur that was celebrated in Algiers and Tunis, however, differed greatly from the Pasteur commemorated on rue Dutot in Paris.

At the Pasteur Institute, speaker after speaker framed Pasteur's contribution in terms of asceticism and piety. A reporter covering the event for Le Temps described a grand tour of Pasteur's apartment, which had been preserved for posterity and shone in "glorious poverty," in the words of Rene Doumic of the Académie Francaise.[132] Visitors were shown Pasteur's "relics"—flasks, microscopes, and lab notes; they were guided in "respectful silence" through the scientist's library and lectured by his collaborators before, "with regrets, leaving this 'temple' (a word used by a pastorian), this temple of work and knowledge."[133] In his speech, Émile Roux immediately evoked Pasteur's origins in "the humble house of a tanner" and contrasted Pasteur's "enormous work ethic" and "absolute faith and courage" in uncovering the truth with his "impassioned adversaries" who refused to change their erroneous views.[134] After listing the various expressions of Pasteur's self-discipline, humility, and work ethic, journalists concluded that the presentation as a whole created an "image of the scientist [which] never ceases to appear in the aura of the most tender and touching family values," connecting Pasteur's professional qualities to a broader model of patriarchal comportment.[135]

A film commissioned by Roux and directed by Jean Epstein and Jean Benoit-Lévy further reinforced this ascetic image. This hour-long docudrama depicted the life and work of Pasteur, culminating in scenes at the contemporary Pasteur Institute. Reviews praised the film for its simplicity and verisimilitude, in keeping with the scientist's modest image: "Nothing was overdramatized. It is the very life of Pasteur, simple and fecund, which unfolds on the film strip."[136] Another review pointed to the way the film focused on Pasteur's instruments—his vials and microscopes—as proof of authenticity.[137] The closing scenes of the film illustrated the two central qualities that metropolitan Pastorians prized. First, the film emphasized continuity between the father and his disciples, as the closing shots focused on Roux and his two *sous-directeurs*, Calmette and René Martin, dressed in black robes, carrying on their master's legacy. Second, Epstein and Benoit-Lévy highlighted Pasteur's peace-loving and humanistic values in contrast to what the authors perceived as a dominating warrior mentality. The final shot of the film, as several reviews noted, featured a title card quoting Pasteur as the fiercest *opponent* of "the law of death," which imagines "new forms of combat" and constantly "obliges people to prepare for the field of battle."[138] Pasteur, in the eyes of Epstein and Benoit-Lévy, represented peace, simplicity, and restraint.

Orators in Tunisia and Algeria, on the other hand, evoked Pasteur as "one of the greatest conquerors that has ever existed," rendering his scientific work not as a peaceful and religious pursuit but as the work of a warrior.[139] This was true both metaphorically, as Pasteur was "the greatest conqueror of all,

who has beat back darkness, suffering, illness, and death," and also in a lit-
eral sense, as the governor-general of Algeria described the bacteriologist
as strengthening the French military by making it impervious to battlefield
injuries from gangrene to "hospital rot."[140] Edmond Sergent, the head of the
Algiers Pasteur Institute, hailed the scientist as an explorer who "discovered,
in our land, a completely new world."[141]

In both Algiers and Tunis, local schools were handed little booklets with
Pasteur's image and select quotations, such as "The grandeur of human
actions is measured by the inspiration that gives birth to them," literally offering him as a role model. Some schools even held a week-long "Pasteur
session," where teachers taught the basics of microbiology as well as Pasteur's
biography based on texts assembled by the Pasteur Institute.[142] These texts,
like their Parisian counterparts, made reference to Pasteur's humble origins
but then quickly turned to emphasize his precociousness and drive: his first
discoveries "already at the age of 25" inspired him with the "power to solve
all scientific questions."[143] Both Parisian and North African celebrations
connected Pasteur's scientific grandeur and work ethic to issues of vitality
and family, to specific models of masculinity that were then set as exemplary
for all future Pastorians. In Paris, Pastorians were supposed to be peaceful
and restrained, in opposition to displaying the military ambitions that seemingly governed the world. In the colonies, however, Pasteur appeared as a
conqueror, an explorer, and a man driven by ambition, power, and the desire
for expansion. The "work of Pasteur [was], in reality, the work of life itself."[144]

Nicolle exploited the public attention during the centenary to strike at
Roux, expressing his ambitions for reorganizing the institute and putting his
own energy in the service of revitalizing the institute as a whole. He confided
to Vallery-Radot, "The goal we are after [is] to transform the necropolis that
extends around your grandfather's tomb into a vital establishment worthy
of his name," again highlighting the lack of virility in the institution.[145]
Publicly, he made his case in a long article, published in *Le Temps*, on the
"peril of microbiological studies in France."[146] Nicolle argued that the institute had become not just stagnant but mortally wounded, with the best days
of bacteriological accomplishments dating from before the war. While public
institutions were stifled by the all-too rigid hand of the state that was funding
them and the teaching obligations of its scientists, the Pasteur Institute itself could potentially show the agile innovation bacteriology required, were
it not reliant solely on charitable donations. Scientists at the Pasteur Institute
were living like monks, from "alms," which prevented them from carrying

out their manly duties. They were *célibataires* out of necessity, or unable to provide for their families. This situation was rendering French science "infertile" in two ways. Scientists already employed at the institute would literally not be able to have children, while the low salaries scared away the next generation. "When the last of us dies," Nicolle concluded, "there won't be any more French microbiology."[147] The future of microbiology, in Nicolle's view, was tied to the vitality of the men working in the institute, and to their ability to procreate and provide. Under Roux's reign, the institute was driven by degeneration, death, and impotence.

In an interview published some years later, Nicolle directly laid the blame on Roux: "He lost confidence in men, and in the future of the house of Pasteur. He procrastinated, reduced expenses, waited for better days. Sick, constantly preoccupied, he saw the institute which he directed in the same manner as he saw himself. Even if in his speeches he maintained the image of an innovator, he dared nothing, he halted the machine."[148] Here, as in his previous attack, Nicolle conflated the state of the institution with the physical state of the man leading it. Decisions made by a physically frail man could themselves be nothing but frail and overly cautious.

Roux's private response, in contrast, highlighted the dangers of unchecked virility against the ironclad discipline of his ascetic masculinity. "Had I started to work in Pasteur's laboratory with a salary of 30,000 fr. instead of 1,800, I might have been tempted to rush out to see what lay beneath dancers' tutus instead of devoting myself tirelessly to my laboratory work. The past shows that the best work has come out of laboratories where researchers were not covered in gold."[149] The scientist was skeptical toward many of the leaders of the overseas institutes, whom he saw as spending too much time on local politics and not enough time on research. On the question of the Athens institute, he had preferred a Parisian microbiologist over someone with tropical experience, and he continually sent Calmette or other scientists at the *maison-mère* to paper over what he perceived as Yersin's "problems with his collaborators" over questions that "had no scientific interest whatsoever."[150] From a distance, outside of Roux's methodical control, the leaders of the colonial institutes appeared hotheaded and capricious.

The interwar atmosphere empowered those Pastorians who sought change and ambition. Writing in the metropolitan press, reformers connected the revitalization of the Pasteur Institute to the revitalization of France. Maurice Barrès, a journalist, thinker, and prominent radical nationalist, began his article advocating for raising the salaries of bacteriologists and firing "mediocre subalterns" with an exhortation against complacency in France: "The danger for France at this hour is to let herself be submerged in the wave of laziness that currently sweeps the world. We will only have properly won the war if we get to work and build on our good luck."[151] He then recalled how Pasteur himself had designated the bacteriological laboratory as the space of "life, fecundity, and power," without which the physical sciences would "become the image of sterility and of death," and scientists "soldiers without weapons on the field of battle."[152] Barrès suggested that it was this legacy of Pasteur that had been forgotten under Roux, who directed the institute without a scientific advisory board, let different laboratories do overlapping work, and deprived scientists of the necessary independence. More important, scientific directors at the institute were "extremely regrettably" avoiding collaboration with industry, in contrast to Germany, where, Barrès claimed, such collaboration flourished.[153] Here, Barrès brought together vitality on the microbiological level (the growth and manipulation of laboratory cultures), vitality on the institutional level (the courage to pass reforms, fire incompetent workers, and collaborate with industry), and vitality on the national level. The Pasteur Institute had to aspire to all three.

Nicolle, along with Vallery-Radot, Calmette, and other colonial Pastorians, made the first steps toward reforming one of the most criticized aspects of the *maison-mère*, the lack of new, young staff. In 1921, the three founded the Association for the Extension of Pastorian Studies, which aimed to provide scholarships for young microbiologists.[154] The grants, Calmette underscored, were particularly important given that "current economic conditions impose[d] particularly on heads of families," and given the "preponderant role of scientists in the Victory."[155] The proper Pastorian, according to Nicolle, Calmette, and other reformists, was a patriot and a patriarch, filled with ambition and power.

Nicolle clearly indicated that he hoped to succeed Roux as the director of the Pasteur Institute, or at least to be made a vice director, like Calmette. After Roux's death, in 1933, Nicolle and his close friend the writer Georges Duhamel publicly lobbied for the position.[156] Nicolle did not succeed, but his legacy lived on through his close friend and ally, Pasteur Vallery-Radot, who was named to direct a new department designed to coordinate the activities of all the overseas institutes, bringing the colonial institutes to new prominence. Vallery-Radot pushed for initiatives he had conceived in correspondence with Nicolle, such as establishing permanent rotations between the *maison-mère* and the increasing number of colonial laboratories, and establishing a colonial pavilion in Paris for researchers returning from the colonies so that they could, if they so desired, continue their research in Paris.[157] The Paris institute remained committed to its nonprofit philosophy, and nothing came of Vallery-Radot's proposal, as World War II interrupted his lobbying. The formation of an official Pasteur Institute International Network would have to wait until 1989, following years of financial distress and recovery. In rhetoric and self-presentation, however, the institute drifted in Nicolle's direction already in the interwar years.

Where Nicolle left the clearest mark, however, was in shifting the contours of the institute's rhetoric. By the time of the institute's fiftieth anniversary celebrations in 1939, the image of the true Pastorian had changed. There, Vallery-Radot, Pasteur's grandson and the coordinator of the overseas institutes, commended the "enthusiasm of the young" researchers, whose "principles of action were guided by the magnificent development of the theories coming from [Pasteur's] genius."[158] Again citing Pasteur, Vallery-Radot chose words that rendered danger, courage, and exploration of the unknown as an age-old Pastorian tradition: "[Pastorians] go in the shadow of our soldiers and administrators to our possessions beyond the seas, accomplishing an often arduous and superhuman task, . . . taking as their motto the words of Pasteur himself: 'life in the midst of danger is the true life, it's a life of sacrifice worth emulating, a fecund life.'"[159] Vallery-Radot repeated this language elsewhere, in articles written for the prestigious literary magazine *Revues des Deux Mondes*, where he published an overview of the Pasteur Institute's history devoted almost entirely to its overseas efforts. Instead of the customary praising of Roux, the longest director of the institute, Vallery-Radot focused on men such as Émie Duclaux, Pasteur's colleague and Roux's predecessor as the director of the Institute, and Nicolle, whose "rabid individualism" was a better fit for the "Latin spirit" of researchers who could not "subject themselves to the discipline of collective labor."[160] Here, too, individual courage was emphasized over calm, communal effort, and the discovery of antitoxins and vaccines was celebrated as a victory of specific ingenious researchers rather than the result of methodical, objective teamwork.

A number of publications from the interwar years reinforced the heroic narrative, turning it into the standard account of the Pasteur Institutes. In these tellings, conflicts over what constituted the proper motivations of microbiologists were written out in favor of an account tracing a continuity of militaristic fervor from Pasteur to Vallery-Radot and onward. In 1922, the Bordelaise doctor and journalist Pierre Mauriac, writing in the *Bulletin of Medicine*, recalled the conflict between Pasteur and the ardent secularist skeptic Ernest Renan in an article titled "Pasteur on the Margins of Official Discourse."[161] Mauriac reminded readers that unlike Renan, who had been unable to see the German threat in the 1860s, Pasteur's had a "way of categorically calling the good the good, and the evil the evil," guided by his patriotic and religious spirit. The conflict with Renan, Mauriac wrote, after all culminated in Pasteur "yelling" that all his works implicitly bore the epigraph "Down with Prussia [*Haine à la Prussie*]! Vengeance, vengeance," concluding that the days of war led the majority of Frenchmen "to side with him, and not with Renan."[162] By the end of the 1930s, this idea of Pastorians as patriots and heroes was no longer on the margins. It had been popularized through books such as Paul de Kruif's *Microbe Hunters*, which spoke of the "heroic age" of bacteriology through biographies of scientists including Pasteur, Roux, and Métchnikoff, through popular films and colonial documentaries, and through the various anniversary events recounted earlier in this chapter.[163] Later biographers have largely reproduced the idea of a "heroic era" of bacteriology, concentrated largely on the prewar accomplishments of Yersin, Calmette, and Laveran, and highlighted the militaristic spirit of the Pastorian community.[164]

In the empire, Pastorian values were summarized by a dedication on the facade of the Dakar Pasteur Institute, built in 1938 in the very center of the city's Plateau, minutes away from official buildings and the palace of the governor-general. Echoing the inscription on the Paris Pantheon, the mausoleum for the "Great Men" of France, the dedication on the Dakar institute read, "To Pasteur, Black Africa is grateful." In this rendition, Pasteur was a genius, up there with the Count Mirabeau, Léon Gambetta, or Victor Hugo; colonial subjects were his supplicants. The heroic ideal triumphed.

Conclusion

The network of Pasteur Institutes expanded and changed dramatically in the decades following the establishment of the Indochinese institutes. Propelled by the potential benefits to colonial agriculture and industry, public health concerns, or the ambitions of individual, well-connected bacteriologists, governments established Pasteur Institutes in Algiers (1894), Tananarive (1898), Tunis (1900), Brazzaville (1910), Tangier (1911), Dakar (1923), and Casablanca (1929). Outside the empire, Pastorians had outposts in

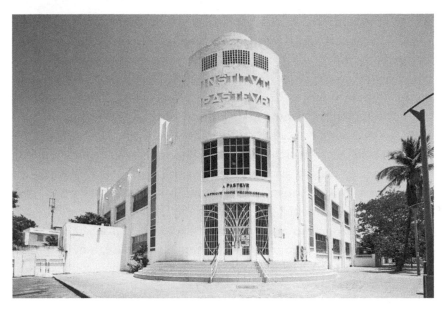

Figure 3.4 Pasteur Institute of Dakar. © MJ Photography / Alamy Stock Photo.

Constantinople (1893), Bangkok (1913), Chengdu (1911), and Shanghai (1938). The overseas institutes were intimately connected to colonial politics and experimented with new funding models as well as new collaborations with governments and industries. The living conditions and social circles in Indochina and elsewhere both attracted more adventurous, less solitary men, and socialized them into a culture that valued independence, courage, and military conquest above all else.

This chapter has proposed a dynamic approach to understanding the relationship between institutional economics, scientific ethos, and masculinity. Bacteriologists' masculine norms could change their economic calculus in certain moments, and shifting economic fortunes could empower new notions of scientific masculinity in other moments. In other words, we cannot understand the emergence of a capitalist ethos of science without understanding conflicts over masculinity, and we cannot understand conflicts over masculinity without understanding changing economic conditions. Yersin's success as a plantation owner, and Nicolle's success as a pharmaceutical mogul were both initially hampered by patriarchs such as Pasteur and Roux, who took them to task for abandoning the proper ascetic and nonprofit motives of the scientist. Colonial Pastorians had to account to their superiors for their hot-bloodedness, their decisions to abandon laboratory science for expeditions or economic ventures, their ambitions to accelerate the expansion of the institute's reach to new territories and new business models. It was not until the experience of the Great War and the declining fortunes of the metropolitan institutes set into question both ascetism as a manly value and the economic ability of Pastorians to provide for their families that the masculine ascetic ideal advanced by the Paris institute began to fracture.

As bacteriological laboratories multiplied across the French empire, and as changes in leadership made it easier for researchers to circulate between the *maison-mère* and the overseas institutes, Pastorian research projects became increasingly ambitious in scope. The following chapters will look at how this circulation was made possible by epidemiological studies, which brought the entire empire into one microbiological space; how Pastorians used the empire to push their own research further; and how colonial actors used Pastorian research to achieve their own political goals.

4

The Making of Imperial Tuberculosis

By 1910, Pastorians had laboratories in French Indochina, North Africa, sub-Saharan Africa, Madagascar, and, of course, metropolitan France itself. Yet many of these laboratories were islands of biomedical science in the middle of vast tracts of epidemiologically unknown territory. Tuberculosis provides one example of this pattern. Before the twentieth century, medical experts and administrators were largely uninterested in the illness in a colonial context, preferring instead to spend their limited resources on unfamiliar tropical diseases, which endangered French colonists—predominantly malaria and yellow fever.[1] The few existing surveys dismissed the danger posed by TB, declaring it an ancient and indigenous colonial disease, rendered impotent by environmental and racial adaptations. In metropolitan France, TB prevention became something of a national obsession in the fin de siècle; in the empire, such concerns simply did not exist.

The Pastorians changed this view. A series of new epidemiological studies commissioned by Albert Calmette in the 1910s reframed tuberculosis as an urgent imperial problem. These studies depicted the colonial environment as a virgin soil, colonial subjects as vulnerable bodies, and tuberculosis as a problem generated by infection through European contact rather than an indigenous affliction mitigated by environmental determinants. Tuberculosis, it now appeared, was not evenly distributed but concentrated in coastal cities, in European schools, and in the military. Pastorians concluded—and administrators were forced to agree—that tuberculosis was a product of French activity, "a disease of civilized peoples" that "spread in lockstep with conquest."[2]

Pastorian tuberculosis studies, this chapter argues, were scale-making projects.[3] They constructed a world in which both disease and disease prevention were imperial, rather than national or colonial, issues. By consequence, Pastorians with their pan-imperial network of laboratories, highly mobile tools of intervention, and sophisticated surveys of the microbiological landscape became the perfect agents for preventing the medical and political dangers that European-borne TB posed in the colonies. Calmette

Pasteur's Empire. Aro Velmet, Oxford University Press (2020). © Oxford University Press.
DOI: 10.1093/oso/9780190072827.001.0001

provided the Ministry of the Colonies with tools to standardize imperial governance in the field of public health and make bold claims about the humanitarian aims of French colonizers.

Calmette's intellectual convictions and a specific set of technopolitical tools molded the shape of this new vision of a Pastorian empire. The reconstitution of the colonial environment as a virgin soil, which Europeans were contaminating, was a product of Calmette's belief that contagion was the primary cause of tuberculosis and of his interest in the colonies as sites of experimentation. Calmette's methods stood in contrast to the dominant discourse in France, which interpreted contagion through a hygienist lens and reinforced visions of large-scale programs of social transformation and bodily discipline. The three technopolitical tools he used to bring his Pastorian vision into being—pan-imperial epidemiological studies, the tuberculin skin test, and the BCG vaccine—all helped to reimagine the colonial environment and the dynamics of TB propagation. They minimized the potential of social hygienic interventions as they were being practiced in France, discredited prior studies, and moved Pastorians to the center of all public health efforts.[4]

The politics of epidemiology had unintended consequences. In 1931, when tensions around the question of colonization had reached a boiling point, scientific experts at the Colonial Exposition at Vincennes found themselves agreeing with surrealist and communist critics at the Anti-colonial Exposition, with African intellectuals writing in journals such as *Cri des nègres* and with Vietnamese political organizers, all of whom deemed the spread of tuberculosis a "defect of 'the civilized metropole.'"[5]

Whether TB rates were indeed rising in those years is a question that is difficult to disentangle from the political history of epidemiology. As Randall Packard has argued for South Africa, changes in colonial societies could indeed increase TB prevalence. Forced labor migration, compulsory military service, and the corvée brought Africans together in closed spaces and weakened their immune systems, making it more likely that TB developed into a symptomatic illness.[6] French experts at the time focused instead on questions of contagion through European contact and its effects on what they assumed was virgin African soil. Still, as David Barnes has argued, "retrospective epidemiology" is a fraught affair, as it would inevitably involve wrenching historical sources from the "categories, preconceptions and concerns of the time." It would mean reading history with presentist eyes for data that epidemiological documents were never meant to represent, while blinding the historian to the wealth of information about how TB epidemiology was understood and what kind of work it performed *at the time*.[7] The paucity of studies in West Africa and Indochina prior to 1920 makes it particularly hard to discuss the "true" epidemiology of TB—other than allowing one to conclude that the colonies were definitely not virgin soils.[8] Instead, this chapter investigates what the explosion of interest in colonial TB in the post-1912 period can tell us about the political and scientific purposes of epidemiological inquiry.

Tuberculosis in France and Its Colonies, 1880–1914

In the fin de siécle, tuberculosis became the central public health concern of metropolitan France, while administrators in West Africa and Indochina effectively ignored the disease. This divergence derived from different understandings of tuberculosis epidemiology—the patterns, causes, and determinants of disease across a defined environment and population. In France, experts described the causes of tuberculosis as both environmental and microbial, with newer, bacteriological explanations still culminating in well-known hygienist exhortations about the importance of avoiding vice and keeping clean. In the empire, experts argued that the disease was ancient and less dangerous than in the metropole. Doctors and scientists unequivocally dismissed dangers of contagion. Instead, experts focused on ecological and racial factors, which they understood to determine susceptibility. These claims served to relieve administrators of public health responsibility and to reinforce the idea that different races "belonged" in different environments to which they had adapted.

Tuberculosis is a contagious bacterial disease, caused by the Koch bacillus, *Mycobacterium tuberculosis*. It is transmitted through air, in droplets expelled through coughing. In people with strong immune systems, the infection is usually localized in lesions in the respiratory tract and is rarely expressed in the form of disease. Most carriers do not know they have it, remaining asymptomatic throughout their lives. When the immune system is compromised, however, whether by poor diet, old age, acute or chronic disease, or any number of other pressures, the disease can become active. Today, the rule of thumb is that about 10 percent of those infected with the tubercle microbe actually develop symptoms of the disease.[9]

In urbanizing France, as elsewhere in the nineteenth-century world, weakened immune systems were commonplace among the working class and the elderly, where malnutrition, low standards of living, and cramped living quarters in urban settings facilitated disease transmission. It is possible that almost everyone who lived in urban areas in the late nineteenth century may have carried the Koch bacillus. In places like Paris or Le Havre, TB accounted for a quarter of all deaths, claiming almost twelve thousand victims in Paris alone in the 1870s, or seven deaths per one thousand inhabitants.[10] Until the 1860s, a majority of consumptives were women. Later, the trend reversed and more men became afflicted, a surprising development, the causes of which remain highly debated. Tuberculosis mortality rates grew steadily until the 1870s, spiked during the Franco-Prussian War and the siege of Paris, and then began a halting yet persistent decline. In 1882, Robert Koch identified the tubercle microbe, facilitating diagnosis and leading to the development of experimental cures, many of which—most notably tuberculin—turned out to be ultimately ineffective.

Although long-term trends showed a slow but clear decline in tuberculosis mortality, anxieties over TB exploded in fin-de-siècle France. Tuberculosis had been a subject of debate and a source of social turmoil since Jean-Antoine Villemin's experiments on infection in 1865. It was only in 1898 when the War on Tuberculosis (*la lutte contre la tuberculose*) began properly, as the problem was taken up by the Academy of Medicine, by government commissions, and by popular movements. More than thirty books per year were published on the disease between 1890 and 1906. The anxieties did not reflect reality, however. Tuberculosis in those years claimed far fewer lives than it had in the 1860s. David Barnes has argued that tuberculosis became a way for the French bourgeoisie to express fears over national decline, the threat posed by the unhygienic working classes, the shifting of moral norms, and the rise of vices such as alcoholism and syphilis, which were all placed, along with TB, under the general heading of "social disease." Defeating TB would mean defending prosperity, national security, and bourgeois morality. So framed, anti-TB efforts became a convenient way for marginalizing and controlling not just the diseased but social deviants of all sorts. The rise of contagionist ideas in the metropole added to this discourse, rendering the underclasses dangerous not simply because of their squalid living conditions and moral failures but because they could potentially transmit the disease to the healthy and virtuous.[11]

In France, the mixture of contagionist and ecological etiologies led to a largely privately run response that focused, on the one hand, on the policing of spittle and, on the other hand, on slum housing and alcoholism.[12]

The importance placed on contagion meant that the primary enemy of the antituberculosis movement was the infected person and, in particular, the habit of spitting in public, which was associated almost uniquely with the working class. Medical reformers suggested drastic measures. Dispensaries, for instance, were considered largely as institutions designed to isolate the ill so that they would not be able to infect others. Housing authorities collected information on unsanitary housing, encouraging owners to make improvements. Antialcoholism movements associated drinking and syphilis with tuberculosis and directed their ire against cabarets, where all three could be found all too easily.[13] In short, bacteriological and ecological understandings of tuberculosis combined to form a discourse that turned TB into a moral issue and implicated both the bodies of workers and their living environments in spreading the disease.

In West Africa and Indochina, however, tuberculosis remained largely absent from the official mind. The supposedly "indigenous" disease fell outside the experts' sphere of interest, largely because it was seen as less dangerous than tropical diseases such as malaria, sleeping sickness, and yellow fever, which ravaged Europeans.[14] Indeed, in annual medical reports to the governments of the Afrique Occidentale Française (AOF) and Indochina, tuberculosis rarely occupied more than a paragraph. In the AOF, year after year, TB was simply reported as being "frequent and widespread" in all regions of the colonies and among both Africans and Europeans, but not destructive enough to warrant administrative action.[15] In Indochina, administrators often categorized tuberculosis as a "sporadic disease," the least important of three categories that included "epidemic" (smallpox) and "endemic" (malaria). This meant that tuberculosis was often excluded from official reports or was mentioned in barely a line.[16]

Epidemiological studies of tuberculosis in the AOF and Indochina were also comparatively rare. Because colonial administrators were uninterested in the disease and ordered no large-scale surveys of the affliction, discussions of tuberculosis were often limited to general studies of "diseases in warm climates," often in doctoral dissertations of aspiring tropical medicos or in publications by doctors working in hospitals in Dakar or Saigon, based on individual case studies observed in their clinical practice.[17] In the fin de siècle, as the War on Tuberculosis began in France, administrators began to look more closely at TB in the colonies. Alexandre Kermorgant, the director-general of the Colonial Health Service summarized and analyzed these initial studies in an influential 1905 report.[18]

One of the central concerns of those French medical experts who did study colonial TB in these early days was whether the disease could have been introduced by Europeans. This theory was not unique to the French context—Randall Packard has documented the importance of the "virgin soil" hypothesis in South Africa. There, the idea that Africans were untouched by this particularly "civilized" disease gave rise to segregatory policies on the grounds of "defending" Africans from the European disease, and became an excuse for ignoring the role African labor conditions played in aggravating tuberculosis.[19] Aside from similarly instrumental concerns over responsibility and segregation, however, French doctors seemed to be genuinely concerned that they were importing what they believed to be a contagious "disease of civilization" into their colonial territories.

In his 1905 review, Kermorgant observed that, as in the metropole, tuberculosis in the colonies appeared to multiply with "agglomeration" (population density) and with "civilization," in other words urbanization and European contact. The doctor declared TB almost completely absent from certain parts of Africa (Madagascar, Djibouti, Somalia). He noted that rates had been rising in some regions of West Africa deemed insalubrious and filled with "miserable populations in cramped spaces," such as the island of Gorée or the port city of Dakar.[20] The metropolitan fascination with links between proletarianization, urbanization, and tuberculosis—the "dark side of modernity"—made colonial experts, too, look for signs of overcivilization, while ideas of contagion reinforced the fear that Europeans might inadvertently be importing the disease to unsuspecting natives.

Yet although Kermorgant considered "civilization" to be a contributing factor to rising TB rates, he categorically rejected the idea of its European origin. He emphasized that tuberculosis had been known in French colonies "since time immemorial."[21] This was a consensus among doctors in Indochina and the AOF, all of whom emphasized its ancient local presence. "If tuberculosis was really of European import," argued one doctor reporting from Cochinchina, "the disease should be even today more frequent in places where the races are in daily contact."[22] This, doctors observed, was not true. Hospitals in Hanoi admitted patients from distant provinces of Annam, Cochinchina, and Tonkin, where they could not have had extensive contact with Europeans, and reports of tuberculosis dated back to missionary reports from the 1860s, when colonization had only just begun.

References to local names provided further evidence of the disease's ancient provenance in both Indochina and West Africa. Experts reported that

TB had traditional indigenous names: it was called *lo beng* in Cambodia, *binh ho lao* in Annam, and so on.[23] Some communities, such as Africans living in the Congo or near the Ogooué River, had "themselves imposed very severe isolation and preservation measures on those afflicted by tuberculosis."[24] This sort of ethnographic evidence was marshaled to demonstrate that tuberculosis had a long history in the colonies and that the French need not worry about the responsibility of introducing a new disease into the non-Western world.

Aside from its ancient provenance, colonial doctors rarely agreed on the affliction's epidemiology. Some doctors in the nineteenth and early twentieth centuries believed in racial determinants, arguing that blacks and orientals carried a biological immunity for tuberculosis, therefore rendering the problem moot altogether. This view had a long history: already in 1840, one Dr. Thévenot remarked that *indigènes* of the West African coast "have a sort of natural immunity against tuberculosis," a statement that was still replicated at the end of the nineteenth century.[25] Other experts speculated that Africans were more, rather than less, susceptible to tuberculosis. One doctor suggested that in regions where TB was endemic, blacks were suffering up to "four times as much . . . as Whites," and another noted that they "pay the heaviest tribute" to the disease.[26] Even Kermorgant, who was generally skeptical about the racial specificity of TB infection, suggested that "it is undeniable that the black race is particularly likely to contract tuberculosis" and that this reflected a broader susceptibility to infectious diseases, including smallpox and measles.[27]

In Indochina, Alphonse Voillot believed that the "yellow races" suffered less from the disease "in spite of their ancient contact with Europeans."[28] This long-standing claim of "practically absolute immunity of the yellow races" was probably bolstered by the belief in the heritability of tuberculosis, which led some doctors to conclude that societies that avoided intermarriage between the "clean" and the "sick" would develop greater resistance to the disease.[29] Even doctors, who observed high affliction rates in almost all parts of Indochina, noted that tuberculosis among "orientals" was milder, with "a slow evolution," "dry," without coughing or the production of sputum, and symptoms were more likely to include "diarrhea and intestinal problems."[30]

Ultimately, however expressed, discourses of racial specificity worked to reinforce the notion that different races were accustomed to specific environments, and that venturing outside those environments would inevitably result in poorer health. "Inhabitants of tropical lands," one doctor summarized, "have a lesser chance of developing tuberculosis than those of temperate European climes or those newly arrived in the tropics."[31] Kermorgant agreed with doctors like Voillot in concluding that "the *métis*, the 'mixed-bloods' appear to have less resistance to tuberculosis than individuals of the pure races from which they have emerged."[32] Voillot himself surmised that, because of racial differences in resistance to tuberculosis, it was in the "interests of tuberculosis prophylaxis to carefully avoid the mixing of races in all agglomerations where there's a possibility of overcrowding."[33] This discourse survived well into the twentieth century, although better mortality statistics from hospitals in Dakar and elsewhere forced Kermorgant and others to admit that racial resistance was not an absolute fact, but rather "only relative."[34]

Others emphasized environmental determinants: for them, cleaner air and the warm, dry tropical climate were responsible for the low rates of affliction. Algeria, in particular, was known for its clean air, which decreased the possibility of infection, with some doctors calling the country's climate the *patibulum vitae*, the life-giving cross.[35] Some doctors even suggested that malaria acclimatized Africans' organisms against certain forms of morbidity, including tuberculosis. Malaria as the disease most "suited" to the African climate simply outcompeted tuberculosis. "Tuberculosis and the malarial miasma are like two pans of a scale, if one rises then the other must lower," wrote a doctor, J. C. M. Boudin, in 1857, suggesting that regions with high rates of tuberculosis suppressed malaria and vice versa.[36] These views persisted into the early twentieth century, reappearing in reports at the 1904 tuberculosis conference. There, researchers speculated that malaria might be responsible for the low rates of tuberculosis among Malagasies and Somalis.[37] At the same time, these arguments became increasingly contested by doctors who showed that malaria could, in fact, accelerate and worsen tuberculosis.[38]

In the first decades of the twentieth century, when more hospitals were constructed in the AOF and Indochina, experts began to argue from admission statistics that tuberculosis in the colonies was perhaps more common than previously believed. Although experts in Cochinchina and Cambodia, for instance, reported low rates of affliction, they suspected that this was due to underreporting, rather than some sort of racial immunity or favorable climate.[39] These doubts and distinctions, however, rarely made it to official reports, which emphasized high affliction rates in urban centers and low rates in entire regions, most notably Madagascar, Cambodia, Tonkin, and Cochinchina.[40]

Colonial legislators ultimately marshaled these numbers to reject the "virgin soil" hypothesis and evade public health responsibility. Officials interpreted low affliction rates as evidence of environmental or racial resistance, which made the situation appear less urgent. Experts took high affliction rates, particularly in the AOF, as evidence that the disease had been present for a long time, and, given the Africans' "traditionally" poor hygiene, nothing could be done to stop it. Kermorgant's report ultimately arrived at a fatalistic conclusion: TB was a long-standing, local problem, and it "had made so much progress . . . that all prophylactic measures would prove illusory."[41]

No wonder then that, enabled by the defeatist argumentation of Kermorgant and others, administrative action on tuberculosis was rare in both the AOF and Indochina. In 1900 and 1904, the Ministry of the Colonies mandated that hospitals and sanitary services across the colonies take precautions against contagion: military establishments were required to regularly disinfect the premises and aerate buildings, while hospitals were required to isolate consumptives from other patients. Yet even here, officials acknowledged that budgetary resources were insufficient for complying with all the demands and implored that, at a minimum, doctors change shirts and wash hands after seeing patients with TB.[42] These efforts remained scant and produced few concrete results, given, as later analysts admitted, that "the imperious struggle against formidable exotic diseases deprioritized the fight against tuberculosis, the menace of which was less immediate."[43] In the prewar years, neither medical nor administrative elites made the case to take tuberculosis in the colonies seriously. Calmette's and his colleagues' epidemiological studies changed this status quo.

The Great War, the Rockefeller Mission, and the Return of Hygienist Ideas

Calmette's interest in tuberculosis began in the late 1890s, after his return from Indochina. Using the profits he made from developing the Amyloprocess, he founded his own laboratory in Lille in 1898. Lille, along with the neighboring towns of Roubaix and Tourcoing, formed the largest industrial region in France, with 250,000 workers employed in metallurgy, chemistry, and textiles in 1900. Tuberculosis levels were particularly high in the region, with more than two thousand recorded deaths annually. Calmette was increasingly unconvinced by the hygienist efforts directed toward education, housing improvements, and limiting spitting. "I could observe, every day, the inutility of insufficience of the poorly coordinated efforts of public welfare institutions and those of private charity," he wrote in his private autobiography.[44] Public authorities in Lille increasingly deferred to the Pastorian's expertise in matters of public health, from the construction of water purification stations, to diagnosing a hookworm epidemic among the miners of Lille. Given the rates of TB in the area, it was no surprise that Calmette, along with his laboratory chief, Camille Guérin, decided to focus their efforts on the prevention of TB.[45]

Initially, Calmette's suggestions blended environmental and bacteriological approaches, in tune with the prevalent opinion of the time. He proposed setting up dispensaries in all French departments that would track tuberculosis rates among the population, assist in early diagnosis and popular education, and guide the infected to the most appropriate form of treatment. Already here, however, one can see Calmette's emphasis on preventing infection over the amelioration of social conditions. His proposed education and sanitation measures, for instance, focused on recognizing the first signs of illness, reinforced the importance of avoiding spitting, the disinfection of clothing, and "distribution of hygienic spittoons, information on how to clean up spit."[46] By contrast, social hygienists would understand education as a broader, moral task, including counseling on moderation in drinking and better nutrition. Calmette did ultimately found the first dispensary in Lille, named the Dispensaire Émile Roux, after his Pastorian mentor, but he focused, for the next decade, on studying the tubercle microbe in the hopes of developing a vaccine.

After a decade-long pause, tuberculosis resurfaced as a social emergency during World War I, forcing the state to act after decades of reliance on charities and private initiative. Mass mobilization, cramped living conditions, and weakened immune systems of soldiers struggling with injuries and disease in the trenches all contributed to the resurfacing of tuberculosis in the army. As some experts noted later, the war may have "sometimes created, . . . often aggravated, but mostly *revealed*" the prevalence of tuberculosis.[47] Out of 9 million enlisted men, around 500,000 were screened for TB, 150,000 were diagnosed, and more than 100,000 soldiers were discharged.[48] Social anxieties created by the epidemic were greater still: tuberculosis suddenly seemed to be everywhere, and the threat it posed to the future of the nation appeared no longer metaphorical but very real indeed. The astronomer and science writer Charles Nordmann declared in a 1919 overview of the Rockefeller mission in the *Revue des Deux Mondes* that "even in the lands most ravaged by it, the war remains less dreadful than tuberculosis."[49]

The state's initial response to the epidemic was haphazard and marred by organizational problems. The Military Health Service (Service de Santé des Armées) was, in its initial years, poorly coordinated, with an understaffed patchwork of units attached to various army corps and regions working with little national oversight.[50] From 1915 onward, a series of circulars and laws

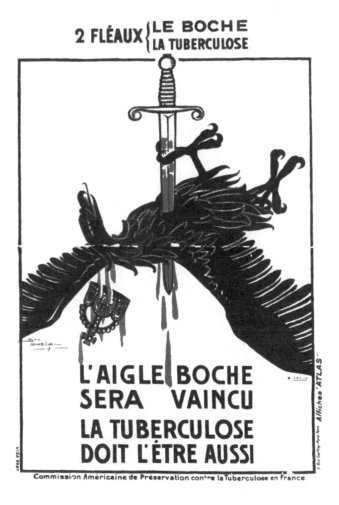

Figure 4.1 "The German Eagle will be defeated. Tuberculosis must be defeated, too." TB propaganda during World War I. Rockefeller Archive Center.

(most notably the 1916 Bourgeois Law and the 1919 Honnorat Law) marked, for the first time, the involvement of the state in the war against tuberculosis. Officials envisioned a national system of preventive education, dispensaries, isolation wards, and sanatoriums that would guide tuberculosis patients from diagnosis to, hopefully, cure.[51] Struggling under the weight of its multitude of tasks, however, the Military Health Service could not implement these steps, leading officials to turn toward civil society to make up for the shortfall. This led to the founding of the Central Committee for Consumptive Veterans (Comité central d'assistance aux anciens militaires tuberculeux), headed by Léon Bourgeois, former prime minister and then minister of work and social security. Finding state support scant, however, the committee contacted the Rockefeller Foundation in the United States, which had already provided assistance with fighting the typhus epidemic in Serbia. This collaboration led to the Wallace Sabine report on tuberculosis in late 1916 and to the development of an antituberculosis plan, which the foundation's International Health Division put into action as the United States entered the war in April 1917.[52]

The Rockefeller initiative, which lasted from 1917 to 1920, focused on public education, collecting statistics, providing technical aid, and establishing dispensaries across the country. Americans created traveling exhibits, puppet shows, instructional films, and awareness-raising posters designed to educate the French, and particularly their children, about the virtues of washing hands, containing spit, and other aspects of good hygiene—all the while reminding them of the role of "the American mission sent to France by Mr. Rockefeller" in this campaign.[53] More than two hundred dispensaries employed "social welfare nurses" (visiteuses d'hygiène) who were tasked with collecting data on TB rates and spreading public health knowledge on how to avoid contagion and maintain proper hygiene. Rockefeller experts also trained nurses and physicians and led coordination efforts between dispensaries, attempting to establish a national public health system, which the French had attempted, but failed, to achieve during the war.[54] While the initiative acknowledged the role of microbes in causing TB, it ultimately continued the prewar focus on "soil" over "seed," an epidemiological vision that emphasized environmental and social conditions, as well as the health of the individual body over a focus on limiting contact between the tubercle microbe and the human agent.

As the foundation handed over the reins to the committee, which had been renamed the Committee for the National Defense against

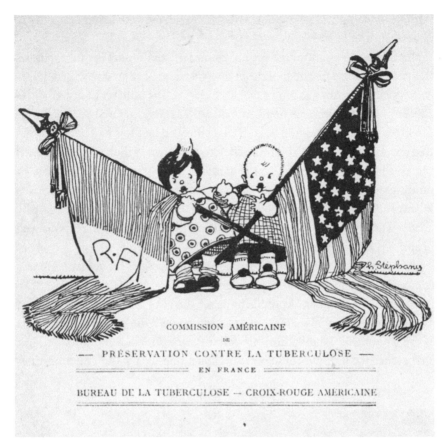

COMMISSION AMÉRICAINE
DE
— PRÉSERVATION CONTRE LA TUBERCULOSE —
EN FRANCE

BUREAU DE LA TUBERCULOSE → CROIX-ROUGE AMÉRICAINE

Figure 4.2 Cover image for a Rockefeller educational publication for French children. Some two million copies of similar literature were distributed during the Rockefeller Foundation mission to France. Rockefeller Archive Center.

Tuberculosis (CNDT), this preventive, sanitary model continued to dominate French efforts in the interwar years. Following the Rockefeller example, the committee raised funds via the selling of thematic stamps that provided easily digestible prophylactic advice such as "neat and clean," "light against tuberculosis," and "kiss of the sun."[55] Experts observed that the diminishment of tuberculosis rates correlated with improved housing conditions and the institution of the eight-hour workday, evidence they argued confirmed the importance of social and environmental conditions.[56] The moral dimension of anti-TB efforts remained central, as the fundraising stamps portrayed well-built, beautiful men and women bathing in sunlight, and medical treatises exhorted the damage caused by alcoholism and promiscuity.[57]

The Rockefeller committee set up a standardized model for tuberculosis prevention at the departmental level that was largely adopted by the CNDT. This systematic work was remarkably successful. The number of dispensaries in France grew from 22 in 1917 to 416 in 1922. By the same year, 1.7 million pieces of literature and five hundred educational films had been distributed around the country, and more than two hundred scholarships had been offered for postgraduate medical students.[58] In 1921, the committee began handing over anti-TB efforts to local authorities, leading to a slowing down of prevention efforts. Institutions put in place during the war years largely survived the transition intact. By 1923, either the state or charities sponsored all anti-TB activities in France.[59]

Calmette, too, was involved with the antituberculosis movement. He was a founding member and vice president of the Central Committee/CNDT and authored a number of publications on the anti-TB fight in the years of the Rockefeller campaign. He, however, interpreted the public health efforts of the Rockefeller Foundation through a Pastorian lens, emphasizing their importance for limiting contagion and collecting data about affliction rates

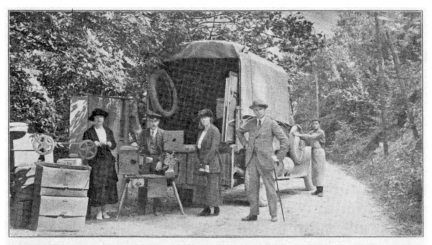

Fig 14 —Traveling unit used by Educational Division, Commission for Prevention of Tuberculosis in France

Figure 4.3 Traveling tuberculosis unit used by the Educational Division, Committee for the Prevention of Tuberculosis in France, 1919. Rockefeller Archive Center.

over social issues such as nutrition, aeration, or alcoholism. In an educational pamphlet published in 1920, Calmette emphasized that the "scientific methods of Pasteur have provided us with efficient means of protecting ourselves," providing a sort of counteradvertising to the public inundated with Rockefeller propaganda.[60] Echoing the language of the day, Calmette argued that the role of the departmental dispensaries was to be "essentially and exclusively social," yet his interpretation of the term "social," again, differed from that of the Rockefeller Foundation. For Calmette, the institutions were to focus on "establishing diagnosis as early as possible" and "to indicate measures for avoiding contagion."[61] While Rockefeller propaganda included education on the importance of proper nutrition, clean air, and protection of the immune system by avoiding alcohol and other social vices, Calmette's notion of avoiding contagion was more restrictive.

This approach set him—and the Pastorian brand—apart from the Rockefeller approach. He elaborated on his notion of contagion in several high-profile studies, most notably in a 713-page magnum opus titled *Microbial Infection and Tuberculosis in Humans and Animals* (*Infection bacillaire et la tuberculose chez l'homme et chez les animaux*). After devoting several hundred pages to the morphology, cultivation, life cycle, chemical composition, and infection mechanisms of the tubercle microbe, Calmette proceeded to demolish the ecological, "soil"-focused public health approach of the day. Listing popular arguments that grounded tuberculosis infections in "ignorance," "alcoholism," "misery," and "insufficient nutrition," Calmette concluded:

> It would be best to not repeat too often these aphorisms intended for the public, since it would detract our attention from the central goal which we need and wish to follow, that is to reduce or render docile the sources of infection. . . . Alcoholism, misery, lack of nutrition, unsanitary housing cannot cause tuberculosis *if the microbe itself is not present*. These are only— and this is already too strong a claim—factors of organic decay which, after the infection has already manifested itself, can paralyze or hinder the organism's natural defensive weapons.[62]

Calmette therefore believed that the broad social campaign against tuberculosis was misguided, focusing too much on the environmental conditions of potential victims and not enough on eradicating the microbe itself. On the one hand, Calmette prescribed the destruction of microbes in livestock, primarily by the heating of milk to seventy to eighty degrees Celsius, the process we now call pasteurization. On the other hand, he argued, "It is hard to imagine the limitation and then extinction [of the tubercle microbe] otherwise than by the *vaccination* of all men and susceptible animals."[63] Vaccination, however, was still purely hypothetical. Calmette did not have a working prototype before 1924, nor was he convinced that his research direction would be accepted by activists increasingly focused on Rockefeller-inspired social interventions.

The Construction of Tuberculosis as a Colonial Problem

While Calmette's approach was out of step with the public health mainstream in France, he had many allies in the colonies, where his own career had begun and where he had mentored a generation of young Pastorians. From 1912 onward, Calmette supervised a series of studies, which sharply reoriented the relationship between the tubercle microbe, the tropical environment, and its French and native inhabitants. These studies argued that the distribution of tuberculosis across colonies, with higher rates in French schools, the army, and urban environments, proved, contrary to prior belief, that the French were in fact responsible for introducing the disease to a virgin soil. They dismissed the conclusions of earlier studies by pointing to their often impressionistic and unreliable evidence, derived from clinical practice and mortality statistics, although the newer studies did not demonstrate radically diverging results. The Calmette era studies should not be seen as "better" or "more accurate" descriptions of tuberculosis epidemiology, but rather as epidemiological devices that constructed an argument for Pastorian medical intervention, by considering the colonies not as ancient habitats for the TB microbe but as virgin soils that Europeans were carelessly contaminating.[64]

Interest in colonial tuberculosis surged further in the 1920s and 1930s, thanks largely to the production of new studies that were coproduced with the extension of BCG vaccination (the subject of the next chapter). This surge was prefigured by Calmette's study of colonial tuberculosis, gathered with the help of local Pastorians and published in 1912, the first systematic attempt to study TB epidemiology across the empire. In the interwar years, nineteen major studies on tuberculosis were published in the AOF alone.[65] Because many, if not most, of these studies were linked to BCG trials, they tended to focus on contexts such as the military and maternity wards in colonial capitals, spaces that were conducive to the kinds of semirandomized trials statisticians in Europe demanded; however, these spaces also produced data that emphasized the role of European contact. For Calmette and his collaborators in the Pasteur Institutes of Algiers, Dakar, and Saigon, these studies were primarily fodder in the battle for legitimating his vaccine research and the colonial space as proper field for experimentation, but they simultaneously produced a new discourse of French responsibility, the evolution of which Pastorians could no longer fully control.

Calmette first turned his attention toward the colonies in 1910, when he and Guérin had managed to cultivate a nonvirulent strain of the tubercle bacterium and a vaccine appeared to be within their grasp. At the same time, bacteriologists had a new tool in their arsenal, enabling them to more precisely diagnose tuberculosis infection, even in the majority of people who were not symptomatic, a major innovation at a time when even symptomatic tuberculosis could easily be confused with other lung diseases such as pneumonia or lung cancer. This tool was the tuberculin skin test, developed by the French doctors Mantoux and Von Pirquet in 1907, which was, in turn, based on the research of Robert Koch. The test involved injecting matter extracted from dead tubercle microbes—tuberculin—and then observing the subject's reactions. A red patch developing at the site of injection within forty-eight to seventy-two hours indicated that the subject had TB antibodies and therefore had been exposed to the tubercle microbe at some point (even if the subject was not symptomatic).[66] The tuberculin skin test was a cheap and easy way of determining the presence of TB in a particular region. It is no surprise that Calmette, anticipating the importance of the empire for his vaccine-in-development, decided to enroll his collaborators in the colonial military and the various overseas Pasteur Institutes to study the prevalence of TB across Greater France.

Calmette furnished his collaborators with free tuberculin developed at the Pasteur Institute in Lille, while Pastorians and doctors in the colonies, sensing an opportunity for furthering their careers, eagerly went along with the plan.[67] The resulting study was published in the *Annales of the Institut Pasteur* in 1912 and became the groundwork for a number of future studies, cited as the beginning of a new epoch by both colonial administrators and later researchers alike.[68]

Calmette's claims to the study's novelty enabled him to obscure the sparse yet nevertheless existing history of tuberculosis prevalence studies in colonies such as Cambodia, Cochinchina, and Senegal. It obscured the degree to which his results did not differ qualitatively from earlier data collected by doctors and hospital workers and summarized by administrators like Kermorgant, while at the same time allowing him to draw radically novel conclusions from the data, arguing that tuberculosis was a disease of "civilization," introduced to the colonies by the French.

The basis for the Pastorian's claim to innovation was the specificity of the tuberculin skin test. Although Calmette and his colleagues recognized the existence of prior studies, they dismissed them as too imprecise and impressionistic to give a true understanding of TB epidemiology. As Marcel Leger argued in his overview of TB studies in West Africa:

> Morbidity and mortality statistics have always only very imperfectly informed us of the frequency of a bacterial infection in a given country. There are, in reality, always a number of subjects in whom the manifestations of illness are completely absent or constantly hidden, yet who are still infected by the microbe. These are the sources of contagion, far more dangerous as they are hidden and ignored.[69]

Other sources besides hospital statistics were even more unreliable: tuberculosis could be confused with a number of diseases, and nineteenth-century doctors regularly disagreed on whether one or another region was contaminated or not.[70] Tuberculin tests could detect latent carriers of TB; equally important Pastorians considered the test sufficiently *precise*. Calmette suggested that the "great precision" of the tuberculin test would make it possible to chart the spread of the disease and develop a "*tuberculosis index* of a particular ethnic group, locality or even of an entire country."[71] The level of detail that could be achieved with tuberculin tests, Calmette argued, would help "public authorities to understand the necessity of defensive and protective measures" appropriate to each location.[72] For Calmette, the tuberculin test meant using a scalpel, where previously only a hacksaw had been available. To that end, the only studies he considered relevant were those that utilized tuberculin, such as those done in the Kalmyk steppes in Russia, or a few studies attempted at around the same time by other Pastorians.[73]

Yet for all the claims to precision in instrumentation, Calmette's statistics were not much more detailed than those collected by Kermorgant ten years earlier, nor did they show a fundamentally different picture of TB epidemiology. It was true that Calmette's collaborators could break down the communities they studied by age (children under one year, one to fifteen, and older than fifteen) and by ethnic group (white, Wolof, Maure, Bambara), rather than extrapolating from mortality rates or simply reporting the disease as "rare," "present," or "dominant," as Kermorgant's study had done.[74] Yet Calmette's study was far from a village-by-village chart of TB rates. The Pastorian's reach was limited by his network of collaborators: Pastorians were based in laboratories in major cities such as Dakar or Saigon but had little access to the less-traveled areas of West Africa and Indochina. This meant his data skewed heavily toward colonial capitals and toward colonies with better infrastructure and more Pastorian presence. In Indochina, Calmette had data from all five colonies, but even there, most of the tuberculin tests were performed in urban areas, in Hué, Saigon, and Phnom Penh, with only a few tests done in rural regions. In the AOF, the vast majority of his data came primarily from the colonies of Senegal and Guinea (3,000 tests), with some 816 tests also completed in Côte d'Ivoire. Saint-Louis, the capital of Senegal, was vastly overrepresented, as was the region of Casamance, which together accounted for nearly 2,000 of the 3,000 tests in the two colonies. In short, Calmette may have been able to gather accurate information on TB infections in regions he could access. Yet the geographical range of his data remained highly limited, and in regions outside colonial capitals, his conclusions remained as impressionistic as those of Kermorgant and earlier researchers.

Nor did his results differ largely from those of previous studies. In Indochina, tuberculin tests showed high rates of infection in prisons and the military (up to 80 percent tested positive), elevated overall rates in Tonkin, Annam, and Cochinchina, where tests skewed urban (average rates of 31 percent, 38 percent, and 16 percent, respectively), while indicating extremely low rates in Cambodia (4.6 percent). This mirrored the general estimates given by Kermorgant and by local studies, which had reported about an eightfold difference in TB rates between Cochinchina and Cambodia, while noting that these statistics were almost certainly undercounting actual rates.[75] In the AOF, tuberculin tests were performed predominantly in Saint-Louis and the Casamance region, which showed 15 to 30 percent positives, edging higher in urban regions, again confirming results of "surprising" prevalence in Casamance already reported by Kermorgant.[76] Calmette's synthetic study confirmed long-observed patterns, although the actual rates differed—unsurprisingly, since infection rates were bound to be higher than morbidity and mortality rates.

Calmette's conclusions, however, pointed in a very different direction. He argued that tuberculosis was "extremely rare among the indigenous populations of the black race, in areas where Europeans have only recently penetrated; but the proportion of contaminated subjects grows with the intensity of commercial exchange and foreign immigration."[77] Calmette further asserted that in such "virgin soil" areas, tuberculosis infection was more likely to develop into symptomatic illness, and such illness would have graver consequences than in regions where tuberculosis was "more widespread and more ancient."[78] Further, since infants in the colonies "never [drank]" cow's milk, the infection could not come from bovine TB.[79] This, Calmette concluded, meant that "Europeans . . . constitute[d] the primary means of infection" and were responsible for the development of "serious forms" of the disease among colonized populations.[80] Questions of nutrition, climate, racial specificity, and other envirobiological factors, which previous researchers had used to explain the variability of TB rates in the colonies, were completely irrelevant to Calmette. He focused on infection, which he asserted came from Europeans. The solution, therefore, had to be bacteriological, one that could halt the spread of the infection both from Europeans to colonized subjects, and from those with a latent infection to those with symptomatic illness. The study, Calmette stated, pointed toward the role of "methods of vaccination" he was studying along with Guérin.[81]

Although Calmette's data were not nearly as comprehensive as he claimed, and largely mirrored results achieved by previous researchers, he managed to construct a new vision of TB epidemiology in the French colonies. The European contagion thesis was rehearsed time and time again in follow-up studies in the interwar years, constructing tuberculosis as an acute and widespread problem, whereas it had been previously considered a marginal issue. After 1924, when Calmette and Guérin had a prototype of the BCG vaccine, epidemiological studies were often coproduced with BCG tests; tuberculin tests were used to justify BCG trials in Dakar, Saint-Louis, Saigon, Hanoi, and other colonial cities. Because BCG injections caused tuberculin tests to return positive (the tests responded to TB antibodies), researchers soon returned to old-fashioned mortality statistics.

In the AOF, the Pastorian Marcel Leger and the doctor-general Lasnet conducted the most comprehensive studies in 1922 and 1927, arguing once again that *indigènes* who had traveled to European countries and Europeans traveling to the AOF were the primary sources of contagion. This was based on observations of high rates of tuberculosis among tirailleurs (once again assuming that the high rate of positive tests had to do with infection from European sources rather than intramilitary contagion within cramped spaces). Lasnet admitted that following repatriated tirailleurs back to their villages of origin was nearly impossible, but this only heightened his concerns about the danger posed by troops bringing the disease over from "a European country."[82] These studies were often conducted in locations convenient for BCG vaccinations—Dakarois schools, maternity wards, and military barracks. Unsurprisingly, these locations were bound to have more European contact and higher infection rates, facts that epidemiological studies confirmed, entrenching the European contagion thesis further in scientific discourse.[83]

Similarly, in Indochina, interwar tuberculosis studies went hand in hand with BCG vaccinations, showing increasing numbers of infections, which in turn reinforced the argument that TB was an acute problem and required immediate action.[84] Here, experts held Chinese migrants as responsible as European contacts, joining both under the umbrella of "civilization." Crucially, not everyone agreed with this assessment. Dr. Gaide noted in his survey of tuberculosis that the "augmentation of observed cases does not necessarily indicate an extension of the illness, but reflects simply the development of our Medical Assistance and the growing confidence of *indigènes* in our methods."[85] These opinions, however, were in a minority, with most experts using epidemiological data to raise the alarm and issue a call to action.

European Contact and Critiques of Imperialism

The most influential aspect of the new tuberculosis epidemiology was the revitalization of the European contact thesis. This argument grew increasingly powerful in France during the 1920s and 1930s, where it cohered with a general discontent around industrial civilization and was embraced not only by the medical establishment and Pastorians but also by more radical, communist, surrealist, and anticolonialist constituencies. These groups drew different lessons from the argument but agreed on the general principle that tuberculosis was a social ill introduced to the colonies by the French themselves. This confluence was most clearly expressed in 1931, when it surfaced in a Pastorian rendition at the Colonial Exposition, in communist and surrealist form at the so-called Anti-colonial Exposition, and in African and Vietnamese activist journals, such as the *Cri des nègres* or *L'Âme Annamite*.

The Colonial Exposition was a lavish, five-month celebration of Greater France, organized in the Bois de Vincennes, the larger of the two major parks in Paris. Organized by Marshal Hubert Lyautey, the famous conqueror of Morocco, and General Marcel Olivier, the exposition had both propagandistic and economic goals. It had to articulate a colonial ideology that would appease a growing chorus of critics, but also to promote the empire to potential investors, a response to the worsening Great Depression. At the same time, the Colonial Exposition also aimed for scientific authority, exhibiting authentic "reconstructions of tropical life" instead of "exploiting the low instincts of a vulgar public," which had brought "discredit upon many another exhibition of the colonial sphere."[86]

This latter goal put the Pasteur Institutes at the center of the project, as the Ministry of the Colonies sought to reorient colonial propaganda. Previous efforts had focused "principally on development and on the economic possibilities," while the exposition was supposed to "make manifest to our citizens the improvements that our administration has brought to the general well-being of indigenous populations, . . . in the social sphere, and in particular in Medical Assistance and public health."[87] This included separate publications and displays of scientific research, which were usually supervised by Pastorians in various colonies.[88] Bacteriologists compiled statistics on the development of the institutes, water purification, malaria, plague, and other diseases and provided photographic material for display at the exposition. The resulting publications generally presented a flattering picture of colonial medical efforts. Still, language contrasting French responsibility for various social and medical ills with the vitality of indigenous culture occasionally made it into official publications.

Tuberculosis was discussed relatively infrequently at the Colonial Exposition, compared with tropical diseases such as malaria or the plague. Still, it formed an important pivot in the "social hygiene" section of the exposition, and most colonies dedicated some space to the issue. Generally, this meant praising the Pasteur Institute for its efforts in distributing the experimental BCG vaccine. At the same time, the reports had to acknowledge new statistics showing an increase in TB cases in most colonies. The exposition's publications noted that in Indochina, as elsewhere, "tuberculosis is far more widespread . . . than previously believed," and that it was spreading "among the higher classes as well as the proletariat."[89] Reports from the AOF noted that the spike in TB rates during the postwar years was the result of the "exceptional situation, created by the return of *indigènes*, tuberculized in European battles, to West Africa."[90] Although these reports emphasized the role of Africans, suggesting that returning tirailleurs spread the disease to far reaches of the colony, with their poor spitting habits and general ignorance, they nevertheless acknowledged the Pastorian dictum about the European origins of tuberculosis. Crucially, some reports emphasized the role of local culture as a barrier against contagion. The exposition claimed that Muslim populations of Senegal "appear to have fewer cases of tuberculosis than . . . those who have converted to Catholicism."[91] This contrast was explained partly by the Muslim ban on alcohol but also by "a certain corporeal discipline" that improved resistance.[92] Underneath rhetorical praise for French medical progress, representations of TB at the Colonial Exposition highlighted institutional neglect, European contagion, and the positive role of indigenous culture.

Speaking outside the exposition, Pastorians were more candid about the French failure to provide preventive hygiene. Calmette authored a number of popular articles highlighting how "tuberculosis, which only some years ago, spared the autochthonous populations of the African hinterland," was now spreading due to the influence of "the civilized people" brought into contact with Africans via "large commercial routes," "the development of railways," and "the recruitment of *indigènes* [to the military]."[93] He was seconded by Pastorians such as Noël Bernard, who noted similar increases in TB rates in Indochina. These publications called for new and aggressive preventive measures, "to urgently organize the fight against this global disease," and highlighted that the scientific and medical staff dedicated to preventive hygiene was "inferior to the needs," echoing the conclusions of some reports at the exposition, which noted that the administration had left social diseases like TB "truly and totally ignored."[94] The Pastorians, in short, used the European origin thesis to leverage popular support for increased funding and expansion of their colonial mission.

At the same time, this new epidemiology cohered with surrealist and anti-colonialist critiques of Western civilization, which saw industrial progress as a harmful and unnatural development to which more "authentic" non-Western cultures could oppose themselves. The idea was equally sympathetic to communists who saw tuberculosis as yet another product of capitalist exploitation caused by the use of forced agricultural and industrial labor. These ideas were made explicit at the oppositional exposition titled Truth about the Colonies and on the pages of African and Vietnamese activist magazines published in Paris during the same period.

Refuting the idea of French civilizational supremacy was particularly important to African writers, who sought to counter French claims that Africans were not ready for self-governance, while constructing a basis for pan-African solidarity. These intellectuals came from interwar activist groups such as the Intercolonial Union and were united in their support for racial solidarity. Over the 1920s, these activists moved ever closer to the French Communist Party, which vocally condemned French imperialism, exploitation. and colonial war, while continuing to draw on, and take seriously, the language of French republicanism in articulating their claims.[95] Even as communist and nationalist ideas were being more forcefully articulated in organizations such as the Union des Travailleurs Nègres, the civilizing mission remained an important target of immanent critique, particularly during a time when the Colonial Exposition leaned heavily on French humanitarianism to make the positive case for empire.

These texts often invoked demographic, sanitary, and moral arguments to expose the emptiness of French claims to civilizational superiority. One intellectual writing in the *Cri des nègres* argued that the trifecta of tuberculosis, alcoholism, and syphilis, the "defects of 'civilized metropoles,'" had led to demographic decline in Africa, thereby proving that colonized societies under French rule were "in a worse state than when they were left to their 'barbarous instincts.'"[96] Tuberculosis, indeed, was a familiar foe to African activists, many of whom had served as tirailleurs during the war. One of the great shifts in power among Parisian anti-imperialists, from the war veteran Lamine Senghor to the student activist Tiémoko Garan Kouyaté, was prompted by the former's declining health due to TB. To the "archaic hygienic conditions of life that civilization has left them," African intellectuals opposed the "beauty of our lands, the fertility of our soil, the skill of our artists."[97] Unwittingly echoing some of the language at the Colonial Exposition, tuberculosis here became a vehicle for demonstrating the corrupting influence of European civilization and the value of African culture and environment. Unlike researchers at the exposition, however, African intellectuals drew more radical conclusions, arguing that such examples of deteriorating living conditions demonstrated that "it is a cynical lie to say that Negroes are incapable of self-governance and that they need the tutelage of European metropoles to prevent them from falling back into barbarity."[98]

A different critique was leveled by communists and surrealists at the Truth About the Colonies counterexposition, mounted at Konstantin Melnikov's Soviet Pavilion at the parc de Buttes-Chaumont, in late 1931. The surrealists, most notably Louis Aragon and André Thirion, put on some of the most sustained protests against the Colonial Exposition, which they saw as both politically and artistically corrupt. Deeply influenced by the legacy of the Great War, they, like many other artists, from dadaists to cubists, were skeptical of the value of industrial civilization, seeing it as corrupt, repressive, and overly reliant on reason.[99] Surrealists distributed flyers condemning forced labor and colonial violence at the Bois de Vincennes itself and aggressively promoted the Anti-colonial Exposition at newspapers such as the communist *L'Humanité* as well as various African magazines—although somewhat unsuccessfully, since the exposition only totaled some five thousand visitors over five months.[100] There, familiar tropes about European-induced hygienic decline joined with critiques of forced labor emphasizing the destructive power of capitalist exploitation rather than a broader and more diffuse cultural notion of "civilization." "Alcoholism, prostitution and tuberculosis" were seen as byproducts of labor exploitation, while humanitarian French civilization of the sort on display at Vincennes was termed a "conceptual swindle . . . giving citizens of the metropole the conscience of ownership they need, to hear the echo of faraway guns without shaking."[101] Here, TB was seen not as a moral consequence of a corrupt civilization but as a social consequence of exploitation, to which the rhetoric of the civilizing mission provided a neat cover.

In this formulation, the surrealists and communists joined Vietnamese critics who, in almost identical language, inspired by communist and nationalist ideas, used evidence of rising rates of tuberculosis as evidence for the ill effects of economic changes.[102] These activists, most of whom were educated in Paris, saw tuberculosis as the product of "horrifying working conditions" created by the alliance of French imperialists and capitalist factory owners.[103] In one instance, tuberculosis was rendered as a metaphor for colonialism itself, where a rhetoric of civilization lulls colonial subjects into a false complacency. "This kind of policy has been compared to tuberculosis," the Vietnamese nationalist intellectual Trần Huy Liệu wrote. "Its germs have already devoured the lungs and liver of the patient, who, nonetheless does not feel any discomfort until the day when he succumbs to the illness without even being aware of his impending death!"[104] While these critics invoked tuberculosis and other social diseases to call for more radical changes, the structure of their critique—social disease as a marker of Western corruption opposed to a robustly healthy indigenous culture—replicated the language used by Pastorians at the Colonial Exposition and elsewhere.

These similarities became increasingly inconvenient for administrators and Pastorians themselves. While bacteriologists were bound by their interpretive frame, they began to note the threat the European contact thesis posed to colonial order. Pastorians conducting studies on TB rates among tirailleurs noted that "the theory which makes the tirailleurs the principal agent of the propagation of tuberculosis can only have regrettable consequences in terms of public opinion and in terms of the direction of the prophylactic fight itself."[105] When this argument was raised in the League of Nations, it appeared to confirm the idea already observed among South African miners that "first contact with civilization" produced higher mortality rates. This caused league experts considerable "anxiety."[106] The new epidemiology of tuberculosis in Africa and Indochina had rendered the colonies fertile ground for Pastorian medical development, but it had also opened the way for broader critiques and medical interventions that administrators and bacteriologists did not entirely control.

Conclusion

It is an old trope in the history of medicine that European scientists saw the colonies as "living laboratories."[107] Yet this was not always obvious to the actors at the time. For many decades, medical experts had no interest in tropical tuberculosis, although they claimed the disease had been present in colonial environments for centuries. Calmette's epidemiological studies reconstructed the tropical environment as well as the relationship of Europeans and the *indigènes* with it. Tuberculosis no longer appeared as a local disease but as a European importation. The tropical environment was reimagined as neutral, not hostile to the disease. The colonial body was no longer seen as racially differentiated but as essentially similar to the European, but crucially particularly vulnerable because of an assumed lack of contact with the disease. Finally, indigenous customs and religions were reinterpreted as providing, if anything, a degree of resistance to the disease that European acculturation was slowly chipping away. Contagion, rather than environment or race, became the focus of expert attention. Pastorians

THE MAKING OF IMPERIAL TUBERCULOSIS   141

used this new epidemiology to advocate for the development and testing of a vaccine that would solve the problem the French themselves had created.

Yet as this new discourse interacted with anticolonial movements, metropolitan disillusionment, and competing antituberculosis campaigns, it soon became apparent that this shift in tropical TB epidemiology had unintended consequences. In the metropole, Pastorians became increasingly concerned with how well the European origin thesis cohered with anti-imperialist critiques of the civilizing mission. In the colonies, a renewed focus on tuberculosis prevention opened the way for other actors to adopt and reinterpret French antituberculosis technologies for their own political ends.

BCG and Technopolitics from
Europe to Empire

What kind of scientific and political work could pan-imperial tuberculosis studies accomplish? By the interwar years, experts in France had generally accepted that TB was a growing problem across the colonies. Yet how this issue ought to be addressed became increasingly controversial. Calmette sought a distinctively Pastorian solution, a microbiological weapon that would prevent the tubercle microbe from ever affecting the human body. By 1924, he had produced something tangible: the bacillus Calmette-Guérin (BCG) vaccine. The road from development to deployment, however, was rocky. Researchers in France, Germany, and elsewhere challenged the safety and efficacy of the vaccine, pointing to unreliable statistics and high-profile accidents such as the "Lübeck catastrophe" of 1929, which left seventy-two newly vaccinated infants dead in one German city. Because the hygienist strategies of the Rockefeller Foundation appeared to be working, the need for a new vaccine was far from obvious.

This chapter explores the scalar politics of BCG trials as they moved between international, imperial, and colonial stages. Put differently, it analyzes how reframing the scale of BCG trials helped scientists, regulators, and activists reframe the scientific and political power of BCG vaccination. Depending on where they were speaking from and what their intended field of deployment was, actors could portray BCG as certifiably safe or unreliable, as a prototype or proven pharmaceutical, and as a technological marvel or a poor substitute for social hygienist projects such as dispensaries and sanatoriums. This play of scales had political effects: BCG vaccination served as a tool for legitimating the humanitarian role of imperialism for politicians in Paris and helped parry questions of labor conditions and rights of speech and association posed by colonial forms of social hygiene. Restaging BCG testing also had scientific effects, as new contexts produced evidence about the efficacy and safety of the prototypical vaccine that could not be achieved elsewhere.[1] Three developments are particularly central to understanding

Pasteur's Empire. Aro Velmet, Oxford University Press (2020). © Oxford University Press.
DOI: 10.1093/oso/9780190072827.001.0001

the evolution of the vaccine: first, the rise of international standard makers, in particular the League of Nations Health Organization (LNHO), on a previously national scientific stage; second, interwar concerns with birth rates and the biopolitical health of the French race, understood on the scale of the empire writ large; and, finally, local political struggles formed in the context of rising nationalist and communist sentiments in colonial Indochina.

In the interwar years, new international organizations sought to establish frameworks for global governance in politics and science alike. The League of Nations, in particular, has recently been reassessed as an "agent of geopolitical transformation" and "internationalization." There, imperial powers had at least to justify their policies in front of a public audience, even if they were not compelled to modify their behavior on the ground.[2] As a defender of the peace, the league may have failed, but in terms of setting the stage for new forms of global order, it succeeded, particularly in the fields of ordering sovereignty and in technical cooperation. The historiographical consensus is that the league's coordinating and technical activities, which ranged from creating standards on air traffic control to combating sex and drug trafficking, gradually "elevated the role of those new international actors, 'the expert' and what we would today call the NGO."[3] Health cooperation—the collection of epidemiological data and the setting of standards for experimentation and drug trials—has, in particular, been interpreted as prefiguring the postwar emergence of global health development initiatives. Ironically, this is at the same time as historians of medicine are revising accounts of postwar health development and emphasizing the interwar, imperial roots of the contemporary field of global health.[4]

This chapter argues that, rather than taking decisive steps toward international expert arbitrage and "statistical modes of thinking," the LNHO generated epistemological anarchy and disrupted national norms of experimental ethics, which, at least in France, relied heavily on personal authority and clinical experience.[5] As the BCG controversy entered the LNHO's agenda, new critics could add their voices to the fray, demanding new standards of experimentation. When medical experts in Scandinavia, Germany, and England challenged Calmette's use of statistics, the Pastorian appealed to the LNHO in hopes that the international body would close the controversy. Instead, he received even further criticism and a set of standards that were next to impossible to meet in a European country.[6]

But Calmette did not have to work in a European country. In the 1920s and 1930s, the microbiologist moved his research into the empire, where it interacted with a different set of political concerns. The problem of birth rates and questions about the "quality" of population growth had brought social hygiene back into the imperial agenda. In 1924, the minister of the colonies, Édouard Daladier, outlined a new, ambitious agenda for improving preventive medicine, neonatal care, and indigenous birth rates, but legislators did not commit funds for real action. In this climate, wide-scale BCG trials, largely sponsored by the network of Pasteur Institutes, offered a simple answer to this rhetorical quagmire, allowing administrators to claim they were living up to the imperial promise while doing very little in practice. Colonial administrators' enthusiasm toward Pastorian technologies, the wider latitude for human experimentation, the existing network of Pastorian laboratories, and far less independent oversight than in Europe—all these factors became resources that Calmette could use to respond to his metropolitan adversaries and secure the success of BCG in France, as well as in the colonies.

On the colonial stage, the introduction of BCG created new kinds of political frictions. In Indochina, tuberculosis prevention interacted with a number of political concerns, such as working conditions, the establishment of mutual aid societies, and freedom of the press. On the one hand, as French charitable organizations made their way to Indochina, Vietnamese elites used their rhetoric to demand rights they perceived as equally medical and social. Yet the French, concerned with the dangers of Vietnamese nationalism and international communism, did not wish to grant them. Here, BCG vaccination became a technopolitical tool that helped the French justify the absence of policies of social hygiene. Although scholarship on clinical trials and empire has continuously emphasized the ways in which colonial power inequalities structured the treatment of human subjects in pharmaceutical trials, less attention has been paid to causality moving in the opposite direction: how medical technologies themselves changed imperial politics.[7] Both the imperial and the scientific dimensions of BCG development need to be historicized.[8]

BCG Scandals, Social Hygiene, and Epistemological Anarchy in Europe

From 1905 until his death in 1933, Albert Calmette dedicated his life to the War against Tuberculosis. The bacteriologist's approach diverged from the general return to social hygiene that characterized both interwar France and

Europe. Wartime campaigns, from the Rockefeller TB mission to France to the founding of the Red Cross, generated new confidence in programs that saw health as embedded in social determinants such as nutrition and quality of housing.[9] Concerns over the quality and quantity of populations, on the one hand, and surging socialist movements, on the other, encouraged policymakers and health experts to consider broader measures to improve the social body. In France, much of the discourse around TB was shaped by the wartime activities of the American Rockefeller Foundation, which built up a powerful system of charities, dispensaries, and education programs, instilling the principles of social hygiene in French medicos and the lay population from primary school onward.[10]

Evidence from the United States suggested that social hygiene was indeed effective. Rockefeller propaganda materials cited in particular the rapid fall of TB mortality in New York after reforms taken by the newly established city health board in the early 1900s.[11] Statistics indicating that mortality rates in New York in 1913 were half (1.92 per 10,000) of what they were in Paris (3.79) made their way from Rockefeller publications to prestigious general interest journals such as the *Revue des Deux Mondes*.[12] Mortality rates in France did decline, though not as rapidly as in the United States, the Netherlands, or Germany. For medical experts, improving demographics reinforced the idea that a proper response to the tuberculosis epidemic would take place largely, and perhaps even principally, in the domain of *social* medicine.[13] Calmette seemed to be addressing a problem that already had a reliable solution, thereby making the risks of vaccination unjustifiable. Here, common wisdom asserted that the "white plague" would "not be cured by drugs, but by hygiene, a particular way of life, by following simple precautions, in a word, that which doctors, never at a loss for neologisms call dietetics."[14]

Calmette, however, was certain that only vaccination would adequately defend against TB. He was committed to what Ed Cohen has termed "a defensive concept of immunity," which rendered the body as a bounded organism, the social environment as an essentially passive milieu, and the microbe as the criminal whose unauthorized permeation of the human domain had to be stopped through vaccination.[15] The Russian bacteriologist Élie Metchnikoff substantially developed this mode of thinking within the Pastorian community through his work on immunology. He gave an account of the role of phagocytes (leukocytes, or white blood cells) as the primary defense mechanism of the organism against outside invaders, providing a scientific basis for the immunity metaphor.[16] By 1921, Calmette and

Guérin had cultivated a tubercle microbe in its 230th passage, which they believed had lost all virulence—even in large doses, the culture failed to produce tuberculosis in guinea pigs.[17] This culture became the basis for the BCG vaccine. Satisfied with their lab results, the scientists proceeded to human trials, injecting the prototype first to infants born to consumptive mothers under the care of Benjamin Weill-Hallé at the La Charité hospital and then to infants in the 6th arrondissement of Paris.[18]

In 1924, Calmette and Guérin reported their results in a series of articles in *Les Annales de l'Institut Pasteur, Bulletin de l'Académie de Médecine*, and *La Presse Médicale*, as well as at a presentation at the academy itself.[19] They argued that laboratory science, animal testing, and two series of human trials with a total of 667 infant subjects demonstrated the safety of the vaccine; to demonstrate its efficacy, they both promised new, "large-scale preventative studies" and promised to send all interested practitioners samples of the vaccine, in return for write-ups of their experiences.[20] From the beginning, the bacteriologists envisioned a multipronged attack to convince the scientific and the lay public of the vaccine's safety and efficacy.

The Pastorians' eclectic approach to winning the public's trust was unsurprising. As Christian Bonah and Clifford Rosenberg have demonstrated, interwar French standards on medical experimentation were in a state of flux, and responsibility for studies remained primarily on the experimenter. Through the late nineteenth and early twentieth centuries, French doctors keenly guarded their expertise and independence. Most doctors were private practitioners, and the medical ethos reinforced their decision-making based on experience and a common honor code, rather than explicit guidelines, regulations, or patient-doctor dialogue.[21] Although no official regulations existed, legal precedents held doctors fully accountable for all mistakes in medical conduct, meaning that researchers generally avoided human trials.[22] By the interwar period, however, this consensus had begun to fracture. Sources of medical innovation had multiplied: pharmaceutical companies, research institutes (with the Pasteur Institute on the forefront), social insurance groups, and international scientific organizations were all reshaping the medical landscape.

Initially, Calmette appealed to the authority and experience of both individual practitioners and collective bodies, as had been common practice for decades. The sheer number of successful vaccinations performed by clinical practitioners of different nationalities demonstrated, the Pastorian claimed, that the vaccine was generally safe and that accidents resulted from contamination or production errors. "If BCG had harmful properties," Calmette stated in one speech, "then the doctors who in France alone have administered the vaccine to over 110,000 children, would have observed and recorded such accidents."[23] Calmette furnished free samples of BCG to all interested doctors in exchange for their clinical reports, allowing him to then cite a number of experimental studies by French and foreign bacteriologists as authorities vouching for the veracity of his own claims. In one defense, Calmette listed Drs. Ascoli, Cantacuzene, Maelstromm, Hembeck, Aldershoff, Malvoz, Silverschmitt, and William Park as just some of the experts who had testified to the safety of the vaccine. He insisted that only experimental evidence could counter the opinions of so many distinguished scientists, and if such evidence was not forthcoming, any incidents would have to be considered the result of an accidental infection.[24]

Still, the BCG vaccine fell under intense criticism, most notably by Joseph Lignières, a veterinarian and a member of the Academy of Medicine. Lignières claimed that the few accidents that had been recorded in infants vaccinated with BCG were not random but resulted from "a series of favorable circumstances," which "under special conditions of sensitivity to BCG can give it a pathogenic power that is difficult to even imagine."[25] At the same time, Lignières claimed, the premunitive power of BCG was negligible, and ensuring the vaccine safe for all subjects in all environments would reduce the vaccine's potency to a degree that would render it essentially useless.

At stake in Lignières's critique was a different approach to the human subject and the scope of medical intervention. Already in his first angle of attack, he distinguished his approach from Calmette's Pastorian fixation on the bounded body and the microbiological enemy, reminding his audience that both the environment and individual variability could shape the subject's susceptibility to the pathogenic power of BCG. In a different text, Lignières outlined his own proposals for containing tuberculosis, which focused on the "participation of the public in hygienic measures," and called to "win over the public to the side of the hygienists," highlighting the importance of not relying on expert authority alone.[26] In practice, his suggestions were more paternalistic than participatory: he called for mandatory fines for crimes against hygiene such as littering or coughing without covering one's mouth, and for measures such as increasing the number of public waste bins and public education. In so doing, he added the force of state authority to the well-known laundry list of hygienic measures France had been debating since the nineteenth century.[27] BCG, in Lignières opinion, disrupted the complex network of trust and authority between the state and the public by creating "legitimate apprehensions" within the medical profession and "disquiet" in the public. In contrast to Calmette's conviction in the authority of medical expertise and experimental results taken as a whole, Lignières opposed a fragile and indeterminate alliance between the state and the public, which had to be maintained through both broad state intervention and the examination of even seemingly exceptional cases. At the end of the day, Lignières called for a "ceasefire" on campaigns of mass vaccination and advocated for "well considered measures of hygiene" in guiding preventive action.[28] Calmette's mode of technological intervention and Lignières's critique offered two different configurations of power between experts, the state, and the lay public.

As part of his campaign of legitimization, Calmette called upon the international scientific community to experiment with BCG and confirm his claims. Yet these connections could also work against him. From December 1929 to October 1930, infants vaccinated at a maternity ward in Lübeck, Germany, began falling ill and dying. By the end of the year, only 43 infants out of the 252 who had received a shot were in good health, and 72 had died.[29] The subsequent investigation became a focal point for journalists looking for a good scandal, with most newspapers in France covering the trial on a daily basis. It resurrected debates over the safety of the vaccine, and in particular the question of authority: Would Calmette's Pastorian credentials suffice to vouch for the safety of the vaccine, or would the incident itself taint Calmette's reputation?

Prosecutors at the trials in Germany interrogated Dr. Alstaedt and Dr. Deycke, the two health officials responsible for the defective vaccinations, and asked why the variety of criticisms leveled at Calmette over the years had not been taken into account.[30] The prosecutors' implication was that rather than weighing the experimental evidence, Alstaedt and Deycke had put too much faith in Calmette's reputation. Indeed, over the course of the trials, many participants suggested that the Pasteur Institute deliberately used its influence to suppress critics. Marcel Reinbert, writing in a German journal, claimed that doctors were covering up cases of BCG-related fatalities "because of their fear of the Pasteur Institute."[31] Another French professor wrote in a letter to the prosecution that "no French doctor dared to raise their voice against Calmette."[32] Calmette, meanwhile, tried to dissociate from the Lübeck disaster and protect his reputation. His supporters insisted that the BCG strain under investigation be referred to as the "Deycke vaccine" or simply "vaccine," but certainly not as the "Calmette vaccine." Calmette him-self refused to appear in Lübeck, on the account that his work had nothing to do with tragedy.[33] Ultimately, his strategy prevailed: errors of produc-tion were judged to be the cause of the disaster, and Deycke and Alstaedt were sentenced to two years and fifteen months in prison, respectively. Yet Calmette felt his reputation was under threat.

Realizing that he could no longer rely on experimental evidence and ex-pert authority alone, Calmette began to marshal statistical evidence to sup-port his new vaccine. Here, however, he was treading even further into the territory of social hygienists. Their reference points ranged from René-Louis Villermé's reports on textile workers to the works of interwar pronatalists studying demographics and mortality rates.[34] Calmette's harshest critics, the head of the Gothenburg Children's Hospital, Arvid Wallgren, and the med-ical statistician at the London School of Hygiene, Major Greenwood, were both steadfast supporters of social reform. For Wallgren, tuberculosis pre-vention was also a matter of modernizing Swedish society and organizing re-lations between social classes and the state on a modern, "communal" basis.[35] Greenwood's association with the International Labor Organization's health section suggests that he, too, harbored visions of populist social engineering.

Both Greenwood and Wallgren published damning critiques of Calmette's use of data, pointing out serious misreadings of existing literature.[36] Calmette had, for instance, mistaken the rate of overall infant mortality in one Danish study for the rate of infant mortality from tuberculosis only, thereby vastly inflating the effect of BCG.[37] Greenwood also questioned Calmette's own statistical methods. He showed, for instance, that when Calmette compared one-year mortality rates among vaccinated and unvaccinated infants, vacci-nated infants were tracked from the moment of vaccination, while unvacci-nated infants were tracked from birth. Because "the greatest proportion of deaths that occur in the first year occur within the first month of life," before BCG vaccination, Greenwood argued, Calmette's statistics grossly underrep-resented deaths in the vaccinated group.[38] Wallgren criticized Calmette for all sorts of omissions, from not properly reporting the number of children who could not be tracked after vaccination to not specifying whether any of the children in the vaccinated group had developed tuberculosis *and sur-vived*.[39] Both critics concluded that in human trials uncontrolled environ-ments would "inevitably come to trouble the experiment." This conclusion reflected the increasingly elaborate conceptual apparatus of statistics but also reflected the belief that the social environment was inherently indeterminate and difficult to control. Wallgren suggested that selecting newborns from TB-infected families, dividing them into a test group and a control group, and separating them from their mothers for two to three months would improve the reliability of statistics. Having proposed this, though, he then immediately admitted that "actually executing such a program is hardly realistic."[40]

As criticisms mounted, Calmette called for the League of Nations Health Organization to adjudicate the issue. In 1928, the LNHO appointed a commission to determine the efficacy and safety of BCG. The problem intersected with a number of priorities of the LNHO, which had been formed in 1921 to capitalize on the rising interest in preventive health in the interwar climate. Led through most of its existence by the Polish bacteriologist and committed socialist Ludwik Rajchman, the LNHO focused on problems of social medicine, following in the footsteps of the Red Cross, the Rockefeller Foundation, and the Inter-Allied Sanitary Commission. Rajchman wanted the agency to focus on the large-scale study of complex health systems, which "no single administration . . . can undertake."[41] This meant gathering data on global epidemiology, the effects of nutrition on health, infant mortality, and rural hygiene, all factors that were social and therefore malleable by human action.[42] It is hardly surprising, then, that tuberculosis, the quintessential social disease, generated considerable interest within the LNHO. Second, the agency saw standardization of data collection, experimentation, and pharmaceutical development as among its central goals. Uniform health data and standards would facilitate the exchange of medical information and bind (often formerly hostile) countries together in their common goal of reducing human suffering.[43]

In practice, the LNHO's activities were much less coordinated and were contingent on limited funding, the interests of partner countries and organizations, and the political implications of its work. The LNHO competed with (but also received funding from) a number of prewar institutions that claimed to have highest authority in matters of public health—the Office of International Public Hygiene, the Rockefeller Foundation, and the Pasteur Institute, to name just a few—and imperial governments were decidedly unwilling to relinquish control over their management of health matters in colonies. At the same time, the LNHO had scant internal resources—its budget was capped at 1 million Swiss francs until the 1930s, and much of its work relied on national collaborators and grants from the Rockefeller Foundation.[44] The advances of the LNHO were often limited to areas that caused little political controversy, and where the potential gains were equally distributed between participating nations.[45] For those reasons, its approach to social hygiene remained grounded in the collection and standardization of data, and it was only during the years of the Great Depression that the agency became more concerned with human welfare writ large.

Luckily, Calmette had quite a bit of leverage at the LNHO, having served as a member of its predecessor, the Provisional Health Committee, in 1922–1923. As the LNHO investigated global TB rates as part of its epidemiological mandate, Yves M. Biraud, a representative of the organization, corresponded with Calmette, discussing the possibilities and limitations of national statistics and ways of standardizing data collection.[46] Setting up a commission of expert statisticians to examine Calmette's questionable data was, therefore, not difficult. After a series of conferences held at the Pasteur Institute in Paris in October 1928, and in Berlin in 1929, the LNHO produced a report proclaiming BCG "a harmless vaccine," "incapable of producing virulent tuberculosis lesions," and concluded that it was potentially, although not conclusively, effective.[47] The experts recommended further human trials, a result that Calmette interpreted as a clear endorsement of the LNHO.[48]

In truth, the LNHO's endorsement was partial at best. The LNHO declared BCG safe but did not rule on its efficacy. The league's experts took issue with Calmette's statistics and demanded further, properly controlled trials rather than widespread use. The committee of expert statisticians recommended experiments in which two groups of children, one vaccinated and one control group, drawn from similar population groups, growing up in similar environments, and exposed to similar risks of infection, would be studied over a long period of time. Essentially, the committee proposed what we would now call a randomized controlled trial (RCT).[49] Yet the statisticians also agreed that it would be nearly impossible to find a location where such a trial could actually be conducted. In New York, for example, TB rates had fallen so low that it was difficult to find children who would qualify as being sufficiently exposed to infection; in France, BCG had become so popular that few mothers would agree to leave their child unvaccinated in the interests of a clinical trial.[50] LNHO experts set out a rigorous set of standards for Calmette to follow but, like his critics in Sweden and Britain, admitted that these standards might be impossible to fulfill.

Calmette responded to his critics by pointing to the "confidence" of "our medical brothers and the families of the over 100,000 children who have been vaccinated with BCG," as well as the expert assessment of the LNHO.[51] When confronted with questions about the unreliability of human testing or the tragic consequences of some vaccinations, most notably the Lübeck incident, Calmette deflected the criticisms by showing that *in laboratory settings*, there was no evidence of BCG reacquiring virulence.[52] Yet this was missing the point of his critics, who argued precisely that there was no simple way to transpose experimental evidence from the laboratory to the much more complicated field of human trials. Rather than seeing authority flowing from the laboratory scientist downward, statisticians and hygienists acknowledged the indeterminacy of the social environment and called for appropriate humility. The lack of control groups in Calmette's studies meant that a number of exogenous variables, especially "the conditions and our knowledge of [improved] sociological measures," could have influenced the reported drop in mortality rates.[53] Rather, critics advocated for "safety," "watchful waiting" for improved techniques of administration in order to avoid errors that "would then be interpreted in a bad light, and the confidence which doctors and the public may have in its correct use would be lost," consideration for "psychological factors" such as levels of public and medical confidence in the vaccine, and other considerations that were difficult to experimentally control.[54]

BCG trials in Europe have been described as "an early example of an international agency dictating the terms on which scientific claims are evaluated" and an important milestone in the emergence of "statistical modes of thinking" in modern biotechnological research.[55] Focusing on the role of the LNHO, however, overstates this shift. Greenwood and the LNHO did push Calmette to consider more sophisticated statistical methods, but, unable to enforce them, Calmette's appeals to authority and experimental evidence remained in play as well. A part of the problem was that different standards of evidence pointed to different concepts of authority and politics. Calmette believed the social environment to be an essentially passive space, and the distinction between laboratory experiment and human trial as being minimal and easily controlled by a professional bacteriologist. Statisticians and social hygienists who dominated in the LNHO and led the antituberculosis charge in Europe and the United States argued that the social environment was fundamentally indeterminate, that experimental evidence could not be used straightforwardly to paper over statistical inaccuracies and exceptional cases. Instead, medical authorities would have to consider social and political factors, including the trust of the public.[56] Neither national bodies, nor the court in Lübeck, nor the LNHO could breach this fundamental divide.

The Lübeck affair was a particularly hard setback: the Netherlands, Belgium, Poland, Switzerland, and Germany all discontinued BCG for a shorter or longer period as the situation unfolded.[57] The controversy caused much anxiety for the Pastorian: his letters to Charles Nicolle from the period were filled with assurances of the vaccine's safety, frustration over the public's lack of confidence in him, and confessions of health issues resulting from the controversy. "This ordeal in Lübeck is making me sick," he wrote in 1930, complaining of "suffering from cardiac troubles since this miserable affair."[58] Yet while Calmette was struggling to get Europe to accept his new vaccine, he found a more receptive audience beyond the continent: in the French empire.

Treatment as Trial: Turn to Preventive Health in the Empire

Officials at the Ministry of the Colonies returned to problems of social hygiene with renewed concern in the interwar years, reflecting broader anxieties in French public discourse. War losses and changing gender roles renewed reproductive anxieties the origins of which dated back at least to the Franco-Prussian War.[59] The French birth rate, historically low compared with that of neighboring countries, and Germany in particular, continued to fall. These changes once again generated interest in social hygiene in the metropole. Solutions, discussed in countless books, newspaper articles, and official committees such as the Conseil Supérieur de la Natalité, ranged from the narrowly biomedical (investing in vaccinations, dispensaries, and primary care) to the eugenicist (social reforms should focus on improving the natality of the most morally and physically outstanding citizens). The majority of commentators fell somewhere in the middle, rejecting outright eugenics in favor of a general improvement of welfare.[60]

Concerns about birth rates also extended to colonial domains. Administrators and experts believed that colonial subjects, particularly Africans, were untainted by civilization and therefore unusually virile and sexually active.[61] While many popular commentators interpreted this demographic claim as yet another danger to the French race, a significant number of experts saw it instead as an opportunity for regenerating the French nation through intermarriage and settler colonialism.[62] The earliest of these measures were adopted by General Gallieni in Madagascar in the fin de siècle, but investigations into colonial demography proliferated after the Great War.[63] Studies of the empire presented at the Congress of Health in 1922 showed high levels of infant mortality, abortion, and sterility, particularly in the AOF.

Because the *indigènes* were "ignorant of the most elementary rules of hygiene," these reports argued, their reproductive advantages were all but lost; "there [were] numerous births, but the number of deaths [was] too high." Researchers called for a renewed focus on "the improvement of both the quality and quantity of the races," recalling pronatalist and eugenicist language spreading in France at the time.[64] Pronatalism in the colonies, however, was more economic-military than social or moral: "All of our colonial problems, from the economic development of our overseas colonies . . . to the recruitment of indigenous troops, depends directly on achieving high population densities in our colonies."[65] For the minister of the colonies, Édouard Daladier, the population problem was primarily a labor problem.

Improving hygiene, however, remained the core strategy for demonstrating imperial humanitarianism. In 1924, Daladier attempted a massive expansion of the colonial health system, refocusing it "on demographic and social questions."[66] From 1905 onward, administrations in Indochina and the AOF had been tasked with building up the Assistance Médicale Indigène (AMI), a health service for subject populations, complete with local medical schools and mobile ambulance units designed to ensure medical coverage even in the African *brousse* (outback). Daladier sought to expand the AMI and the Health Service, allowing them to fulfill their original functions, which he argued had remained essentially powerless since their founding.[67] Daladier's second goal was orienting colonial medical services more toward social hygiene. He imagined reforms like popular education, the training of midwives and construction of maternity wards, improvement of sanitation and potable water in the cities, and finally the prevention of infectious diseases, particularly those that tended to threaten infants and expectant mothers.[68]

Daladier's plans created conflicting demands on colonial officials. After World War I, France's imperial policy moved, in rhetoric, from "assimilation" to "association." The former principle portrayed local authorities—chiefs and mandarins—as tyrants, emphasizing the importance of French investment and the mission civilisatrice, which would socialize subject populations to French values through education, economic development, and public health. In theory, assimilation promised large-scale investments and a focus on economic development, while postwar association involved investing limited consultative power in local notables and the *évolués*, who would then gradually distribute French values throughout the rest of colonized societies.[69] In practice, the distinction between the two policies was largely illusory.

Development funds were meager during assimilation and remained so under association as well; and consultative bodies, to the degree they existed, were products of necessity—the French simply did not have enough men on the ground to rule on their own—and limited in their authority. Large-scale investments to transform the colonies in France's image were not going to be forthcoming, and political transformations were going to be equally limited.

Daladier's medical reforms remained constrained. While European experts debated the values of large-scale education campaigns, social welfare questions, working conditions, and rural hygiene, imperial officials focused on reorienting existing institutions and capitalizing on modest technical improvements under the rubric of social hygiene. In 1924, the governor-general of the AOF, Jules Carde, ordered the AMI to push staff toward indigenous maternity services, hoping that in addition to delivering babies and administering care, midwives and nurses would also impart hygienic education to new mothers.[70] From 1926, colonies were required to report demographic data, although these numbers were wildly inaccurate and often based on little more than guesswork.[71] Daladier ordered increases in indigenous personnel and the creation of mobile infirmaries to ensure the spread of hygienic knowledge—along with basic medical care—to the farthest reaches of the empire. To a limited degree, these attempts bore fruit. Medical schools in Dakar and Hanoi trained increasing numbers of indigenous doctors, the number of maternity wards in the AOF grew from 23 to 130 over the interwar years, the number of infirmaries more than quadrupled, and the number of indigenous doctors with biomedical training grew sixfold in some regions, such as Côte d'Ivoire. Yet these resources were a tiny fraction of the health infrastructure available to the population of the metropole.[72] Ultimately, rather than focusing on public education and the improvement of social conditions and the urban environment, Daladier and colonial officials interpreted social hygiene to mean primarily the physical eradication of "social diseases"—the most important of which was tuberculosis.[73] This feat alone, administrators argued, would improve the social and moral situation as well.

The Pasteur Institute helped provide both the rationale and the practical tools for Daladier's reforms. Pastorians were already collaborating with colonial governments in a number of preventive endeavors: they produced smallpox and rabies vaccines and performed analyses of potable water in cities like Dakar and Saigon, lending force to the ministry's focus on technical improvements. Calmette's studies had demonstrated the pan-imperial reach of tuberculosis, turning it from a marginal disease to an acute social ill that required action. Further, he had reframed tuberculosis as a problem that not only affected children and newborns in particular but also directly implicated the colonizing process, helping to push it to the forefront of health reformers' agenda.

In 1924, Calmette enrolled the Ministry of the Colonies as a supporter of BCG trials. Daladier sent out circulars to governments-general in Madagascar, Indochina, and West and equatorial Africa, ordering them to collaborate with Pastorians.[74] Two arguments, in particular, convinced the minister. The first was the European contact thesis, which he reproduced in his letters to the governors, noting both the "particular exposure" of colonial troops to contagion during their stay in the metropole and the vulnerability of populations living on "virgin soil."[75] Calmette's new epidemiology did indeed impress the urgency of the tuberculosis problem on the ministry. Second, Daladier was concerned about "other problems of colonial demography," namely, infant mortality and population density.[76] At the same time, Calmette lobbied through his pan-imperial Pastorian network. He wrote to his collaborators in Tunis, Dakar, and elsewhere, convincing them to spearhead vaccination campaigns and collect data that would help his crusade to legitimize BCG in Europe.[77] The fact that Pasteur Institutes assumed the cost for producing vaccine made the proposition all the more appealing to the ministry.

Over the course of the 1920s and 1930s, Pastorians in Algeria, Tunis, West Africa, and Indochina produced and distributed the BCG vaccine to local populations. Though these programs were supposed to be *trials* of the vaccine, which remained controversial in Europe, both Pastorians and colonial officials soon began to describe BCG as a proven and efficacious vaccine. From 1929 onward, the Ministry of the Colonies referred to BCG as a reliable vaccine, citing evidence from the 1924 trials, although these were still highly contested in European metropoles.[78] In specific colonies, the experimental nature of BCG disappeared even faster. Already in 1925, doctors in Cholon and Phnom Penh were discussing the "importance of convincing, first of all, the indigenous *milieux* of the innocuity of this procedure as well as its prophylactic importance."[79] In meetings of health councils, bacteriologists did occasionally emphasize the "uncertain efficacy" of the procedure, but they ultimately concluded that it remained "the only applicable [method] in our arsenal, given the state of things," and the problem of efficacy quickly disappeared in official vulgarizations, replaced with references to "encouraging results" in official correspondence.[80]

In West Africa, BCG vaccination was less expansive but more amenable to the kinds of experiments Calmette needed to defend the vaccine against European critics. The vaccine was not easily conserved, which restricted its use to locations that were well connected to the site of production by rail or high-quality roads. In the AOF, this effectively meant that vaccination was limited to Dakar, Saint-Louis, and a few locations in Guinea, near the Pasteur Institute of Kindia. Still, "in accordance with the orders of the Minister of the Colonies," by 1929, the Pasteur Institute of Dakar was dutifully distributing the vaccine to maternities and schools in Dakar and, most important, conducting both tuberculin skin tests and semirandomized BCG tests on the tirailleurs sénégalais.[81]

The AOF lacked not just the *état-civil* but also the infrastructure to roll out BCG across the colony. Constant Mathis, director of the Dakar Pasteur Institute, therefore focused on testing the vaccine on the tirailleurs sénégalais, senegalese troops stationed in Dakar before their tour of duty in metropolitan France. First, Mathis performed tuberculin skin tests on a total of 1,873 tirailleurs over the course of five months. About half of those tested did not react to the test and were therefore considered fit for the study. These tirailleurs were divided into an experimental group of 513 and a control group of 507, both of whom then left to serve in France. Mathis imagined that in addition to showing the safety of BCG, comparing symptomatic TB rates in these two groups would also allow Calmette to demonstrate the efficacy of BCG. In practice, both tasks turned out to be more difficult than first imagined. A number of soldiers in the experimental group developed fever and cold abscesses, which raised doubts about the safety of BCG. Finally, it turned out that following all members of the two groups was more difficult than imagined, and ultimately the only members of the two groups to develop TB were from the experimental, vaccinated group. Other than these cases, there were no statistically significant differences between the two groups—simply too few soldiers had fallen ill, and none had been conclusively diagnosed with TB. The study, therefore, could tell nothing about the efficacy of BCG.[82]

The main purpose of the tirailleurs' study was to provide evidence of the safety of BCG, but, crucially, the study simultaneously rehearsed the European origin thesis of colonial tuberculosis. Because the tirailleurs were drafted from all different regions of the AOF, Mathis argued, tuberculin skin tests could be used to determine the prevalence of TB in the home regions of the tirailleurs and compared with previous studies, such as those conducted by Calmette in 1912 and follow-up studies from the early 1920s. The results were deeply concerning. In 1912, 7.7 percent of tuberculin tests in Tivaouane, for example, came back positive; by 1929, this had risen to 57 percent. The average TB infection rate had risen from 15.2 percent to 41 percent across Senegal, from 16.7 percent to 38 percent in the city of Bamako, from 8 percent to 46 percent in Côte d'Ivoire, and so forth. Increases were particularly dramatic after 1925. As Mathis noted, "In less than four years, the proportion of infected has almost tripled in Senegal and more than quadrupled in Sudan and Upper Volta."[83] This increase was explained by "the return of demobilized tirailleurs to their home regions, of whom many were certainly contaminated during their time in Europe."[84] Those demobilized tirailleurs were, in Mathis' view, a particular danger because they had acquired a degree of immunity to the disease, while Africans living on the virgin soil of Guinea, Upper Volta, or Sudan were particularly susceptible to infection, allowing for the fast spread of the disease. The European origin argument, originally articulated by Calmette (and referenced by Mathis), was seemingly confirmed by studies of the tirailleurs. The solution to this problem, naturally, was vaccinating not only all the tirailleurs headed to France but "also the largest possible number of newborn Africans."[85]

Although the vaccination of the tirailleurs sénégalais was closer to an experimental study than Calmette's previous strategy of simply comparing mortality statistics in regions where BCG had been applied to regions where it had not, it was a far cry from the sort of statistical rigor the LNHO demanded. The expert statisticians' committee required that the experimental groups and control groups live in comparable social settings, in demographically similar families, and be observed regularly over a long time.[86] To appease the LNHO, Calmette turned to his friend Edmond Sergent, head of the Algiers Pasteur Institute.

By the interwar years, administrative record keeping had existed in the northernmost regions of Algeria for nearly a half-century. The state had records on genealogical trees, marital records, births, and deaths; Algiers also had extremely high levels of tuberculosis, particularly among the Muslim population, several tuberculosis treatment programs, and a Pasteur Institute.[87] The first trial vaccinations were performed in the Algiers Kasbah in 1931, and by 1935, the Algiers Pasteur Institute had begun a full RCT involving forty thousand subjects and following the LNHO guidelines to the letter (the team, in fact, included Yves Biraud, the director of epidemiology at the LNHO). The trial ran for twenty-six years and provided encouraging yet far from definitive proof of the vaccine's efficacy. As elsewhere, the trial did not preclude simultaneous mass vaccination in Algiers. Calmette (who died in 1933) and his associates continued to claim that the vaccine's safety and efficacy had already been proved beyond a reasonable doubt. For the Pastorians, the RCTs simply added to a mounting body of evidence, rather than providing a conclusive or distinctly compelling source of proof.

The variable legal, political, and ecological conditions in the empire allowed Pastorians to gather different kinds of evidence in order to respond to the broad variety of criticisms they were encountering in Europe. First, the different understanding of social hygiene, which focused on the technical, top-down containment of "social diseases," empowered Pastorians to experiment without oversight and efface the distinction between trial and prevention. They could marshal different kinds of evidence from different settings, pointing to the broad use of BCG in Indochina—more than one hundred thousand vaccinations in 1930—the experience of clinical practitioners, and the level of trust among the local population as proof of the vaccine's safety.[88] Pastorians could use vaccination trials in the maternity wards of Dakar and among the tirailleurs sénégalais when challenged on the unreliability of using mortality statistics to prove the efficacy of BCG.[89] Finally, the Algiers trial met the LNHO guidelines, although, ironically, it did so at the expense of the concerns many statisticians had expressed in their reports—the serious consideration of the trust and consent of participating families.[90] However, imperial administrators also benefited from the introduction of BCG in specific ways. Concerns around tuberculosis and social hygiene acquired particular political valences in different colonies, and BCG offered a way for officials to dodge many uncomfortable issues raised by this new paradigm. The following section examines one such situation in colonial Indochina.

Technopolitics of Tuberculosis Prevention in French Indochina

The most expansive BCG campaigns took place in Indochina. With the exception of the North African colonies, Indochina had the best-developed health system in the empire, with a medical school in Hanoi; Pasteur Institutes in Saigon, Nha Trang; and Hanoi; and infrastructure that, while far from perfect, nevertheless allowed the AMI to access some of the more remote areas of the colony. Several critical requirements were met: there were several laboratories where BCG could be produced, roads and railways ensured that the vaccine could be distributed fairly widely before it expired, and technical staff trained in Hanoi and elsewhere ensured that the shots could be properly administered.[91] As a result, the French reported high vaccination numbers from the beginning of the trials. In 1924, a total of 1,717 infants were vaccinated in the maternity wards of Saigon-Cholon and Phnom Penh.[92] By 1928, the Pasteur Institute was distributing more than sixty thousand doses a year to maternities in twelve cities, and the number increased to more than one hundred thousand annual doses by 1931. From 1929, the Government-General made the War against Tuberculosis a part of the institute's mission and a separate line item in the colonial budget.[93] Indeed, Laurence Monnais has used BCG vaccination as an example of the colony marching ahead of the metropole in providing preventive health care and responding to local needs.[94] Yet a closer look suggests that there was, in fact, much debate over the proper means of combating TB in Indochina. The consensus that emerged between colonial officials and Pastorians had more to do with BCG's political rather than humanitarian potential.

When tuberculosis, owing largely to Calmette's research, became an imperial problem, it was not just the Pastorians who came to the rescue. The CNDT, which spearheaded the social hygienist response to TB prevention in France, sought to expand to Indochina, organize stamp sales, fund dispensaries and sanatoriums, and provide public education. Its concerns, which emphasized improving living and working conditions and the importance of associational life, intersected with those of Vietnamese doctors and local notables, who could use the language of social hygiene to discuss controversial political issues around labor and organizing. The rise of hygiene talk around tuberculosis, then, created a number of political concerns for French officials. The enthusiasm for BCG therefore needs to be seen in the context of rising political tensions in interwar Indochina.

For administrators, political radicalism posed the greatest threat to French rule during the interwar years. Intellectuals educated in francophone schools in Indochina or in the universities of France created a new, vibrant culture of public debate. Nguyễn An Ninh, Trần Huy Liệu, and Bùi Quang Chiêu founded newspapers and journals, such as La Cloche Felée and Đông Pháp Thời Báo, as well as revolutionary groups such as the Young Annamites and the Secret Society of Nguyễn An Ninh. These movements eventually drifted ever closer to communism and built a small but active following among

Vietnamese students, workers, and soldiers in France, as well as among the urban dwellers of Hanoi and Saigon. As various incidents—the arrest of Nguyễn An Ninh, the Yen Bay rebellion, to name just two—escalated and led to mass boycotts and strikes, French officials clamped down on associational life, believing it to be a road to radicalization.[95] Repressions peaked in 1930–1931, when French forces responded to peasant riots by machine-gunning protests from the air, burning down "communist" villages, and executing those suspected of seditious activity.[96]

Meanwhile, workplace rights rose to the top of both Vietnamese and French concerns, driven largely by increases in plantation labor and the concerns of French industrialists about the detrimental effect of poor health on labor productivity, but also by the efforts of the Vietnamese themselves in calling attention to abuses and violence. Problems of industrialization only exacerbated more general problems of malnutrition and outright famine, which consistently threatened wide areas of Tonkin. By 1928, the workforce on French plantations had ballooned to nearly one hundred thousand laborers, a small fraction of the expanding Vietnamese population but economically significant nonetheless. Colonial health officers noted that the establishment of *hévéa* (rubber) plantations by companies like Michelin had brought about unprecedented epidemics of malaria.[97] Responding to episodes of mass worker desertion, such as at the Mimot plantation where three hundred workers deserted their posts in response to mistreatment, the French government sent out experts to study the conditions of labor and life in rubber plantations. These studies became the basis of official and popular exposés that uncovered unsanitary housing conditions, routinely violent managers, undernourishment and starvation, and forced hiring, all of which were compounded by malaria.

Vietnamese workers quickly learned how to take up the language of medical science in making claims against their employers. In the late 1920s, mandarins like Bùi Bằng Đoàn inspected plantations and chronicled instances of abuse, and Vietnamese council members criticized the French medical system for catering only to the rich and to urban dwellers. In the age of rising nationalism and anticolonial sentiment, Vietnamese doctors and activists increasingly articulated concerns over epidemic disease, labor conditions, and the inadequate medical response as specifically anti-Vietnamese in nature.[98] In 1927, the Government-General set up a Department of Labor and issued a series of decrees that reformed labor law, set up retirement funds, and strengthened public health provisions.[99] As usual, these laws looked better on paper than in practice. Around the country, however, more and more Vietnamese came to see health as a political issue.

The arrival of the CNDT in 1926 brought questions of social hygiene and TB prevention into the center of Indochinese politics. The construction of new dispensaries and sanatoriums was largely financed through the sale of stamps, as in France. As the society's finances lagged behind its expanding reach, representatives of the CNDT wrote to officials and medical experts in Indochina, encouraging them to join the "defence against the social danger" and become a part of the charitable network.[100] Indochinese administrators initially rejected the idea, since it proposed creating nongovernmental Franco-Vietnamese associations, which officials saw as potentially dangerous. The first proposal of Senator André Honnorat was returned with a note saying, "This does not concern local affairs and deals with an issue not immediately useful to the Annamite people."[101]

The reluctance of the Government-General, however, was superseded by pressure from both above and below. The CNDT's proposal aligned perfectly with the Ministry of the Colonies' new emphasis on social hygiene, leading the minister to pen a strongly worded reminder to the Indochinese governor-general about the "capital demographic importance" of the TB problem.[102] Meanwhile, CNDT propaganda began to spread in Vietnam, largely due to Camille Guérin's efforts to raise awareness about the role of childhood infection in the development of TB and to highlight the importance of proper prophylaxis and maternal care. The propaganda discussed the cost of tuberculosis to "the social capital," the importance of better living and working conditions, and the need for collective action to combat the disease—the hygienist aspects of TB prevention, largely copied directly from metropolitan French examples.[103] Such brochures were quickly translated into Vietnamese and distributed in schools and hospitals in Saigon, Cholon, and elsewhere.[104] Soon, a corps of Vietnamese doctors and officials expressed support for extending anti-TB prophylaxis, constructing dispensaries, and organizing anti-TB social movements in Indochina itself. Joining forces with French doctors and medical officers, these activists founded a number of associations dedicated to selling TB stamps and building a movement for social hygiene. By 1930, these included the Central Committee for Mutual Aid, the Anti-Tuberculosis League of Tonkin, the Masonic Fraternité Tonkinoise, the Pierre Pasquier Dispensary, the Anti-Tuberculosis League of Cochinchina, and the League of the Friends of Annam.[105]

Vietnamese doctors quickly learned to speak the language of social hygiene and used even marginal cases of infection to lobby for the expansion of workers' rights and improvement of working conditions. In 1939, Dr. Hoang Mong Luong filed a report with the resident of Annam, demanding greater attention to tuberculosis among the giáo sư (secondary school teachers) in a township near Hué. The number of recorded cases turned out to be very low—only ten over three years among a population of 215 teachers—but, as Luong argued, the social danger posed by the disease was much greater. Infected teachers could spread TB in the classroom before developing symptoms, but crucially, the rise in confirmed cases signified "deplorable hygienic conditions in which our giáo sư live: lack of physical exercise, poor nutrition and probably overworking."[106] To combat tuberculosis, Luong suggested a number of measures ranging from the clinical—regular checkups and X-rays for suspected cases—to the social, namely, limiting the number of students per teacher to fifty, reducing working hours, raising wages to "improve nutrition," and organizing a free "center of vacation for tired teachers, whether at a beach or a hill station."[107] Here, the expert language of hygienist tuberculosis control enabled Vietnamese doctors to pivot toward basic labor concerns.

Other Vietnamese activists used the language of social hygiene to request government subventions to support the work of voluntary associations, which drew most of their funds from the sale of anti-TB stamps, following the model of the CNDT in France.[108] These projects were extremely successful: more than five hundred stamps were sold in 1929 in Cochinchina alone, netting nearly 4,500 piasters or 56,000 francs. By 1932, the sum had grown tenfold, to 43,000 piasters.[109] This financial success combined with endorsements from the CNDT gave the Vietnamese considerable leverage in negotiating contributions from the colonial administration. The Indochinese administration had to take these organizations seriously and formed a committee in 1932 to study the best use for the funds raised by the stamp sales.

Most French members of the committee suggested modest initiatives, ranging from expansion of BCG vaccination to the construction of a few new dispensaries. One Dr. Bourgin, however, joined two Vietnamese experts, Dr. Lan, and Dr. Cua, in proposing a thorough overhaul of the TB prevention system. Their proposal focused on three pillars: "Protect—Instruct—Cure," again drawing from the CNDT's hygienist lexicon. They proposed a nine-year plan for radically expanding TB facilities, constructing new isolation

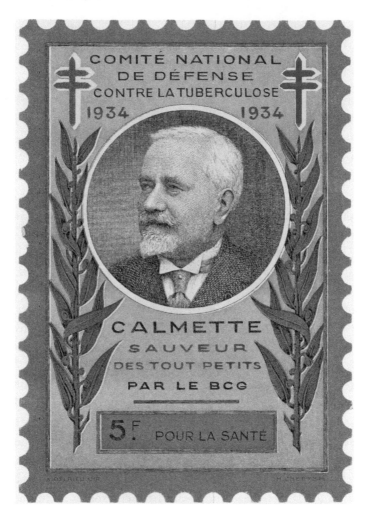

Figure 5.1 Anti-TB stamp of Albert Calmette, "savior of the newborns with BCG." © Institut Pasteur / Musée Pasteur.

wards within existing hospitals, producing popular educational and propagandistic films, building seaside resorts for Vietnamese children, buying mobile dispensary units, and, in the last stage, constructing seaside and high-altitude sanatoriums for adult Vietnamese patients. This proposal would have required a vast expansion of state funding for anti-TB efforts—the estimated budget, as one councilor noted, was more than 360,000 piasters, nearly ten times the money raised by the sale of stamps, creating immediate opposition among administrators.[110]

Yet there were other, political reasons for the French to resist such proposals. Often Vietnamese hygienists' plans would have further empowered voluntary associations and Vietnamese labor. In order to secure the trust of the population, experts such as Tran Ham Nghiep argued, it was crucial to staff the new dispensaries with "annamite nurses, women of excellent general education, high technical skill and exceptional moral values."[111] Others suggested training Indochinese doctors in every province and equipping them with a mobile sanitary unit, to improve anti-TB propaganda.[112] Finally, Bourgin and others recommended using money from the sale of stamps to construct "larger and more hygienic housing" for the Vietnamese in cities like Saigon, Hanoi, and Hué.[113] While always couched in the language of social hygiene, Vietnamese doctors' and their French allies' recommendations sought to increase the power and social standing of Vietnamese professionals, address the social injustices in the domains of labor and housing, and direct more power to voluntary associations.

These proposals threatened the entrenched colonial order of things. Beyond the challenge to French policies on labor and housing, authorities in the late 1920s and 1930s were even more troubled by their potential to empower associational life, as voluntary organizations were seen as hotbeds of seditious activity. As communist and nationalist movements became increasingly fused, and the Great Depression of the 1930s brought about a new surge in protests, strikes, and popular movements, colonial authorities feared communist organizers working with nationalist activists would produce new, ideologically coherent, well-organized terror organizations. Voluntary associations came under particular scrutiny as potential loci for radicalization, particularly if these were engaged in labor rights, religious affairs, or any kind of activity that could be tied to Freemasonry or other sorts of "secret societies."[114]

In contrast to the metropole, where much of TB prevention was done on a charitable basis, administrators in Indochina therefore actively discouraged private initiative in combating tuberculosis. When one health officer in Tonkin attempted to coordinate the activities of various voluntary anti-TB organizations in 1936, he received strict orders from the inspector-general of hygiene ordering him to ensure that all private activity remained under the control of the administration: "It is the Administration that has to ensure the coordination of the war against tuberculosis . . . abandoning the fight solely to private enterprise can result in a lack of coordination and the loss of effort and money."[115] The inspector-general outlined a model that subjected all voluntary associations to direct administrative control, named representatives of the Government-General to their boards, and created a rigid hierarchy for activities—such as the organization of dispensaries or the collection of donations—deemed efficient and permissible. One such organization, the Anti-Tuberculosis League of Tonkin, was closely monitored by the *police des associations*, and the local resident-general expressed repeated concern that discussions of hygienist TB prevention could spill over to politics, such as social welfare or public education. When asked to approve the constitution of the society, the resident reminded that, in particular, "all religious and political discussion is strictly prohibited. . . . If [the league's] publications are in quoc-ngu or in foreign languages then the league has to, additionally, conform to the rules of the Indochinese press."[116] Yet, as previous examples have shown, this was precisely what the language of social hygiene achieved: it blurred the boundaries between "political discussion" and "medical discussion" by rendering questions like those related to working hours, salaries, or the quality of housing medical questions that were subject to legitimate *medical* debate.

In response to the political problems raised by the CNDT's social hygiene model of TB prevention, the government relied on medical expertise of its own. Officials consistently argued that the use of the "progressive" BCG was sufficient to protect against tuberculosis, therefore obviating the need for further reforms or for the expansion of associative life. Here again, experts conveniently forgot about the experimental nature of the vaccine as well as the logistical limits to its proliferation and portrayed it as a robust and proven vaccine of the future. When the Anti-Tuberculosis League of Tonkin applied for the government to approve the society's constitution, the resident superior ordered a *medical* expert to offer his opinion on the mission of the association. The local director of health broadly disapproved of the wide mandate of the society by leaning on Calmette's contagionist thesis. He noted that, unlike in France, working conditions had little to do with the spread of TB because the movement of air and the availability of space on plantations made contagion more difficult: "Workers are less affected since they lead an active life in open air and they live in *paillottes* open to all kinds of bad weather; agricultural workers are even less affected for similar reasons."[117] In this rendition, the low quality of Vietnamese housing and the harsh conditions of the *indigenat* (the separate legal system for colonial subjects) became virtues instead of factors that contributed to disease.

Instead, the doctor argued, the real problem was infant mortality, which could be solved uniquely with the help of the BCG: "The War against Tuberculosis has its only weapon in the form of antituberculosis vaccination with BCG; other means, without meaning to neglect them, have only a secondary importance. In fact, with the exception of vaccination, no other prophylactic measure can take hold among this carefree population completely ignorant of the laws of hygiene."[118] Noting that "all other efforts would lead to useless waste," the doctor combined scientific rhetoric of contagion, moralist language about the Vietnamese constitution, and a technical insistence on the reliability of BCG. The health director ultimately convinced the administration to curtail the permitted range of activities of the Anti-Tuberculosis League, limiting its ability to purchase real estate and to publish educational material, and placing it under close police surveillance for years to come.[119]

Officials also used BCG as a trump card in the committee for distributing the anti-TB stamp funds. Countering the demands for widespread development of dispensaries, educational programs, and improved industrial hygiene, administrators emphasized that BCG was the colony's "first line of defense" and was provided for free by the Pasteur Institute. Colonial officials proposed using the anti-TB stamps to further fund the TB laboratories of the Pasteur Institute, helping extend BCG vaccinations further. The growing number of immunizations already done in Indochina (from fifty-nine thousand in 1927 to more than one hundred thousand) was brought up as evidence of the success of the vaccine, rather than simply consequences of expanding an ongoing trial. As the president of the ad hoc committee argued: "In order not to disperse our efforts, we ought to focus them on BCG, because BCG represents the future."[120] At the end of the day, the ambitious proposals of Vietnamese doctors were all rejected, with a single concession to provide more public propaganda, but only if it was limited to advertising the benefits of BCG.[121]

This was a political move, which, ironically, Pastorians were quick to notice in other contexts. In 1936, Dr. Morin, the director-general of the Indochinese Pasteur Institutes, noted that the British and the Japanese were taking an increasing interest in BCG in their colonial domains: "Because they consider it impossible to fight against tuberculosis by improving the living conditions of coolies, [the British and the Japanese] are taking an active interest in BCG vaccination."[122] For that exact same reason, so were the French. While administrators, pressured by the Ministry of the Colonies and the CNDT lobby in France and in Indochina, floated ideas of more expansive sanatorium programs, mobile dispensaries, improved housing, and better labor protections, they ultimately went with the "way of the future"—BCG. The high numbers of vaccinated infants recorded in the yearbooks of the Pasteur Institute were considered proof positive of the vaccine's efficacy. Although Calmette's epidemiology and consequently rising concerns over colonial TB rates had opened up the path for debating labor and associational politics under the rubric of health, the technopolitics of BCG vaccination once again closed these debates shut.

Conclusion

In Europe, in the empire, and in Indochina, tuberculosis raised questions about the implications of social hygiene for politics and gave rise to technopolitical solutions for managing the fallout. What tuberculosis meant for politics, however, depends on where one looked. In France and much of Europe, expert statisticians, League of Nations officials, and medical reforms saw BCG as an unnecessarily dangerous and fundamentally untestable vaccine that relied on outdated models of vertical expert power that disregarded the fundamental unpredictability of biomedicine, ethics, and politics outside the laboratory. In the corridors of the Ministry of the Colonies, BCG represented the possibility to make good on the promises to decrease infant mortality rates, address the problem of colonial demography, and put into action a new program of preventive medicine despite continuously shoestring budgets. In Indochina, BCG provided an answer to calls for better labor protections, broader opportunities for Vietnamese specialists, and more associational life that were prompted by the rise of plantation labor. These shifting meanings also shifted Calmette's relative power as his BCG trials expanded beyond the metropole almost immediately after the vaccine's discovery in 1924: if, in Europe, he found widespread criticisms both within, but especially outside, France, in the empire, the colonial administration stood firmly by his side.

Ironically, while his European critics accused Calmette of not properly considering his ethical and democratic responsibilities toward patients and their families, it was precisely because of the fundamentally undemocratic nature of imperial governance that Calmette could meet League of Nations criteria for RCTs and leverage data from West Africa and Indochina to his advantage. In Indochina and elsewhere, Pastorians and officials blurred the line between "trial" and "prevention," arguing that doctors were distributing a completely proven, effective, and progressive vaccine, rather than a highly contested, experimental drug. The West African trials were made possible by the fact that the tirailleurs sénégalais could be ordered to comply with vaccination programs and tracked because of the hierarchical nature of military service; in Algiers, as Clifford Rosenberg has noted, Pastorians benefited from illegal access to the personal records of patients in the kasbah, as well as their abject poverty, which made them less likely to resist vaccination.[123] This sort of "ethical variability" across the empire proved another major resource for the Pastorians.

Calmette regularly invoked the large numbers of vaccinations in Indochina, as well as the Algiers RCT and trials with African tirailleurs in defending his invention in Europe. Yet up until World War II, European experts remained skeptical of the vaccine's utility. After the war, when mass vaccination campaigns in Eastern Europe prevented TB breakouts that were thought to be inevitable in postconflict situations, the efficacy and safety of BCG were finally confirmed beyond a reasonable doubt. Many countries, from the Soviet Union to France itself, made the vaccine mandatory in the immediate postwar years, though most have now discontinued these programs. Currently, the World Health Organization—the successor organization to the LNHO—recommends the use of BCG in regions with high TB endemicity. In this case, worries about the safety of the vaccine proved unfounded, although social hygienists were most likely correct in claiming that improvements in living standards did far more than the vaccine to curb TB rates. The BCG trials, however, demonstrated to the Pastorians how the strategic use of imperial mobility and the politics of scale could be used to avoid ethical and practical obstacles. In the case of the yellow fever vaccine, these strategies had far graver consequences.

6

The Racial Politics of Microbes
in Colonial Dakar

Pastorians designed their technologies and policies for universal application. In practice, they were shaped and constrained by political and scientific debates in very specific and circumscribed settings, even if these places claimed to represent "international" or "global" forums. BCG vaccination did not mean the same thing for the investigators of the Lübeck trial as it did for the statisticians at the LNHO; it did not mean the same thing for the tirailleurs senegalais as it did for Vietnamese doctors. Throughout this process, technological artifacts—the tuberculin skin test, Calmette's epidemiological studies, and finally the BCG vaccine itself—made it possible to imagine new scales of operation and allowed Pastorian expertise to travel. These devices helped to reimagine TB as an imperial problem rather than a metropolitan or narrowly colonial one; because of them, Pastorians could become experts of some importance in debates over Vietnamese labor or associational rights.[1] The costs of Pastorian universal projects were distributed locally and unevenly. Scaling TB up to an imperial problem could rally anticolonial activists as well as administrators; more often, the unexpected consequences would be borne by colonial subjects, whether the soldiers who became imperial subjects or the activists who found their arguments for reform countered with references to BCG. The technopolitical power of Pastorian inventions lay precisely in making the costs of universalism invisible. The previous chapters have attempted to make them visible again.

Intertwined with both universal Pastorian models and their emplaced technopolitical practices is the underlying biological reality of microbial interactions. Complex ecologies of humans, vectors, microbes, viruses, and many other biological agents interacted differently in Senegal than they did in Saigon. This chapter looks at the role of microbes and viruses themselves. We return to where we began: to the third plague pandemic, which directed the Pastorian focus toward technical solutions, namely, disinfections, vaccination, and deratization, and shaped French containment programs across

Pasteur's Empire. Aro Velmet, Oxford University Press (2020). © Oxford University Press.
DOI: 10.1093/oso/9780190072827.001.0001

the empire. In the AOF in the 1910s, plague epidemics shaped the politics of contagious disease containment for many years to come, as Myron
Echenberg has argued.[2] But what happens if the agent of contagion changes?

Pastorian plague programs came to Senegal, as they did to Tunisia,
Morocco, Madagascar, and other French colonies, with ships, rats, and fleas.
Yet, as in Indochina, enacting "progressive" Pastorian methods in Dakar
turned out to be difficult. The surrounding political conflict pressured both
French and African leaders to embrace dramatic interventions, which relied
ultimately on quarantine, segregation, the wholesale destruction of African
housing, and relocation of subject populations into what is now known as
the Médina. Over the course of the 1910s, repeated experiences with plague
outbreaks reinforced the conviction in French authorities that containment
efforts had to be coercively directed primarily at Africans. As administrators
saw it, Africans refused Pastorian measures such as vaccinations and sanitary passports, and therefore deserved being whipped into line.

The different disease ecology of yellow fever, I argue in this chapter,
disrupted this political dynamic. The French case for focusing on African
communities rested on the fact that these were usually far harder hit by the
plague—French houses had better insulation, and fewer inhabitants, who, in
turn, had stronger immune systems. Yellow fever, in contrast, struck French
officials, Syrian and Lebanese traders, immigrants, and others who did not
grow up in areas of yellow fever endemicity and had therefore not acquired
childhood immunity. These communities often had more political capital and would not put up with the kind of coercive measures French health
authorities were used to enacting during plague outbreaks. This novel situation created an opening for African leaders, who used the yellow fever
outbreak of 1927 to call out French hypocrisy and racism over disease containment writ large.

What began as a French attempt to tame the Yersinia pestis became a public
health system uniquely vulnerable to the yellow fever virus. Understanding
why the virus could upend decades of French policy in a little over a year,
however, requires us to observe the virus not isolated in a laboratory,
separated from its environment and history. We must put yellow fever
back in its place—in twentieth-century Dakar, shaped by histories of prior
epidemics, by anxieties of doctors who had lost their ancestors to the tropical
blight, by migratory flows that shaped the virus's spread and generated panic
within the city, and by political forces seeking to use the epidemic to achieve
their own ends. Only then can we understand why the Pasteur Institute's

proposal to contain yellow fever in the laboratory again suddenly seemed so attractive.

Meanings of Epidemic Disease and Public Health in Colonial Dakar

The plague is central to understanding the history of disease containment in the AOF. Dakar, one of France's *anciens colonies* in West Africa, and capital of the federation from 1902, suffered from many afflictions. These ranged from cholera and malaria, perennial guests in tropical port cities, to yellow fever, spirochetosis, and sleeping sickness. It was the plague epidemic of 1914, however, that remade West Africa's public health system, reconfigured colonial politics, and changed the very landscape of Dakar itself. The epidemic also claimed nearly fifteen hundred victims. In a city with a population of roughly thirty thousand, this was a frightening 5 percent of the population.[3]

Prior to the twentieth century, European scientists had recorded no plague outbreaks in Senegal or in the surrounding areas. As a result, the 1914 epidemic was all the more surprising and destructive. Public health authorities in Senegal were well aware of Pastorian containment measures, which had been developed in Indochina, and which medical experts considered civilized and progressive: steam disinfection with Clayton machines, the destruction of rats using a bounty system or by the sulfuration of sewers, and preventive vaccination with the Haffkine lymph. A serious outbreak in Madagascar in 1902 and a milder one in Tunisia in 1907 demonstrated the potential effectiveness of Pastorian measures, although they were always combined with more "classical" measures, such as sanitary cordons around infected areas and quarantine.[4]

Accordingly, state authorities responded to the first confirmed cases in Dakar with relative calm. Officials imposed sanitary cordons around "indigenous districts" and ordered both Haffkine vaccinations and disinfections.[5] Some experts, notably Pastorians working at the Dakar bacteriological laboratory, continued to advocate for vector control and vaccination measures throughout the epidemic.[6] Municipal and colonial administrators, as well as competing experts, however, quickly began to call for more dramatic and racially oriented control measures, using language familiar to anyone who had experience with the Hanoi epidemic a decade earlier. Vaccination, disinfection, and vector control were expensive, the technology was not always available, Africans were not being cooperative, and desperate times called for desperate measures.

On 14 May 1914, Dr. Huot, head of the Senegalese medical service, convened the sanitary council of Dakar and issued a decree mandating harsh measures to stop the disease. While Huot theoretically accepted standard bacteriological explanations of plague etiology alongside Pastorian prescriptions for containment, he cited previous examples from Haiphong, Indochina; Nouméa, New Caledonia; and the Gold Coast as conclusive evidence that the destruction of "insalubrious housing" was a crucial part of an effective response.[7] Finally, the sanitary council concluded, it was simply more financially efficient to destroy low-quality *paillotes* (African huts) than to spend a considerable amount of labor and money on disinfecting them with Clayton apparatuses.

Yet as many critics even within the health service itself observed, vaccination efforts failed not because Africans rejected vaccines out of fear or misunderstanding but because the French lacked the manpower to service all the demand. Incineration, meanwhile, was actually not as cost-effective as Huot had claimed, since indemnities for destroyed housing ate up the majority of the colonial public health budget for several years after the epidemic.[8] Why did French officials remain so committed to measures they knew were ineffective?

From the deliberations of the sanitary committee, it appears that French commitment to ineffective but highly visible and quickly realizable measures was *precisely* a product of the committee's awareness of its own limits.[9] The lack of manpower, the presence of swindlers peddling vaccination cards, and the inability to enforce quarantine and sanitary cordons led to a sense of palpable impotence at the committee meetings, while growing panic and climbing death rates demanded some kind of forceful action. The farther the epidemic spread, the more members called for "immediate action," to "put an end to the disastrous situation as soon as possible." The committee chose to focus on the "only measure of diverting the threat of a *dangerous return* of the disease"—the incineration of housing.[10] Put differently, health officials chose to focus on spectacular and drastic measures in a performance of state power against a seemingly overwhelming disease. Officials rationalized these measures as preventing a future outbreak of the disease while inventing new obstacles—the "dangerous rituals" and "inveterate filth" of the Africans—to justify their inability to commit to prophylactic action against the current one.[11]

The politics of performance over prophylaxis, spectacle over safety, and violence over vaccination all crystallized as the default approach of the colonial state to disease containment. While subsequent epidemics never proved quite as disastrous, officials constantly feared the return of the chaos of the early days of the infamous 1914 outbreak. When the plague reappeared in Dakar in 1919, Governor-General Martial Merlin suggested that the "same elements of the population" that had refused to cooperate in 1914 were doing so again. This led authorities to once again conclude that precautions should be taken to prevent chaos in the next epidemic—"segregation, the absolute separation of native and European quarters, will remain an absolute necessity."[12] Indeed, with each subsequent epidemic, the French preference for spectacular but ineffective quarantine measures was inscribed farther into the physical layout of the city. As authorities destroyed more African *paillottes* and relocated their inhabitants to the Médina, quarantining African districts became logistically easier, since the French no longer had to deal with the awkwardness of imposing quarantine in neighborhoods where European and African populations mixed.[13]

For many Africans, the French medical response became a symbol of the unequal struggle for fair treatment and political rights, as Echenberg has argued. Dakar played a unique role in colonial politics, since it was, alongside Saint-Louis, Gorée, and Rufisque, one of the Four Communes of Senegal endowed with voting rights. Those "originating" from these regions, irrespective of their race, were not colonial subjects but citizens (though with many restrictions). Voters in the Four Communes could elect mayors and representatives to local councils and the General Council, as well as vote for a representative in the National Assembly in metropolitan France. Though, in theory, Africans could hold any of these posts, most remained in the hands of either French or mixed-race politicians throughout the nineteenth century.

In the early twentieth century, French politicians in the AOF began to restrict voting rights. Governor-General Ponty wanted to limit citizenship to those Africans who had rejected Islam and accepted French civil law, the model that had been used effectively to limit representation in Algeria.[14] Recognizing the growing concerns of citizenship rights of the African elite, a successful Sereer customs official named Blaise Diagne returned to Dakar after a twenty-year absence to campaign for a seat in the National Assembly. Supported by the oppositional newspaper *La Démocratie*, Lebou elites in the Dakar assembly, and other African *évolués* in the French bureaucracy, Diagne soundly beat a crowded field of French-backed opponents. On 10

May 1914, he became the first African representative to the highest legislative body in France.[15]

The fact that the plague epidemic coincided with the election of Blaise Diagne, both in mid-May, gave rise to numerous conspiracy theories. Activists building support for Diagne spread rumors that the coercive containment measures of the French were in fact retributions for the election of the African deputy.[16] These suspicions were entirely rational: during the election campaign, French merchants had refused credit to African customers known for supporting Diagne, and the mayor of Dakar had threatened to cut off water and electricity to Africans campaigning for the future deputy. There were rumors that African civil servants would be dismissed if Diagne won.[17] Jean d'Oxoby, editor at *La Démocratie* and a prominent Diagnist, wrote a long polemic titled "Things Come to a Head," in which he suggested that the medical crisis was an entirely fabricated retribution, since after all the sanitary cordons, unwarranted incineration of housing, and arbitrary searches of African homes, not a single rat cadaver had been found in Dakar.[18] Finally, Blaise Diagne himself mysteriously disappeared for several weeks after the declaration of a medical emergency. As a result, more rumors circulated among Dakarois, suggesting that the French were trying to assassinate the newly elected deputy by infecting him with Yersin's microbe.[19] The election of Diagne and the medical response to the plague outbreak became intertwined in the minds of Senegalese voters. It was only when Blaise Diagne returned to the city and cooperated with Governor-General Ponty, which combined with the retreat of the plague and the relaxation of containment measures, that order returned to the city.[20]

The 1914 epidemic politicized disease containment for Africans and French alike. Blaise Diagne realized that he exercised considerable power in such situations, as his name could both fire up African protests and calm them down when needed. The Government-General needed his help in getting Africans to accept the drastic containment measures, and Dakarois activists realized that they had more agency over the medical response than they initially thought. Africans may not have been able to convince the French to call off the forced destruction of housing, but they were able to extract important concessions such as greater indemnities and ownership over the makeshift housing in segregation villages. In future epidemics, Africans were quick to call the Government-General to account over previous injustices. In 1919, Lebou activists could demand that sanitary measures exclude the destruction of housing. Meanwhile, colonial administrators suspected that some activists were purposefully spreading rumors intended to alienate the Lebou and the administration, so that Blaise Diagne could ride in and play the hero.[21]

Yellow Fever as an "Event" in Dakarois Racial Politics

Changing ecological realities soon changed how French and African actors conceived of biomedical disease containment. The yellow fever epidemic of 1927 forced administrators and public health experts to rethink their overreach-and-retreat policies. The epidemic was, to use William Sewell's term, an "event" in Dakarois public health politics—a rupture with routine practice, which amplified and reverberated across various fields of social life, resulting in a transformation of established social structures.[22] The outbreak made entrenched rituals of disease control unthinkable and escalated the conflict between Africans and French Dakarois beyond its usual confines and into the metropole, spurring new interventions, the highlight of which was the Pastorian vaccine project.

A disease exists only in a specific time and place. In early twentieth-century Senegal, the biological effects of the yellow fever virus, transmitted to humans by the *Aedes aegypti* mosquito, were inflected by many historical, environmental, and social factors. These included a history of deadly epidemics, a disease ecology that gave many Africans, who grew up in endemic regions, childhood immunity while rendering Europeans vulnerable, and the politics of race, which privileged European victims and policed non-Europeans, often aggravating their suffering. To illustrate, take a health commission report from 1932, a year mostly without major yellow fever outbreaks. It describes an incident at the "Cultures Tropicales" concession, a plantation with seven European managers and more than two hundred African laborers. The report highlights how the disease experience was shaped by ecology and society alike.

The illness was first reported among the European staff, with one Mr. P and Mrs. P falling ill within days of each other. Their symptoms were quite typical: fever, muscle pain, backache, shivers, loss of appetite, nausea, and, of course, jaundice, which gives the disease its name. Mr. P's symptoms eased somewhat four days after they first appeared, only to return, characteristically accompanied with bleeding from the mouth and death less than twenty-four hours later. Mrs. P fared better: on the fourth day of her illness, she was transported to a separate lodging, near the plantation director's house, where her fever quietly subsided, and she was declared healthy a week later. The houses of Mr. and Mrs. P were disinfected with sulfur, the nearby brush was cleared, and samples from both patients were sent to the Dakar Pasteur Institute for analysis.

Weeks later, health officers discovered that the disease had also ravaged the African population of the plantation, but no French manager had noticed. In the two weeks following the first case, six African workers had fallen ill, and four of them had perished. The local doctor responsible for monitoring the health of African workers had not recorded their deaths, since he lived away from the workers' community and simply did not realize what had transpired. Upon learning of these incidents, officials isolated the African village for several days and put traffic to and from the village under "severe surveillance."[23] In contrast to the response to European cases, the "Cultures Tropicales" retaliated against the entire village, imposing additional hardship on African families.

Equally significantly, Africans working at the "Cultures Tropicales" were migrant workers, so they were more likely to be vulnerable to infection by the *Aedes aegypti*. Often, though, adult Africans suffered less from the disease than European colonizers. Similarly to measles or mumps, yellow fever, when contracted in childhood, is milder and confers lifelong immunity. Because this rendered many adult West Africans immune, while Europeans generally were susceptible, the ecological specificity of yellow fever created a very different dynamic between the two communities than diseases such as the plague. Indeed, many contemporary scientists believed, falsely, that blacks had genetic immunity to the disease, the same way some Africans had genetically acquired resistance to malaria.[24] Yellow fever outbreaks left little room for the usual arguments about the danger of "filthy" African neighborhoods, as the disease spread mostly in European districts. This peculiarity was the first reason that made the 1927 epidemic transformative.

The second reason had to do with the history of yellow fever epidemics in Dakar. Although no major outbreaks had been recorded in the twentieth century, memories of terrible outbreaks went all the way back to the eighteenth century and colored the entire history of French colonization. During the Haitian Revolution, in 1892, the disease claimed the lives of some fourteen thousand British soldiers and twenty-nine thousand Frenchmen stationed on Saint-Domingue. The medical historian Erwin Ackerknecht and others have suggested that the epidemic may have facilitated the Louisiana

Purchase from Napoleon and prevented an invasion of North America by the French emperor.[25] Dakar had suffered a particularly tragic outbreak in 1878, which claimed the lives of 769 of the 1,474 European inhabitants at the time, including twenty-two of twenty-six doctors.[26]

The epidemic left a mark on entire generations of colonial doctors and military men. Take, for instance, the Mathis family. Michel Mathis, a thirty-eight-year-old naval doctor, first class, perished in the epidemic. His son, Constant, dedicated his life to tropical medicine and became the longest-serving director of the Pasteur Institute of Dakar, coordinating the scientific response to the 1927 epidemic. Constant's son, Maurice, in turn proceeded to study the epidemiology of the yellow fever virus under Émile Brumpt in Paris and dedicated his doctoral dissertation to his grandfather's memory.[27] In short, for Europeans, yellow fever became a symbol of the deadly tropics, while leaving Africans relatively untouched.

Let us return to Constant Mathis. In 1927, the year of the epidemic, the bacteriologist was preparing to expand his laboratory beyond the confines

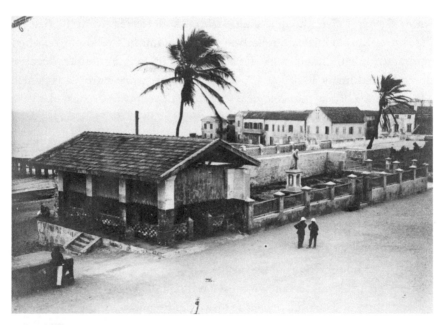

Figure 6.1 French constructions in Dakar. The two men are standing in front of a memorial to those who perished in the 1878 yellow fever epidemic, ca. 1928. Rockefeller Archive Center.

of the former maternity ward, where it had been housed since its relocation from Saint-Louis in 1913.[28] Under his direction the Dakar laboratory became a beacon of European hygiene and civilization, at least compared with the abysmal state of official sanitary services.[29] The arrival of yellow fever opened up new possibilities for the institute.

In May 1927, just before the start of the rainy season, two villages, Tivaouane and M'Bour, both around seventy kilometers from the capital, began to report yellow fever cases. The first village suffered a total of twenty-one cases, with eleven fatalities, while in M'Bour, officials recorded twelve cases and seven deaths.[30] This was gravely concerning. Local administrators reacted quickly, demanding the hospitalization of all suspected cases and imposing curfews. They also sent out sanitary teams to check that European houses were adequately equipped with mosquito nets and that their surroundings had been debrushed. Finally, officials demanded that Europeans, Syrians, and Moroccans—the trading population of the two villages—avoid venturing inland, where they would be unable to get medical assistance should they contract yellow fever in the brush.[31]

These measures, while standard when applied to Africans, had a different effect when applied to the privileged European and Middle Eastern populations of Tivaouane and M'Bour.[32] They caused a scandal in M'Bour serious enough to require an investigation by the governor-general himself. In particular, Syrian businessmen filed a series of complaints against one Dr. Lemonnier. They complained about the poor living conditions in isolation wards, accused Lemonnier of medical neglect, and protested his "imperious and arrogant" tone—he reportedly called Syrians "pigs" and "savages." The Syrians refused treatment and organized demonstrations against the insolent doctor, leading the mayor of M'Bour to call for help first from the lieutenant governor of Senegal and then from Governor-General Carde himself.[33] Administrators described the situation as "deplorable," the population as "up at arms" and requiring "immediate reaction."[34]

Yet even the governor-general failed to ease tensions. In August, European merchants organized two meetings where they demanded freedom of movement. As the harvest season approached and more Europeans needed to make trips inland to meet with suppliers, merchants demanded that they be allowed to move beyond the quarantine city, provided that they wear mosquito nets. Sanitary teams coming to isolate suspected yellow fever cases routinely found themselves facing squads of men protecting the patients in danger of hospitalization.[35]

This crisis illustrates how yellow fever disrupted habituated forms of epidemic control and created an atmosphere of excessive caution among administrators. With plague outbreaks, administrators could apply initial harsh emergency measures, knowing that with the help of Blaise Diagne and other African activists, they would be able to calm things down later on. Yellow fever, however, required the policing of Europeans and Syrians. These constituents had greater economic and political power than Africans and could stir up trouble all the way up to the governor-general. At the same time, administrators were aware that they were ill-equipped to actually deal with yellow fever epidemics: the number of doctors was limited, sanitary teams could not be formed in time, and there was not even enough metal for manufacturing mosquito nets. Harsh emergency measures, as the mayor of M'Bour quickly learned, represented a considerable danger, without a comparable payoff: while these measures did little to actually contain the spread of yellow fever, they were likely to upset powerful constituencies who did not want to see their freedom of movement limited.

It should be no surprise, then, that the mayor of Dakar resisted declaring an outbreak until the last possible moment.[36] In July, the disease broke out in the village of Thiès, with particularly bad outcomes: out of twenty-two recorded cases, twenty-one ended in death. In the second half of July, the disease surfaced in Dakar proper. It ravaged the city until the end of year, resulting in eighty-one confirmed cases and fifty-one fatalities, with an additional thirty suspected cases and twenty fatalities. Municipal authorities of Dakar, however, waited until mid-October before declaring the city contaminated and enforcing emergency measures.[37]

The lack of official response, combined with increasing reports of hospitalizations in the city and the terrifying memory of the deadly 1876 epidemic, exacerbated rather than counteracted the atmosphere of panic. Increasingly, soldiers and merchants stationed in Dakar started requesting repatriation.[38] Mathis, writing to his friends in Paris, was displeased too: "It reminded me of the Dreyfus affair: those who dared to speak of yellow fever were considered to be bad Frenchmen. Us doctors, we were treated as defeatists, until the number of deaths multiplied, and then we were considered to have been talking too candidly."[39]

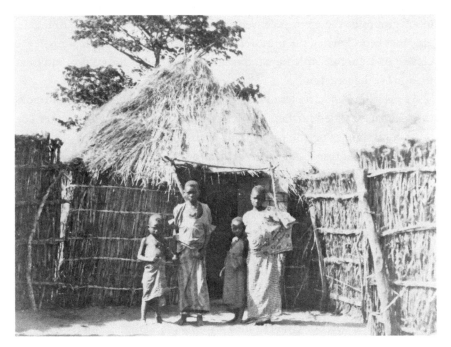

Figure 6.2 An African homestead in Thiès, Senegal. This building would have been incinerated in case of a yellow fever outbreak. Rockefeller Archive Center.

Escalation to the Metropole

Faced with the administration's indecisiveness, both European and African actors appealed to metropolitan authorities. Europeans had three principal means of pressuring the government: petitions, journalism, and personal connections in the National Assembly. These activities were highly coordinated. The Dakar police reported several meetings of civil servants, bankers, and merchants in the coffee shops of Dakar in early September. These meetings of more than a hundred people got increasingly vocal—on occasion, someone would call for the group to protest at the Government-General's office.[40] Administrators received petitions from the Dakar Chamber of Commerce, the union of public servants in Dakar, the head of the Colonial Union, and Senator François-Marsal in Paris. All petitioners lamented the slow reaction of the Dakar sanitary committee and urged the government to take action, in order to "conserve the so-far excellent morale" of the Dakarois merchants.[41] Public servants demanded curfews starting at 6 p.m. as well as the repatriation of women and children.[42] National Assembly members and lobby groups in the metropole were bombarded with complaints, to the degree that Léon Perrier, the minister of the colonies, himself sent a missive to Governor-General Carde demanding a report on what the colony had done to improve the situation.[43]

As the letters and articles of disgruntled Dakarois reached the metropole, the scandal escalated further. Magazines in the metropole and in other colonies took stances on the issue. Some accused the government of denying the outbreak because it did not have the proper resources to combat it. "The AOF belongs on the same list as Madagascar, where diseases are fought with circulars, decrees, and paper more often than they are fought with syringes and serums.... Our plans are devised on a large canvas, but we execute them on a footstool," wrote one commentator.[44] Others pointed out the effectiveness of aggressive sanitation measures—the draining of swamps and destruction of larvae—that had been carried out elsewhere, in Cuba, Nigeria, and the Gold Coast, wondering why the government of the AOF was not following suit.[45] Time and again, journalists recalled the disastrous epidemic of 1878, which had killed half of the Dakarois population, underscoring the potential costs of inaction.[46]

Some journalists looked for scapegoats. Syrians and Africans were the most common targets. Blamed, too, were the "Black Frenchmen," by which commentators meant Frenchmen who "acted like Africans," those who have "only a vague understanding of their responsibilities, won't cede an inch of ground with regards to their rights, and if they're not outright hostile to elementary rules of hygiene, they are at least very indifferent."[47] The most political and inflammatory statements blamed African suffrage for the crisis, arguing that empowering an uncivilized class made it difficult to impose sanitary measures, since the disruption of unsanitary African customs would no doubt come back to haunt legislators at the polls.[48] However, the majority of critics directed their ire against the colonial government and put responsibility on it for creating a situation that interrupted commerce, broke down solidarity, and put French women and children at risk.

Africans, too, attacked the colonial government. *La France Coloniale*, Blaise Diagne's newspaper, led the charge in Senegal, with articles that contrasted the restrained response of Dakar's public health apparatus to the aggressive measures taken by the US government in Cuba. One article highlighted the new sanitary measures in Santiago, which kept the streets in pristine condition and imposed tougher regulations on housing stock. "This, to me, sounds like a fight held with vigor.... [In Dakar] too, there is no lack of energy, but the results are left wanting. . . . If our streets remain like boon-docks, filled with greenish water."[49] It was not due to a lack of options that the colonial government was not acting, writers in *La France Coloniale* argued. Something else was at play.

This something else was racial prejudice, as Blaise Diagne argued in an interview in one of the most widely circulated Parisian newspapers, *Le Matin*: "Indigenous districts, which have been properly surveilled, and where inhabitants have had to submit to the rules of hygiene, have been spared from the disease. By contrast, Europeans live in houses that are often defective, but inviolable. And I can say without fear of contradiction, that all recorded cases of yellow fever have been in the European parts of Dakar."[50] Diagne took particular offense at the suggestion that African suffrage was to blame. He argued that the disease had spread far beyond the borders of the Four Communes, to Niger, Sudan, and elsewhere, where the iron fist of French sanitationists would be felt without fearing a backlash in the polls. Indeed, the deputy appeared to deny the epidemic altogether, pointing out that casualty rates were nowhere near as high as during the 1878 and 1900 outbreaks, and insinuating further that the real problem lay with the outsize privileges of the European elite, who had flouted the rules of hygiene and were now paying the consequences.[51] The series of interviews set off a minor firestorm, with numerous rebuttals by outraged colonialists appearing in *Écho de Paris*, *La France Militaire*, *Annales Coloniales*, and *Le Journal des Coloniaux*.[52] By and large, these responses shifted blame back to either insalubrious Africans or the migrant population of Syrians and highlighted the importance of more forceful government action. Diagne's interview had certainly hit a nerve.

By October 1927 the colonial administration in AOF, from the mayor of Dakar to Governor-General Carde, had lost the trust of all of its constituents. Since yellow fever hit Europeans, and because it carried with it memories of devastating past epidemics, the disease created a level of panic among the white population of Dakar that plague outbreaks had been unable to muster. Africans accused the government of privileging European privacy over public health and refusing to apply the same measures on French residents that it had been so casually forced on Africans during plague outbreaks. Both of these claims were made possible by the disease ecology of the virus, which rendered the racial prejudices of standard containment practices visible. The government, as one hygienist later put it, was "caught between two fires. If, for every suspected case, it took prophylactic measures, it would be accused of alarmism. If, on the contrary, it did not make a precise diagnosis, the epidemic would spread further."[53] Now, in the face of attacks from all corners, and pressure from the Ministry of the Colonies, the colonial lobby, and individual parliamentarians, it was finally forced to act.

On 27 September and 15 October, the governor-general passed decrees tightening emergency measures and creating a new sanitary regime called "the state of imminent danger," which was imposed on all of Senegal. Under the most restrictive rules, all cafes and bars were forced to close at 6:00 p.m., car traffic was banned from 9:00 p.m. onward, and all houseowners "of the white race" were required to cover entrances and windows in mosquito nets between 6:00 p.m. and 6:00 a.m.[54] People in surveillance zones were required to carry sanitary passports, which had to be updated every three days, and hospitalization was mandated even for relatively mild and common symptoms such as fever. The Dakar municipal budget was given a 3 million franc boost for the funding of sanitary teams and cleanup projects.[55] The new rules enabled the government to punish miscreants with fines ranging from 500 to 5,000 francs, imprisonment of up to three years, or immediate deportation, if the culprit was not a French citizen or subject.[56] After a thorough scolding from the minister of the colonies and facing political unrest at home, the Government-General was hoping to restore its lost confidence.

The new situation proved particularly favorable to the Pasteur Institute, as the government was eager to seize on any opportunity that might make it appear proactive. Dr. Mathis proposed as early as August that the Dakar bacteriological laboratory might serve as a resource for curbing the epidemic. Yet it was only when the government found itself increasingly under attack by all constituents that it sought to capitalize on the Pastorians' perceived neutrality. Carde enthusiastically promised to fund the travel of top Parisian bacteriologists to Dakar to study the disease, gave them prominent seats on the sanitary council, and bankrolled an international conference on yellow fever in the early months of 1928. "The Governor-General Carde demanded the creation of a [yellow fever] mission by the Pasteur Institute. . . . My little telegram set in motion an action that I could not foresee," wrote the surprised scientist to his friend Mesnil.[57]

As the bacteriologist Émile Marchoux explained the intricacies of yellow fever epidemiology to the news-reading public in Paris, two other Pastorians, Jean Laigret and Auguste Pettit, set sail toward Dakar. What the Pastorians encountered on arrival was more than a little stunning:

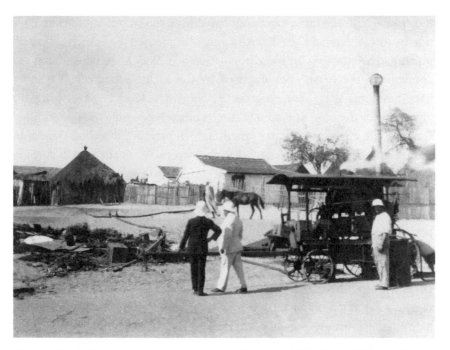

Figure 6.3 A Clayton apparatus at work in Dakar in 1927. Rockefeller Archive Center.

Maritime trade with the West coast was interrupted. The large trade ships no longer sailed. . . . [In Dakar], I was greeted by an unforgettable sight: a totally paralyzed city, the harbor bereft of ships, merchandise abandoned on the pier, fear in all the faces and utterings of the inhabitants. . . . the city deserted, the streets completely empty, the doors and windows of all the houses shut as soon as the sun set, the prohibition to be outside under pains of an eight-day confinement in quarantine.[58]

The Pastorians distanced themselves from the colonial administration both rhetorically and in practice. In newspaper interviews, they condemned the administration for both its initial lack of action and its later overreach. Marchoux, in an interview with *Le Matin*, noted that "the hygiene service needs to be not an advisory organization, but an executive body with the necessary staff and budget," and that sanitation activities had to be undertaken "without being vexatious. Under no circumstances should they cause additional trouble for the *indigènes*."[59] With these statements, he was attempting to appease both the Europeans, concerned over the lack of authoritative action by the government, and the Africans, who accused the French of disproportionately harassing the black population of Dakar. Elsewhere, Marchoux condemned the harsh fines imposed by the October decrees: "Penalties have never made hygiene progress; it's the worst kind of advertising. To give a doctor the power to forcibly enter a household and write out criminal charges, is to close the door to hygienists."[60] In private, Pastorians were even more candid: Laigret reportedly called the government's attempts at curbing the epidemic "nothing but bluff and lies," resulting in an official complaint to the minister of the colonies.[61]

As an alternative to the government's coercive methods, Pastorians proposed what they deemed a scientific approach, focused on vaccination and sanitation, and drawing on research and best practices from abroad. They envisioned a variety of innovations. The bacteriologists could study the curious immunity of the blacks to yellow fever. They could take advantage of a Pastorian outpost in the jungles of Guinea and experimentally infect monkeys with the disease. They could collaborate with other colonial governments struggling with the disease in Nigeria, the Gold Coast, and elsewhere.[62] Journalists and European Dakarois praised the involvement of the Pasteur Institute to no end.[63] Even Blaise Diagne "expressed his joy at the departure of the Pettit mission" and praised Governor Carde at finally taking personal command of the emergency.[64] It appeared that with the arrival of the Pastorians, a long-term solution was finally in sight. It did not hurt that with the end of the rainy season, the number of yellow fever cases fell markedly: in November, the number of confirmed cases dropped by half to twenty-three, and in December, only six new cases were registered in the entire colony of Senegal.[65]

Parisian Pastorians were not the only new arrivals to the diseased port city. The fight against yellow fever unexpectedly took on a transnational dimension. When Jean Laigret disembarked in Dakar and observed the deserted city with its curfews, locked doors, and closed windows, he also noticed an out-of-place foreigner observing his surroundings with evident curiosity. Years later, he wrote of this encounter: "One morning a passenger disembarked, came straight to see me and introduced himself: 'Watson Sellards, professor at Harvard University in Boston.' . . . It was the start of a friendship that was to last fifteen years."[66] This encounter signaled the degree to which Franco-African fights over the politics of disease containment participated in a larger, global history of yellow fever. This history, which encompasses

Rockefeller missions to Latin America, Anglo-American projects in British Nigeria, a South African scientist working in New York, a Pastorian rivalry reignited in Tunisia, and imperial rivalries played out on the pages of popular and specialized science magazines, forms the subject of the next chapter.

Conclusion

The Rockefeller Foundation had been investigating the possibility of setting up a West African yellow fever commission already since 1920. On numerous occasions, its representatives had visited both French and British territories, as well as Liberia and even parts of the Belgian Congo.[67] Yet despite numerous visits to Dakar and Conakry and lunches with the governor-general and various health officials, the Rockefeller advance guard reported progressively declining enthusiasm. If, in their initial reports, French territories appeared as some of the most promising locations for their base, by 1925, Rockefeller scientists experienced a skeptical reception on the part of the French. One report described French attitudes as follows: "It was intimated that yellow fever is not of particular interest in the French African territories as they do not consider it endemic there, but imported from British possessions."[68] Three years later, the French dramatically shifted course and launched their own research program. The Pasteur Institute's yellow fever vaccine project was at time in competition, and at times in collaboration, with parallel efforts in Britain and at the Rockefeller Foundation.

Understanding how the AOF went from a region with little interest in yellow fever to being the hub of Jean Laigret's vaccine project requires understanding not just the changing epidemiological reality but also its connections to the historical and political reality of the AOF. It was not obvious that the yellow fever epidemic would become such a catalyst for French science. After all, the plague epidemics of previous decades had claimed far more lives. Nor was it obvious that the Pasteur Institute would be the right organization to lead the countercharge. After all, during plague outbreaks, administrators often ignored Pastorian advice in practice, even if they celebrated it in their rhetoric. Yellow fever mattered because it struck Europeans rather than Africans. It upset far more powerful constituencies than the plague and evoked images of historical epidemics, which were entrenched in the memories of many Frenchmen stationed in Dakar. It escalated political conflicts because it provided African leaders with prima facie evidence of

French hypocrisy and racism—it proved that Africans were not less hygienic than Europeans and that the French were unwilling to impose on themselves the kinds of measures they had forced on Africans. Microbes and viruses do not exist outside of history, politics, and culture. In this instance, changes in microbiological conditions precipitated changes in the political and scientific fields.

Yet the precise implications of new microbiological conditions depended on the tools with which they were apprehended, and on the politics through which their impacts were evaluated. The yellow fever virus is made visible through its effects on the human body—through jaundice, fever, and diarrhea—but also through scientific observation and technological manipulation. In 1932, Georges Stefanopoulo's new seroprotection tests revealed the presence of yellow fever antibodies in Africans. As the next chapter will show, experts and officials then refocused their attention on the *indigènes*, whom they now saw as "reservoirs" of disease, as invisible and therefore perhaps even more dangerous carriers. Viruses could change politics and science, but microbiology itself was fundamentally unstable. How French and African observers understood microbiological reality depended itself on the tools of observation and the location of those doing the observing. All three factors—the microbes themselves, the technology of observation, and the spaces of observation—shaped the Dakar vaccine project.

7

Africa in the Global Race for a Yellow Fever Vaccine

In 1952, a quarter-century after the Dakar yellow fever epidemic, British medical experts invited Jean Laigret to Lagos, Nigeria, to get his opinion on an unexpected development. An outbreak of yellow fever in Lagos had prompted British authorities to mandate mass vaccinations with the Dakar strain, the vaccine Laigret had helped develop in the 1930s. By that point, more than thirty million doses had already been distributed in French West Africa, and the vaccine had become the standard weapon against the deadly tropical disease.

Laigret observed a disturbing development in Nigeria. Hospitals in the southern region were admitting increasing numbers of Africans, most of them children, with encephalitic symptoms: high fever, headache, confusion, and convulsions. These cases were frequently deadly. In one instance, thirty-two out of eighty-two children perished. Even more concerning was the one trait all patients had in common: they had all come from the Enugu township, by the River Niger, which had no history of yellow fever. Recently, however, all patients had been vaccinated with the Dakar strain as part of the public health campaign.[1]

Laigret realized that he had seen similar symptoms before. During the trial phase of the Dakar yellow fever vaccine, the bacteriologist had frequently observed severe neurological side effects, although never fatal ones. The year 1934 "was the first time, when I observed meningoencephalitis after yellow fever vaccination. I have now observed more than ten such cases," he admitted in 1953.[2] Later studies confirmed his suspicions: the Ibo deaths were caused by the Dakar vaccine itself. Most likely the vaccine virus, which was cultivated in the brains of lab mice, had mutated in the process of production. This was a possibility that Pastorians had discussed already during the development of the vaccine. As cases of fatal encephalitis accumulated over the years, the Dakar vaccine was eventually discontinued from use with children under the age of ten in 1960, and production stopped completely in

Pasteur's Empire. Aro Velmet, Oxford University Press (2020). © Oxford University Press.
DOI: 10.1093/oso/9780190072827.001.0001

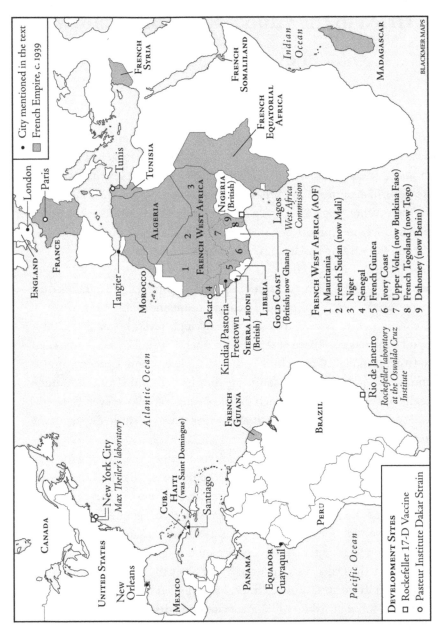

Map 3 Yellow fever vaccine laboratories.

1980. The vaccine was replaced with the safer 17D vaccine developed at the Rockefeller Foundation. Yet the question remains: If Pastorians knew of the dangers posed by the Dakar vaccine already in the 1930s, why did they not address this issue until several decades later?

The tragic end of the Dakar strain is but a coda in the vaccine's long history, layered with contradictory meanings and unexpected political consequences. The vaccine project was born in Dakar, in the throes of the political conflict during the 1927 epidemic, as described in the previous chapter. It then became a weapon in a battle for imperial and national prestige, as Pastorians raced against British colonialists and scientists at the American Rockefeller Foundation in developing a viable vaccine strain. For a brief moment, in 1930s Paris, the vaccine became the subject of an ethical controversy surrounding its neurological effects, but these concerns were quickly effaced, as Pastorians moved the development and deployment of the vaccine back to Africa, where other priorities prevailed. For nearly two decades, the Dakar strain was the symbol of effective, Pastorian public health. Teams of soldiers vaccinated millions of Africans in the AOF in the late 1930s and early 1940s. It was only in the 1950s and 1960s, when decolonization disrupted old networks of authority and expertise, that the dark side of the vaccine became visible once again.

Understanding how this vaccine became the basis for mass vaccination campaigns despite the Pastorians' own concerns over its safety requires using all the tools of analysis developed in the previous chapters. We need to take a global lens and follow the vaccine project as it traveled across countries and continents over its decade-long development cycle. The Dakar strain was shaped by microbiological contingencies, by technological obstacles, by unexpected political and scientific debates that emerged in transit, and, finally, by the visibilities and occlusions produced by the laboratories' and public infrastructures, which constituted the foundation of the vaccine's development and deployment. At its core, this chapter highlights the Pastorian politics of scale and mobility: the role physical and imaginative spaces played in solving the political and material problems that emerged during the vaccine's development. The ambiguous success of grand Pastorian projects has long fascinated scholars. Noémi Tousignant has written about the failures of Eugène Jamot's mission to eradicate sleeping sickness, and Guillaume Lachenal has analyzed the politics of failure in the postwar fascination with Lomidine. This chapter highlights the pan-imperial and international web of uneven regulations, unequally equipped laboratories, and wavering rivalries that surrounded such African campaigns.[3]

In the first section of the chapter, mobility emerges as both the source of and the solution to various microbiological problems. Pastorians in Dakar and Rockefeller scientists in Lagos sought to transport a sample of the yellow fever virus to better-equipped laboratories outside of Africa, but neither could find a suitable host animal. For Pastorians, epistolary mobility helped solve the problem of viral immobility: In Lagos, A. Watson Sellards's colleague Adrien Stokes sent a letter to Dakar shortly before his own death, describing how rhesus monkeys could be used to transport the yellow fever virus. Yet if rhesus monkeys worked for moving the virus within a network of laboratories (from Dakar to Paris), then producing the vaccine at an industrial scale required a different beast. Here, too, research networks across institutions and across empires proved fruitful. Different imaginations of scale and space simultaneously created and solved problems for the Pastorians.

The second section focuses on how spaces of debate inflected the problems of ethics and engineering that emerged in the vaccine's production. In France, the vaccine became entwined in a broader debate over the prestige of French science and emblematic of colonial rivalries with the British Empire and scientific rivalries with the Rockefeller Foundation. Much like BCG, different versions of the Dakar vaccine were challenged on the account of safety. As some Pastorians began to imagine Africans, and not Europeans, as the primary recipients of the vaccine, however, this ethical calculus changed. When human testing of the vaccine moved to Tunisia and French sub-Saharan Africa, concerns of individual safety fell by the wayside, replaced with concerns about hidden "disease reservoirs." Several engineering decisions made in this period likely amplified the ill effects of the vaccine.

The final section of the chapter looks at the mass vaccination campaigns in the AOF, undertaken even as some members of the Pasteur Institute harbored suspicions about the vaccine's safety. Here, I highlight the ways in which the imperial management of vaccine politics was *infrastructural*, in at least two senses.[4] First, the advantages of the Pastorians' colonial alliances rested literally in existing infrastructure: in the laboratories built with colonial subventions, which enabled Pastorians to harvest and study samples of the virus; the Pastoria field site in Kindia, which supplied monkeys for experimentation; and the shipping lines that moved researchers between Dakar, Paris, and Tunis. These infrastructures allowed Pastorians to switch research sites as needed and gain access to more sophisticated technologies. Second, the management of vaccine politics manifested itself in the systemic *absence* of infrastructure, which provided the kind of low-constraint environment the Pastorians needed to roll out their vaccine. A lack of public record-keeping, medical infrastructure, and adequate personnel meant that outside of the hospitals of Dakar, African patients could not be properly monitored, certainly not for the twelve to fourteen days it took for the vaccine's harmful effects to manifest. The inability of metropolitan critics to travel to Africa, or of Africans to participate in medical debates, meant that Pastorians could operate with wider latitude in the AOF than they could in the metropole. Infrastructures, as Susan Leigh Star and Karen Ruhleder have argued, are embedded and transparent; they are nested within other technologies and work "invisibly."[5] When infrastructure works, its users do not have to think about it. The same is often true for a lack of infrastructure. If scientists do not notice the hospital infrastructure, the dense web of medical and lay journalism, and the institutions of accountability, all of which render ill effects of drugs visible to the population at large in France, they similarly may not notice how the absence of these infrastructures renders vaccine dangers invisible in Africa. This aspect of colonial power has often been overlooked in scholarship, largely because colonial archives tend to reproduce these inequalities—one needs infrastructure to build archives, too.[6]

Microbial Actors and International Networks

The arrival of A. Watson Sellards pulled the French state and the Pasteur Institute into an ongoing international conversation both had thus far mostly ignored. Sellards was the head of the Harvard Medical School and a longtime collaborator with the Rockefeller Foundation, both organizations with long-standing interest in yellow fever. The disease was common in the Caribbean and South America, and it occasionally made its way to the southern United States, most notably Louisiana. The foundation had been involved in sanitation efforts in Brazil and Cuba and had long sought to establish outposts in West Africa, widely believed to be the "native" home of the disease. Once researchers in Dakar began serious work on the disease, they had to contend with the Rockefeller Foundation: both as a source of authoritative knowledge and experience and as a direct competitor. The foundation's own yellow fever commission in Lagos was also working on a vaccine, and a number of questions about the etiology and epidemiology of yellow fever remained unanswered. What microbiological agent caused the disease, how it was transmitted, which population groups had immunity and why—all these questions were being debated in 1927. Providing answers, not to mention a vaccine, could yield substantial scientific prestige.

The development of the Dakar strain needs to be situated within this international and imperial context, where American, British, and French organizations stood to lose or gain institutional and national prestige, and rival empires worried about being dependent on a different foreign power for public health needs. Here, Pastorians and Rockefeller Foundation scientists oscillated between competition and cooperation, as they shared a scientific and public health problem in need of a solution, and were divided by institutional and imperial rivalries. In this complex political environment, unexpected microbiological events played key roles in nudging the relationship between Pastorians and Rockefeller scientists from competition toward cooperation. In the complicated environment where scientific allies could also be imperial competitors, biological contingencies could often determine the difference.

The Pasteur Institute and the Rockefeller Foundation had a long history of both cooperation and competition. Beyond the uneasy relationship around tuberculosis prevention, which was explored in chapters 4 and 5, the institute and the foundation had also crossed paths in yellow fever research. For decades, the main French reference point for bacteriology in the Americas had been Brazil. In 1898, Oswaldo Cruz, a prominent Brazilian bacteriologist trained at the Pasteur Institute, established a microbiological laboratory in Rio de Janeiro to produce Yersin's plague serum and the Haffkine lymph, in order to protect the country against the spreading plague pandemic.[7] In 1900, following an outbreak of yellow fever in Senegal, prominent Pastorians Paul-Louis Simond, Albert Salimbeni, and Émile Marchoux traveled to Rio de Janeiro in the hopes of learning more about the disease during an active epidemic. That mission established the already prevalent prejudice of black "racial immunity" as a virtual fact in French medical science.[8] Nearly two decades later, the Oswaldo Cruz Institute found new collaborators at the Rockefeller Foundation and began an extensive public health campaign to eradicate mosquito habitats, improve sanitation, and install mosquito nets, greatly decreasing incidents of yellow fever infection in Rio. Pastorians in the AOF, who traced their research back to the work of Simond, Marchoux, and Salimbeni, were well aware of the Rockefeller Foundation's success in

Brazil—and were they to forget, critics of the AOF government's indecisive response would not hesitate to remind them of the comparison.[9]

Much like the Pastorians, the Rockefeller Foundation's interest in yellow fever grew out of imperial politics. The US South, most notably New Orleans, regularly suffered yellow fever outbreaks, and although most long-time residents had acquired immunity through childhood exposure, new populations were exposed to the risk of disease as migration to the United States increased. Mariola Espinosa has argued that fear of Cuban outbreaks spreading to the US South in part motivated the US war with Spain and the occupation of Cuba in 1901. There, US medical forces undertook a massive campaign to eradicate mosquito breeding grounds in hopes of halting the spread of the disease. The Platt Amendment to the Cuban constitution, which ended the occupation, mandated that the island nation retain the sanitary standards put in place by the United States. This set a model for the practice of US involvement in the sanitary politics of nearby states, as well as a model for yellow fever eradication—the destruction of mosquito breeding grounds.[10] This model was adopted by General William Gorgas, a founding member of the Rockefeller Foundation, who further tested the efficacy of eradicating yellow fever by destroying "key centers" of mosquitos before the opening of the Panama Canal in 1914. Finding the exercise successful, he directed the foundation's International Health Division (IHD) to the cause and took the eradication campaigns first to Guayaquil, Ecuador, and then to Brazil. Drawing from high-profile successes in Cuba and Panama, Gorgas was confident that yellow fever campaigns would establish the foundation as a major player on the international stage.[11]

Yellow fever quickly became the central focus of the IHD, consuming between 40 and 60 percent of its budget in the interwar years. After campaigns in Ecuador, Mexico, Peru, and Brazil, the IHD looked toward West Africa. In 1920, the division commissioned a report to study potential sites for establishing a research center. Dr. Juan Guiteras, the lead investigator, proposed three locations: Dakar in the AOF, Freetown in Liberia, and Lagos in British Nigeria. All three were close to sites of minor outbreaks, but Dakar and Lagos offered additional advantages. Both were "great commercial centres of the Coast," with already existing laboratories and good communication with the interior and the exterior. The sites also had large European populations, which the Rockefeller scientists assumed were more susceptible to the disease.

Dakar, in particular, was attractive, since it was well-stocked and easily ac-
cessible by sea, with a large population of mixed-race citizens whom Guiteras
considered "a better touchstone than the Negro."[12] At the same time, yellow
fever outbreaks were markedly more common in British colonies, particularly in Nigeria and the Gold Coast, which recorded an epidemic almost
every year from 1910 onward.[13] In 1925, Dr. Henry Beeuwkes traveled to the
three cities, meeting with colonial officials, local bacteriologists, and other
elites and hoping to secure a site for the new project. Yet the enthusiasm of
AOF administrators had waned. Dr. Lasnet, the head of the sanitary service
in particular, dismissed Beeuwkes's interest, suggesting that the disease was
mostly a problem for the British and that the AOF had not suffered a single
major outbreak in the twentieth century.[14] Beeuwkes also corresponded with
Calmette, who had just unveiled the BCG vaccine and had similarly limited
interest in working with his primary rival.[15]

The British were more accommodating: having secured the support of the Colonial Office in London, Beeuwkes and his partner, Henry
Hanson, approached authorities in Nigeria and soon set up a settlement
of six well-equipped buildings, six acres of land, and around ten American
bacteriologists with many more local subalterns in a compound on the out-
skirts of Lagos.[16] From there, Beeuwkes and his collaborators organized
missions inland. They observed epidemics in progress, charted the ende-
micity of the disease, and studied whether other mosquitoes besides the
Aedes aegypti could transmit the illness.[17] The region quickly became the
largest recipient of Rockefeller yellow fever funding, after Brazil. From 1925
to 1928, the foundation dedicated about half of its roughly $500,000 yellow
fever budget to West Africa.[18] When new cases were reported in 1926, the
Rockefeller West Africa Commission, which at the time was led by the ambitious British bacteriologist Adrien Stokes, was ready to investigate.

The Pastorian vaccine program, then, was a late arrival. Indeed, Rockefeller
scientists were generally unimpressed with the French response. When
Beeuwkes attended the French yellow fever conference in Dakar following
the 1927 epidemic, he wrote back to the director of the foundation with a
blunt critique of health officers' "sketchy" epidemiology, the "deplorable"
sanitary conditions, and in particular the lack of antilarval work of the sort
promoted by the foundation in South America. In terms of vaccine development and bacteriological research, Beeuwkes was skeptical as well: "The
papers read by the French were not particularly illuminating, and as we did
not wish to ask embarrassing questions, we are not clear as to all steps taken

to combat the epidemic."[19] Beeuwkes, Stokes, and others in Nigeria did indeed seek greater cooperation with the Pastorians, expressing hope that "one or more of their better men might visit [Lagos] at our expense." However, higher-ups in New York cautioned against an overly cavalier exchange of information, reminding the scientists in Lagos that it was "unfortunate that news of your work has spread by the grapevine telegraph to the French in advance of its publication."[20] While taking an interest in their work, Rockefeller scientists considered Pastorians inferior competitors. The feeling, no doubt, was mutual.

Two unexpected biological problems brought the two institutions closer into each other's orbits. The connecting link was Sellards, a Harvard bacteriologist who had rejected a position at a Rockefeller-funded public health laboratory in Manila on the account that the work there was too "routine" and "practical."[21] After a brief stint in Brazil, he traveled to Dakar, in search of the biggest epidemic, and began working with Laigret and Mathis on a potential vaccine. The three bacteriologists soon isolated the yellow fever virus

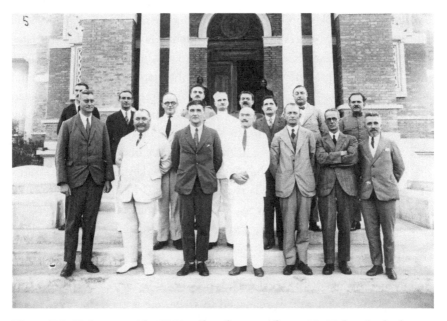

Figure 7.1 Delegates at the 1928 yellow fever conference in Dakar. In the first row, third from the left, is Jean Laigret, third from the right is Henry Beeuwkes, first from the right is A. Watson Sellards, and second row third from the right is Constant Mathis. Rockefeller Archive Center.

from samples taken from a Syrian patient, François Mayali, in 1928. Quickly, however, they faced a new problem: the Dakar facilities were not properly equipped for developing a vaccine, and the virus had to be transported to Paris for further study. But how could the scientists keep the virus alive for the duration of the trip?[22]

Alas, the only man with the answer was a direct competitor. In Lagos, Adrien Stokes struggled with the same problem. Yellow fever outbreaks often occurred far from Lagos, and access to patients was limited. In order to study the virus, and to develop a vaccine, it would have to be preserved and cultivated—but how? Stokes's answer was to have "as many varieties of monkeys as he could" shipped over from Hamburg and London, in the hopes that one of the species would be susceptible to yellow fever and could therefore be used as a vehicle for cultivating the virus. His experiment was a success: the Indian monkey, *Macacus rhesus* was successfully infected, both with injections of contaminated blood and by way of captured mosquitoes that had recently fed on yellow fever victims. Soon, more specimens were shipped to Lagos to keep the Rockefeller experiments going.[23]

Handling monkeys was a dangerous business. It may have been a chimpanzee bite that Stokes suffered when handling the monkey, or a later bite by one of the Indian monkeys that was subsequently exposed to infected material. It might have even been a stray mosquito feeding on one of the lab animals that made it past the nets or, quite simply, a laboratory accident. What is certain is that on 16 September 1927 Stokes came down with high fever, headache, joint pain, and, soon after, jaundice. His colleagues immediately suspected yellow fever, sent him to the hospital, and isolated the laboratory to protect other scientists and workers. Stokes himself, ever the scientist, demanded that his blood be injected into monkeys so that new strains of the virus might be recovered. Two days later, his health seemed to have improved. Stokes asked for new reading material and planned for returning to work in the coming days. Knowing the standard progression of yellow fever, though, his colleagues remained cautious—and, alas, their concerns were founded. Less than a day later, Stokes began vomiting blood; he died quietly on the night of 19 September.[24]

During his illness, Stokes managed to write one letter. He sent it to his friend in Dakar, A. Watson Sellards, describing in detail the process by which the yellow fever virus could be transmitted to, and then cultivated in, rhesus monkeys. Building on Stokes's research over the next few months, Sellards, Laigret, and Mathis acquired monkeys first from Paris and then from the institute's zoological station in Pastoria, Guinea, and infected them either through injections of blood drawn from infected patients or through subcutaneous insertions of organ tissue drawn from the autopsies of patients who did not survive the infection.[25] Using rhesus monkeys as vessels, Pastorians then transported the virus back to Paris, where the full power of the *maison-mère* could be brought to bear on its study.

The Paris team, which expanded to include Auguste Pettit and his student Georges Stefanopoulo, experimented with a number of ways of inducing immunity in test animals. Ultimately, they succeeded thanks to the help of another Rockefeller scientist, Max Theiler, an old friend of Sellards's. Theiler discovered that the virus could be cultivated in the brains of lab mice—a cheaper, faster, and altogether more successful alternative to other, larger animals such as rhesus monkeys. Sellards quickly wrote his colleagues at the Pasteur Institute in Paris and invited them to New York to learn from Theiler's technique firsthand.[26] Armed with the Dakar strain and Theiler's technique, Sellards, Pettit, Laigret, and Stefanopoulo cultivated a murine yellow fever virus, which at its 125th passage conferred immunity to rhesus monkeys with only mild neurological side effects. Sellards's international connections had once again allowed the Pasteur Institute to move its research on the Dakar strain one step forward.

Excited by the prospects of a viable vaccine, Sellards volunteered to be the first human test subject of the vaccine. Here, however, he hit a wall: Émile Roux, the director of the Paris institute, unequivocally denied him permission. This was not an unreasonable response, given that several researchers in the anglophone world, from Stokes to Theiler, had contracted yellow fever in the laboratory. The disease had a reputation for getting out of control.

Institutional and national rivalries then motivated Sellards, Laigret, and others to proceed without Roux's consent. In the United States, Sellards was finding increasingly less support for his research, as the Rockefeller Foundation concentrated yellow fever researchers in New York, while Sellards was unwilling to leave his job as the head of the Harvard Medical School. "Harvard is humoring Rockefeller, who wants to have an *exclusive monopoly* on the studies of yellow fever, and has indicated Sellards that he should not be counting on getting research funds in the future. . . . It is for this reason that he wants to return to Paris," explained Constant Mathis to his friend Félix Mesnil in early 1931.[27] The Pastorians, too, felt the ongoing rivalry between them and the Rockefeller Foundation, as well as the importance the project had for France's imperial prestige. At one conference in 1935, Laigret gently corrected a delegate who suggested that the yellow fever vaccine was at the heart of an "Anglo-French rivalry" by saying that the competing process was "not English, but American" and adding that "the time is near when even the Central and Southern American countries will follow the lead of French colonies."[28] Those were, of course, countries that had collaborated with the Rockefeller Foundation, and where Pastorian superiority would have to be reasserted. As Sellards and others were looking for a colonial location to carry out the human trials Roux had vetoed, one man, ever keen to enter into conflict with the *maison-mère*, was happy to oblige. In 1931, Charles Nicolle invited the yellow fever researchers to experiment in his laboratory in Tunis, kicking off the next phase of development.

As the yellow fever experiment moved beyond Dakar, Pastorians plugged into an intricate system of international and imperial networks. They navigated personal relationships, institutional rivalries, and various colonial and metropolitan laboratories. Yet the contours of their travels were shaped as much by local biological contingencies as by strategic scientific and political decisions. The lack of yellow fever outbreaks in the AOF motivated health officials to decline the Rockefeller Foundation's offer of collaboration in the 1920s; the major outbreak in Dakar prompted A. Watson Sellards to choose it as his site of investigation. Adrien Stokes's illness prompted him to mail his research findings to Sellards, who brought them to the attention of the Pastorians, initiating a collaborative phase between the two laboratories during a period of rather intense rivalry. From this perspective, the circulation of the Dakar yellow fever program appears less like transnational grand strategy and more like a series of desperate attempts to manage unexpected, dramatic, and costly biological events. Stokes, Sellards, and others wished to bend the yellow fever virus to their will; the reality may have well been the reverse.

War of the Vaccines

Once Nicolle had invited Sellards and Laigret to Tunis, the Pastorians' research agenda split into two competing paths, one led by Stefanopoulo in Paris, the other by Laigret in Tunis. Both parties took advantage of the AOF government's generosity and conducted field testing in West Africa, but they nevertheless came to drastically different conclusions about what kinds of research to pursue. As the two teams were faced with problems concerning the safety of the vaccine, on the one hand, and building a simple and cheap de-livery mechanism, on the other hand, the contrasting engineering decisions they pursued had distinctly technopolitical ends. In the 1930s, Stefanopoulo conducted seroprotection tests in the AOF, which returned Africans to the center of yellow fever epidemiology as potential "reservoirs" of the disease and set the scientific basis for a series of different choices in vaccine design. Which choices the Pastorians pursued and how they turned theoretical knowledge into practical technology ultimately depended equally on bio-technological limits and political assumptions about the value of different kinds of life.

In Paris, Stefanopoulo and Pettit decided to continue experimental work on their own strain, without proceeding to human trials. They combined the vaccine prototype with a serum, hoping that the injection of yellow fever anti-bodies would reduce the danger of infection. Preliminary testing on animals was promising, but since the Paris institute was running out of monkeys, and Roux maintained the ban on human testing, the research of the Paris team ran into an impasse.[29]

Suddenly, a minor outbreak of the disease in the AOF prompted the co-lonial government to commission a thorough study of yellow fever ende-micity in 1931. Stefanopoulo became the lead investigator of the study. His job was to chart the number of people in different regions of the AOF who had contracted yellow fever in their lifetimes. The Pastorian method for de-termining this involved a seroprotection test, a new tool made possible by re-cent research on yellow fever antibodies. Researchers could draw blood from a random sample of indigènes in a region and then inject the serum collected from the sample together with a small dose of the murine yellow fever strain into lab mice. Having calculated the precise ratio of doses of the live virus to the serum, Stefanopoulo could predict that if the mouse died within ten days, then the sample did not contain yellow fever antibodies. This outcome meant that the indigène whose blood was injected to the mouse had not been exposed to the disease. If the mouse survived, then the serum did contain antibodies, meaning that the subject lived in an area where yellow fever was endemic and had acquired immunity through childhood infection.[30]

During his five-month expedition in late 1931 and early 1932, Stefanopoulo traveled to nearly all of the West African colonies: Senegal, Sudan, Upper Volta, the Ivory Coast, and Guinea. He collected 782 blood samples from fourteen different regions and performed the seroprotection tests at the Pasteur Institute in Paris. Much to the dismay of the AOF government, he confirmed that yellow fever was endemic in a number of previously un-suspected locations, most notably in areas of Upper Volta.[31] However, the expedition proved transformative for the Pastorian yellow fever vaccina-tion project for a different reason. The identification of yellow fever anti-bodies in African blood led Stefanopoulo to conclude that Africans could act as reservoirs for the yellow fever virus. This insight raised the question of whether vaccinating only the Europeans traveling to West Africa would suffice to protect those populations and eradicate the disease in the French colonies.[32]

The supposed genetic immunity of Africans to yellow fever had been a dominant, although contested, stereotype among Europeans at least from the eighteenth century, when yellow fever epidemics imported from West Africa began to spread in Caribbean slave plantations and later in the US South.[33] Pastorians reformulated this hypothesis themselves, most notably during Paul-Louis Simond's mission to Brazil in 1902. However, cases of yellow fever observed among Africans during the 1927 epidemic had begun to crack this consensus. Still, Africans clearly suffered much less from the disease, which proved so deadly for French settlers in the four communes. Stefanopoulo's serotherapy tests showed that many Africans harbored yellow fever antibodies, although only a small number claimed to ever have exhibited symptoms consistent with the disease.[34] However, mild fevers were common among African children, and Africans who had moved from parts of the colony without yellow fever to endemic areas suffered from disease just as badly as Europeans did. This, Stefanopoulo concluded, meant that yellow fever had to be a disease much like the measles or mumps—benign in child-hood, deadly in adulthood, and conferring lifelong immunity if the victim survived the initial infection. Moreover, it meant that Africans, and African children in particular, constituted a "reservoir" for the disease, as mosquitoes biting asymptomatic carriers could nevertheless spread the disease to suscep-tible Europeans and Africans without immunity. This had huge implications for public health, leading Stefanopoulo to conclude that "all the measures conceived by the 1927 decrees, prescribing surveillance measures and non-observation penalties to 'all members of the white race or with white her-itage,' be applied immediately in all their rigor on the entire population of the AOF."[35]

Metropolitan medical journalists quickly picked up the hypothesis of Africans as disease reservoirs. Articles on the phenomenon underscored the urgency of vaccine development and shifted the emphasis away from the vaccination of Europeans toward the possibility of a colony-wide mass vaccination campaign. Developing a policy for Africans and Europeans alike not only would eliminate yellow fever once and for all but also would show the French empire in all its humanitarian glory. "Only the Rockefeller foundation," lamented *Le Temps Colonial*, "has, thanks to the generosity of its founder, the resources to undertake such expensive projects," while the budgetary difficulties of the AOF government prevented large-scale deswamping and mosquito-killing expeditions from being realized.[36] Other commentators highlighted that a colony-wide sanitation effort had become more feasible, now that Stefanopoulo had shown that only certain areas in the AOF harbored the yellow fever virus. The AOF would no longer have to pay for scrubbing the entire territory but only the locations where the virus was endemic.[37]

Stefanopoulo's discoveries, combined with Anglo-American advances, further amplified the institutional and interimperial rivalries. In London, Rockefeller-sponsored scientists George Findlay and Ernest Hindle, following a similar process as the Pastorians, arrived at their own method of serovaccination, similar to Stefanopoulo's prototype. Unlike Roux, however, officials at the Wellcome Laboratories allowed them to proceed to human trials, and by 1934, Findlay and Hindle had successfully vaccinated more than two hundred volunteers in London and published several articles. Both the specialist and general presses in France were outraged by what they perceived to be an excess of caution, which had almost robbed the French of an important discovery. An opinion piece titled "A Discovery the French Did Not Wish to . . . Discover" published in the popular magazine *Le Nouveau Cri*, succinctly summarized the implications of Roux's caution:

> Here is the news . . . , a French scientist discovered and developed a vaccine for yellow fever. The effects of this serum are undisputable. . . . I sincerely believe that this news has some importance. . . . We would stop discussing the principles of "colonialism" if these "imperialists," the colonizers, knew how to save the colonized from all the scourges, the miseries, the hereditary slavery which burdens them. . . . One can colonize to empower, and not to subjugate.[38]

The writer blamed both the AOF government and the scientific community for being overly cautious, holding back a clearly viable vaccine for two years. As a result, "we are now using English materials and paying them their price.

But these are vaccines, not candy we are talking about."[39] The approval of the vaccine for human trials and subsequent use in the colonies was not only a question of medical ethics; it was a question of national prestige and imperial autonomy.

Colonial administrators understood the urgency of the problems: they were sensitive both to the potential new outbreaks and to the fame that using a French vaccine strain instead of an Anglo-American one would lend the empire. In 1934, Charles Nicolle's lobbying of the Ministry of the Colonies paid off. AOF officials invited Laigret, who had been developing a pure, live attenuated vaccine without serum in Tunis, to test his vaccine in Dakar and its surroundings. At the same time, Stefanopoulo was invited by the government of an adjacent French colony—French Equatorial Africa—to test his more conservative, serotherapy-protected vaccine on its territory. As Laigret's vaccine showed troublesome side effects, and Stefanopoulo's vaccine proved technically difficult to administer, the resulting war of the vaccines pit medical ethics against technological efficiency. Colonial racial politics determined the outcome.

Now that the vaccinable population included Africans in the AOF, colonial Pastorians developed new criteria for research, focusing more on efficiency of delivery than on individual safety. Throughout the first human trials on twelve volunteers in Tunisia, the much larger testing phase on more than two thousand subjects in Dakar, and a twenty-thousand-person trial in West Africa in 1935, Laigret and Sellards consciously tailored their vaccine for the tropical environment. They decided to develop a live neurotropic vaccine without an injection of serum, believing that without external antibodies, the body's own immune system would have more time to react to the virus vaccine. This procedure would produce a stronger, more consistent and durable immunity than the serovaccination process. The latter, developed by both Stefanopoulo in Paris and the Rockefeller Foundation at the Wellcome laboratories, showed reduced immunity already six months after vaccination.[40] Pastorians also developed a host of technical changes that made the vaccine more practical for use in the colonies: "It can be applied by all doctors. Not involving an injection of serum, there is no danger of allergic reactions. It conserves well, and can be transported by plane; test flights from Tunis to the center of Africa and back showed that tested samples remained active."[41] Moreover, a neurotropic vaccine did not require large quantities of immunized horse serum, which made its production both easier and less costly. Because the vaccine conferred long-term immunity, was cheap and easy to administer, cheap, and could be transported quickly, it was the perfect candidate for wide-scale use in the colonies. Only one problem remained: the vaccine required two booster shots to confer full immunity, a feature it shared with Stefanopoulo's serovaccination. This was not a problem when it came to vaccinating Europeans, who could get their shots in France, prior to departure, or simply return to the Dantec hospital in Dakar for revaccination. For the kinds of mass vaccinations both Pastorians and colonial officials envisioned after Stefanopoulo's discovery of the "African disease reservoir," this deficiency was critical.

Laigret soon developed a solution. By increasing the dose of the neurotropic virus in a single injection thirtyfold, and by coating the virus in egg yolk, Laigret managed to increase the absorption time of the virus vaccine and reduce the number of required injections from three to one.[42] Tests conducted by the Pasteur Institute in Dakar showed that individuals vaccinated with the coated virus quickly developed immunity that remained present well over a year later.[43] The Laigret-Sellards method seemed perfect for the sanitation projects envisioned for the AOF. There was just one problem: the new, stronger vaccine produced new, stronger side effects.

The first series of human trials with the Laigret-Sellards vaccine strain were successful: all five volunteers tested positive for antibodies and showed no harmful reactions to the vaccine. The second round of testing was more problematic: three out of seven volunteers in Tunis developed severe side effects, which included high fever, neurological symptoms (meningitis), and bloody sputum.[44] Laigret made efforts to further reduce the virulence of the neurotropic virus, and the side effects became increasingly rare in trials using the method of three consecutive injections with vaccine-viruses of increasing virulence. The vaccine nevertheless remained very unreliable: in the first round of trials in Dakar, which involved 2,164 European volunteers, test subjects regularly experienced high fevers of up to forty degrees Celsius. Two patients developed serious symptoms: intense headaches about a dozen days after vaccination, followed by a loss of movement in the extremities, stiffness of the back, and delirium.[45] Once Laigret began using the neurotropic vaccine coated in egg yolk, he proudly reported a complete loss of side effects but neglected to mention that he had only tested the coated vaccine on a small number of people—89 subjects in Paris, far too few to conclusively show that the vaccine's potential dangers had been abated.[46] Meanwhile, Mathis, who continued testing the same, coated vaccine in Dakar, was not nearly as successful: he tested the vaccine on 450 subjects, 50 of whom were African. In Europeans, the coated vaccine produced mild side effects in seventeen cases out of one hundred, moderate side effects in thirteen cases, and severe reactions—fevers of up to forty degrees Celsius and meningoencephalytic symptoms—in 9 out of 100 cases (all in all, more than a third of European test subjects had some sort of adverse reaction).[47] These effects, assured his friend Mesnil, were "nothing but normal reactions," yet they were concerning enough that Mathis warned his Parisian colleagues to expect the Laigret-Sellards vaccine to fall under heavy criticism.[48]

They did not have to wait for long. The strain was attacked by scientists at the Wellcome Institute in London and at the Rockefeller Institute, as well as by, perhaps most surprisingly, the medical inspector-general of the colonies, François Sorel in a damning report to the Office of International Public Hygiene. The basic danger, critics claimed, lay in the fact that in order for the immunity to develop, a significant quantity of the neurotropic virus had to circulate in the patient's bloodstream for some time. This created the possibility that the "barrier between the circulatory system and the central nervous system [the brain-blood barrier] is ruptured, and that the virus passes into the nervous system and causes meningoencephalitis."[49] Crucially, critics argued, serious side effects usually appeared with a considerable delay, normally ten to fourteen days after vaccination. In addition, most of the testing of the Laigret-Sellards strain was done in West Africa, where follow-up visits were difficult and tropical diseases abound, so that side effects could be confused with other common ailments. This context demonstrated to critics that, if anything, the French were underreporting the number of problematic cases.[50] While Stefanopoulo's serovaccination procedure, too, had caused one much-discussed incident of severe meningoencephalitis, it still appeared to be a safer, more consistent alternative, with the serum limiting the amount of time the live virus circulated in the peripheral bloodstream. Both Rockefeller scientists and Findlay concluded: "For all these reasons, we consider serovaccination as the only usable procedure at this stage."[51]

Parisian scientists tended to agree. The Society of Exotic Pathology held a hearing after a particularly difficult case of meningoencephalitis suffered by Jacqueline B., who developed symptoms after being vaccinated against yellow fever. Eleven days after the injection, her temperature jumped to forty degrees Celsius. She developed narcolepsy, slowed reflexes, hallucinations, and mild meningital symptoms, ultimately losing consciousness for several days before finally recovering, more than three weeks after being admitted to the Pasteur Hospital.[52] At the following meeting, the officers of the society suggested that, in all likelihood, the severe case of meningoencephalitis was caused by the mutation of the yellow fever virus cultivated in the brains of mice, the basic building block of the vaccine. "This provides, in any case, the certainty of danger for any vaccination based on nonsterilized mice brains. Increasingly the mouse appears to us as a dangerous animal," the rapporteurs concluded.[53] The Ministry of the Colonies, which conducted its own inquiry, came to a similar conclusion, with Medical Inspector-General Sorel suggesting that due to the difficulty of long-term observation in West Africa, the number of neurological side effects was likely to be much higher than reported. Monitoring, he suggested, was necessary "not only in the days following inoculation, but in the following several months," concluding that it would be "desirable and cautious not to plan systematic, widespread application of a procedure still under study."[54]

To counter these criticisms, Laigret emphasized the specificity of the West African setting in shaping the results of human testing. He contrasted Parisian laboratory knowledge with African practical knowledge, and individual cautiousness in Paris with collective opportunity for Africans. While Findlay and others suggested that the tropical environment may have masked some of the vaccine's side effects, Laigret made the opposite argument: he accused Findlay of "giving a new interpretation to certain troubles which are very common in the tropics, and constitute a regular part of medical observation."[55] In essence, he accused Findlay of not knowing the tropical environment, and argued that the kind of hypersensitivity appropriate in laboratories in London or Paris was not suitable for West Africa.

He pursued this contrast between hypercautious laboratory scientists and the real experts in West Africa in another line of attack. Laigret argued that Findlay's criticism, particularly his fear of the neurotropic virus mutating into a viscerotropic strain, were based on animal testing, while the thousands of vaccinations Constant Mathis was already performing in West Africa suggested that the vaccine was perfectly safe:

Neither the frequency nor the extent of the risk [of a meningoencephalitic reaction] can be judged from experimental vaccination on monkeys. In the case of humans, the risk is limited to a reaction of about 1:5,000 odds and that, up to now, has always completely healed within a few days. . . . The work has left the laboratory, it belongs to practitioners now.[56]

Finally, Laigret shifted the debate from individual risk to collective protection. He argued that the risk of individual side effects was low enough already and was likely to be even lower among the African population, who would form the basis of a mass vaccination campaign. For Laigret, the collective protection of both Africans and Europeans achieved by the eradication of yellow fever far outweighed the risks of individual harm. "If the large application of our method is approved in regions where yellow fever epidemics are suspected, we can hope that the final reservation, which refuses this benefit to the indigenous masses, can be lifted."[57] In a speech to the Colonial Union, Laigret contrasted the risk of individual side effects with the "cost on economic and social life in Africa that the fear of yellow fever imposes," following it with a tragic story of a young doctor, Clovis Duris, who died in Zinder a day before the arrival of the vaccine.[58] Laigret concluded: "Adverse events following yellow fever vaccination cannot be compared for an instant to the dangers of yellow fever."[59]

Here Laigret used a technopolitical strategy to overcome a seemingly insurmountable problem: he reframed the question of vaccine safety as a cultural issue, which focused on the misunderstanding of colonial context by metropolitan scientists. Engineering a fix to the problem of vaccine safety would have meant a radical shift in Laigret's research agenda. If the neurological side effects were indeed a consequence of the vaccine virus's cultivation in the brains of mice, then resolving this issue would have meant, as some critics had suggested, attempting to cultivate an attenuated vaccine in a different animal, such as the guinea pig. This would have added years to development, without providing a certainty of success. Instead, Laigret reframed the terms of the debate. First, the safety of the vaccine was best determined not through an extrapolation of potential dangers identified in animal testing but through wide-scale practice of vaccination in the tropical environment itself. Second, in the tropical context, the most important criterion was public health at the level of the population, not risk assessment at the level of the individual. Laigret's reframing won him the support of the AOF government, which was concerned about a recurrence of a yellow fever epidemic. Crucially, the AOF government had asserted the importance of collective prophylaxis over individual treatment for years.[60]

The future of the vaccine was in West Africa: further testing, according to Laigret, could only take place on a large scale and in an endemic region, and it was in the interests of the colony to approve large vaccination campaigns. Scientists in Paris softened their stance, and the AOF government powerfully backed Laigret's research, allowing him to begin mass vaccinations in West Africa. As Mathis at the Dakar Pasteur Institute continued to vaccinate using the coated Laigret-Sellards strain, he declared in the middle of 1936: "The battle for the yellow fever vaccine has been won."[61]

Some metropolitan Pastorians and Rockefeller researchers remained concerned. Stefanopoulo, in particular, was very troubled, since the apparent success of Laigret's vaccine and the lack of attention to its defects were rendering his own serovaccination project obsolete. "[The vaccine] is unfortunately supported . . . by the authority of Mr. Nicolle, a member of the Institute, and by characters who are not afraid to kill some of their fellow creatures to gain experience and particularly to infect negro populations who remain outside of 'statistics,'" wrote the researcher to his colleagues at the Rockefeller Foundation in 1934.[62] He highlighted the severity of neurological reactions in lab animals (nearly all rhesus monkeys that developed encephalitis after receiving the pure vaccine had ultimately died). He feared that the vaccinations may have caused unrecorded deaths and wanted to take up the issue at the Office of International Public Hygiene. As the AOF's plans to expand human trials in Senegal advanced, Stefanopoulo became ever more concerned. "My dear Doctor Sawyer," he wrote to his Rockefeller colleague (his own salary at the Pasteur Institute was partly funded by a Rockefeller grant), "please, I beg you, come over here to support me for a few days. Alone, my voice is too feeble."[63] His Rockefeller colleagues rebuffed him, suggesting that he focus on a different line of research and leave developing an alternative vaccine to the Rockefeller team. Sawyer, director of the Rockefeller Foundation's yellow fever program, responded that "it begins to look as if the danger of the [Laigret] method in the experimental animal is much greater than the danger in man," and promised that the foundation was making progress in developing even safer strains.[64] Years later, Rockefeller scientists acknowledged (and quite possibly shared) the sense that the success of Laigret's vaccination campaign depended on a colonial relationship with the recipients of the vaccine. One report on the potential uses of the Dakar vaccine in South America read as follows:

In dealing with native populations in Africa . . . vaccination by the French method and with the French neurotropic strain may be permissible. It is the feeling, however, in Brazil that it would not be advisable to apply a method, which might, though rather rarely, give rise to encephalitis. A strong feeling of the rights of man prevails in Brazil, as I believe it does in most South

American countries, and if serious reactions were prone to occur as a result of the vaccinations, it might readily become impossible to vaccinate.[65]

In colonial West Africa, the ethical calculus was rather different. There, scientific prestige and projection of imperial power trumped strong feelings for the rights of man.

Imperial Infrastructure and the Fall of the Laigret-Sellards Strain

Large-scale trials, Laigret's confident argumentation, and unwillingness to rely on anglophone countries for public health commodities gave the AOF government the confidence to approve the Dakar vaccine strain for mass vaccination in 1938. The campaign began properly in 1939 with the help of the colonial military and local administrations. The vaccine was made compulsory under the Vichy regime in 1941, a time when yellow fever outbreaks in military garrisons in Bamako once again raised the specter of destructive epidemics. The campaign concluded in 1946, when the Pasteur Institute claimed 14,300,735 successful vaccinations—close to total coverage in the colony with an estimated population of 16 million.[66] The Rockefeller Foundation's 17D vaccine strain, developed concurrently in the 1930s from a virus sample recovered in the Gold Coast, produced similar, although milder, complications: encephalitis in the case of one set of subcultures, and delayed jaundice in some vaccinated subjects. These harmful effects delayed its mass production until the war (although limited campaigns were conducted under the supervision of the Oswaldo Cruz Institute in Brazil). During the war, outbreaks of yellow fever in North Africa accelerated the vaccine's use.[67] Despite the existence of this alternative in the postwar years, governments in French Africa continued to use the Dakar strain, which was better suited for delivery in a colonial setting, claiming more than forty-two million vaccinations by 1953.[68] Neighboring regions—British Nigeria and the Belgian Congo—also began using the Dakar strain. Laigret's project was a success.

Over the course of the 1950s, however, more and more doctors began to notice serious, sometimes fatal complications, particularly in young children, following injections of the Laigret-Sellards vaccine. One vaccination campaign in Nigeria, conducted in 1952, produced eighty-three serious cases of meningoencephalitis and thirty-two fatalities, mostly in children under the age of ten. Another vaccination campaign in postindependence Senegal in 1965 led to 235 hospitalizations and twenty-three deaths, without accounting for those who did not seek medical attention when the neurological symptoms appeared. Reactions to the Laigret-Sellards neurotropic vaccine turned out to be particularly severe in children. Experts have estimated that a child had a one in five hundred chance of developing meningoencephalitis from the Laigret vaccine.[69] The scholar Hervé Bazin has extrapolated that mass vaccination campaigns in the AOF may have led to the deaths of up to three thousand Africans.[70] In 1958, the World Health Organization officially recommended the improved Rockefeller 17D strain as the preferred vaccine, and most countries stopped using the Laigret strain, particularly in children under the age of ten. By 1982, the Pasteur Institute of Dakar stopped manufacturing the vaccine altogether.

Laigret, Sellards, Nicolle, and Mathis were all aware of the controversy surrounding their vaccine strain since the production of the first prototype. Yet they nevertheless advocated for its use in West Africa. A number of factors contributed to the vaccine's perceived success and the erasure of the risks associated with it in the years of the first mass campaigns. First, Pastorians saw the African recipients of the vaccine in fundamentally different terms than European patients, focusing on the collective benefits of vaccination rather than on individual health risks. Second, the onset of World War II and the effects of mass mobilization vastly accelerated the pace of vaccinations, making efficient delivery even more of a priority. Finally, the infrastructural conditions on the ground, the meager resources at the disposal of the vaccination teams, and the chaotic process of rounding up patients and delivering the shots in poorly connected areas of the AOF made it nearly impossible to conduct follow-up visits and record adverse effects. Even so, official Pastorian documents recorded enthusiastic African reception and no health issues.

The differential treatment of Europeans and Africans made encephalitic consequences both more likely to happen and less observable in African recipients. European recipients were required to undergo a thorough medical examination *prior* to receiving the inoculation and were then monitored for several days after. For "the natives," "clinical examination was to be reduced to a minimum."[71] When vaccinations were made compulsory in 1941, official orders listed far more exceptions for Europeans than they did for Africans. In the case of Europeans, official instructions specified a series of contraindications: acute illness, ongoing fevers, chronic illness, liver or kidney problems, and "in general terms, any condition that diminishes the resistance of the subject."[72] For Africans, the only reason for "temporary contraindication" was "acute fever."[73] Prior clinical screenings and contraindications likely weeded out many recipients at risk of health complications, while for Africans, the primary concern was mass coverage. Early reports of vaccination campaigns noted that successful efforts in scaling up the process "permit to imagine the possibility of sterilizing this important reservoir of the virus represented by the population of West Africa."[74]

The vaccine itself was modified for the African campaign in ways that made delivery more efficient but reduced transparency and the likelihood that negative reactions would be observed by French authorities. Doctors reporting from the field commented on the great enthusiasm of Africans in receiving the vaccine.[75] This claim, however, omitted important details. To further simplify the delivery of the strain for mass campaigns, Laigret had combined his vaccine with the smallpox vaccine and made it deliverable through scarification.[76] This process was familiar to many Africans and probably made them more positively disposed toward vaccination teams. Most likely, many Africans were not even aware that they were receiving a new, controversial medication. One vaccinator noted that inhabitants of the village of Brinndoukrou refused to travel to get the Laigret vaccine, since they had recently been vaccinated against smallpox. The villagers, "having been vaccinated some days earlier, did not understand why they were being forced to travel again."[77] Often, vaccinators ordered village chiefs to round up people in a predetermined location, without specifying what sort of vaccination they would be getting. Africans, such as the villagers in Brinndoukrou, could not distinguish between yellow fever and smallpox vaccination, since they did not receive sufficient information and the procedures were functionally identical. This must have made the campaigns much easier to conduct but also made it more difficult for subjects to associate adverse effects with the vaccination process. For Europeans, the Health Service specifically prohibited "mixed vaccinations" against both smallpox and yellow fever and excluded children under the age of five altogether.[78]

The yellow fever campaign has to be seen as part of a broader series of vaccination efforts, which accelerated with the start of World War II, when the mass mobilization of colonial troops made preventive health a priority for colonial authorities. The most famous example is probably the mass therapy campaign against trypanosomiasis (sleeping sickness), conducted by the Pastorian Eugène Jamot, which has been the subject of both hagiographic and critical studies.[79] Reports of the Sleeping Sickness Service were full of examples of harmful side effects—the arsenical drugs used in the campaigns could blind people or strengthen trypanosomes, rather than killing them. Here, Pastorians used examples of therapy gone wrong to defend their preferred relationship to the colonial state, one where they were fully in charge and free from administrative oversight—not unlike the maneuvering the Pastorians had successfully used during the 1927 yellow fever outbreak.[80]

The Health Service of the AOF also conducted meningococcal vaccinations on African tirailleurs in 1939 and early 1940. This campaign, too, had a cost. On 29 February 1940, a hundred African recruits were vaccinated against meningitis in Ouagadougou by indigenous medical auxiliaries. Within the next four to eight days, forty-eight of the vaccinated soldiers reported sick with cramps and spasms, and were ultimately diagnosed with tetanus. The director of the Dakar Pasteur Institute, Dr. Durieux, flew in to observe the situation and reported forty-one deaths by the time he returned on 18 March. In his report to the Health Service, Durieux argued that the vaccine could not have been contaminated in the process of production, transport, or delivery, and he suggested "research in other directions" to determine the cause of the catastrophe. Ultimately, the episode concluded with Pasteur Vallery-Radot, the coordinator of the colonial institutes, sending a circular to researchers emphasizing the importance of maintaining the sterility of the vials in which the vaccines were stored. Repeated puncturing with syringes in the process of vaccination could contaminate the vials and lead to the kinds of infections that caused the disaster in Ouagadougou. Nevertheless, both Durieux and Vallery-Radot assured that the Pasteur Institute could continue and even expand in its role as the champion of preventive health.[81] Wartime conditions, the need for expediency, and the doubly subordinated status of the recipients—as both recruits and colonial subjects—clearly shaped the cavalier responses of medical experts.

Mass mobilization similarly accelerated the pace of yellow fever vaccinations. In the first months of 1940, the Pasteur Institute supervised seventy-five thousand vaccinations in the Ivory Coast and the Sudan, almost as many as the one hundred thousand vaccinations that were performed during the entirety of 1939. Pastorians continued to modify the vaccine in order to increase its shelf life (from one month to two months).[82] The German occupation of France and the arrival of the Vichy regime in the AOF vastly reduced the Pasteur Institute's operational capacity and nearly eliminated its research program, forcing it to focus on "practical activities," namely, vaccination. It is telling that even having lost much of the institute's personnel and with very few new resources coming in from France, the Pastorians still reported more than three hundred thousand yellow fever vaccinations by the end of 1940.[83]

Finally, the enthusiastic official reports delivered by the Dakar Pasteur Institute contrast with reports from vaccinators, who were often frustrated and reported various difficulties such as problems with rounding up people, keeping records, communicating with local chiefs, and organizing follow-up surveys. Official reports from 1941 mentioned there were "no side effects among the natives," but several cases of high fever and neurological reactions among recipients "of the white race."[84] Yet if many Europeans were excluded from vaccinations, and still suffered complications, is it really plausible that African subjects, who received the vaccine in almost all states of health, did not develop any reactions? More likely, the Pastorians' optimistic reports reflect not the safety of the vaccine but the difficulty of actually conducting reliable follow-up surveys in the challenging settings of the West African brush.

The Pasteur Institute first conducted control tests on a small number of subjects in the Dakar marina and at schools in Dakar and Rufisque in 1938. Pastorians reported that these tests showed that up to 90 percent of subjects had received immunity without complications. This claim overlooks both the tiny number of control tests under long-term surveillance and the fact that the test subjects in Dakar and Rufisque likely had better nutrition and stronger immune systems than the subjects farther out in the brush. Further control tests took place in various regions of Senegal in 1939, with test groups more similar to the actual populations that would be vaccinated in the upcoming campaigns. The tests included both regions where yellow fever was endemic and populations that likely had childhood immunity, as well as regions without recent outbreaks. The number of control tests, however, was small, as Dr. Peltier, the head investigator of the project, admitted, since, having received the vaccine, Africans traveled back to their homes and "had a hard time understanding the reasons for control tests, and spent little effort in participating in such efforts."[85] That year, the Pasteur Institute vaccinated close to one hundred thousand subjects in Senegal but performed only 1,630 control tests. The tests, in turn, relied on the availability of subjects rather than proper randomization. Finally, the control tests were performed ten days after the original inoculation, while neurological effects, as previous cases had shown, usually presented themselves about two weeks after individuals received the vaccine.[86] The timing of the tests, their small number, and the lack of proper randomization made it impossible for Pastorians to convincingly claim that the vaccine produced no side effects. They made this claim anyway.

For an example of the frustration experienced by vaccinators on the ground, take, for instance, the 1941 vaccination campaign conducted on the Ivory Coast. This was the first such campaign undertaken in a poorly developed region, far away from the vaccine's site of production. Peltier reported that vaccinators saw no ill effects in vaccinated Africans during the campaign, and that the campaign demonstrated the "safety, efficiency, and rapidity of execution of this new method, which is surely a prelude to its generalization to all the colonies of the AOF."[87] In practice, however, the procedure was so ad hoc that if any harmful effects did result from vaccination, they would have been difficult to observe *regardless*. On the Ivory Coast, local administrators and African intermediaries were required to notify villages of the upcoming vaccinations. Local chiefs were then tasked with rounding up the people to a central location, often upwards of ten kilometers from their village. Sometimes, villagers might refuse to present themselves, in which case mobile vaccination units would be sent to their location. In other cases, the villagers simply chose to ignore French orders, and vaccinators found nearly empty villages. Often a team of vaccinators would receive, for example, sixty-nine doses of the Laigret vaccine, but only five people from a distant village would present themselves to get the shots. Sometimes the vaccinators themselves had to "play *gendarmes*" and forcibly bring in people to get vaccinated.[88] Recording vaccine safety under such conditions was difficult to imagine: vaccinators had trouble keeping an accurate count of how many injections they had made per day. Vaccinated subjects quickly returned to their native villages, and vaccinators themselves had to move on in order to keep pace with their own schedule. The sheer scale of the project, combined with the lack of administrative and physical infrastructure, made it impossible to properly monitor the consequences of vaccination. One vaccinator described his mission as filled with "all kinds of difficulties," including "a total lack of preparation, except in rare cases" on the part of the African intermediaries.[89]

Pastorians in Dakar, however, took these early campaigns as prima facie evidence "that it is currently possible to vaccinate a mass of individuals against yellow fever in a minimum of time," and that "no reaction, even light, could be observed."[90] The campaign's perceived success became an important argument in making the vaccine compulsory in 1941. Yet, in reality, the

Pastorians knew very little of its actual effects on Africans outside of the privileged regions of Dakar.

After the war, when the French had already vaccinated more than fourteen million Africans in the AOF, the United Nations Relief and Rehabilitation Administration tested the vaccine on six hundred French soldiers, most of whom were told to stay away from military activity and to rest for a week after having received the vaccine. Still, some 12 percent of them had some sort of "febrile or cephalitic reaction." One group, however, "because of an error," went on a fifteen-kilometer march in open sun after being vaccinated. More than 35 percent of the soldiers in that group had some sort of reaction to the vaccine.[91] These conditions were surely closer to (and yet still far more privileged than) those endured by African subjects.

Conclusion

The transnational networks and infrastructures of the Pasteur Institute served as a way of managing local biological-material events and their political and scientific consequences. The ability of Pastorians to navigate between scientific networks in British territories, the United States, and the French empire, and to take advantage of laboratories in different ecological and political environments (the politics of scale) gave them a flexibility many of their adversaries lacked. Though Blaise Diagne and other well-connected Dakarois could lobby the National Assembly, Africans in Kaolack or M'Bour could not seek a second opinion from a hospital in Paris (or, for that matter, Dakar) when they developed encephalitic symptoms after vaccination. Critics at Rockefeller or in Paris could not observe vaccination programs in the African brush and had to take the Pastorians at their word (a situation that World War II further complicated). Roux denied Laigret the permission to conduct human trials, but he could not prevent Nicolle from permitting them in Tunis. These moves were rarely premeditated and often carried unpredictable consequences. Taken together, they provided colonial Pastorians and the imperial state with a distinct advantage.

In this process, the costs of the yellow fever vaccine were distributed according to an imperial technopolitical logic. Laigret and Sellards were developing a vaccine *for the colonies*, and their research trajectory and engineering choices were determined by colonial concerns. The vaccine had to be easy to apply in a colonial setting: leading them to amplify the dose of the live murine strain and to use scarification rather than injection as the delivery method. Safety of the individual patients was not a primary concern, since, in the empire, what mattered was the effect for the population as a whole. Finally, these arguments would have mattered little had the Pastorians not had their expansive networks or the infrastructural cover for their actions in the AOF.

"No tie can be said to be durable, and made out of social stuff," Bruno Latour once argued.[92] "It's the power exerted through entities that don't sleep and associations that don't break down that allow power to last longer and expand further."[93] In the case of the yellow fever program, it was the imperial infrastructure of overseas laboratories, combined with the fiscal, political, and legal ties to colonial governments, that continued to shaped the Pastorians' research, even as international institutions and metropolitan critics pushed them to take better stock of the ethical dilemmas inherent in their work. In this instance, the weight of colonial infrastructure superseded the voices of scientific critics.

The French scholar Hervé Bazin has discussed the yellow fever vaccine in the context of medical ethics: Should vaccination programs banish risk and be applied only when completely safe, or should problematic vaccines still be used if they deliver population-level immunity?[94] It has not been the purpose of this chapter to provide a normative answer to his question. What it has shown, however, is that scientists facing this issue in the interwar years did not engage deeply in such reflections but evaded responsibility for this dilemma altogether. They did so by taking their research to a location where ethical concerns were not aired, and by applying it to a population whose voices were denied a hearing: the African subjects of the French empire.

Conclusion

Pastorian Origins of Global Health

In the age of bourgeois empires, Pastorians built a network of laboratories in Africa, Indochina, and elsewhere, intending to empower public health experts, improve the *mise-en-valeur* of the colonies, and lift indigenous populations out of hygienic barbarity. They did not succeed. The Pasteur Institutes did not become palaces where bacteriologists could determine the fate of peoples and states as would-be kings, as Albert Calmette envisioned in the 1890s. But neither did Pastorians engage in medical nihilism, responding to public health crises in ways that, in the face of their own powerlessness, emphasize the "acceptance, rationalization as necessary, organization, and moral valuation of inaction."[1] The institutes were not projects of deferral and denial. They were not simply pretty facades hiding the naked exploitation of African and Indochinese lands and peoples. Bacteriology definitely was a form of government. The monopolization of Vietnamese rice wine using a logic of Pastorian modernity structured Franco-Vietnamese relations for decades. BCG vaccinations changed the politics of hygiene in both Indochina and France. Pastorian yellow fever research shaped urban politics in Dakar, biopolitics in West Africa, imperial politics between Britain and France, and international scientific competition and national prestige between the French Pasteur Institute and the American Rockefeller Foundation. What we need to specify are the contours of Pastorian government, its power, and its limitations.

Pasteur's empire was technopolitical. A great deal of colonial policy-making relied on translating political claims into the seemingly objective language of hygienic need or bacteriological efficiency and enacting these claims through the deployment of biotechnology. Bacteriology made it possible to argue for the monopolization of the Vietnamese rice wine industry not because French businessmen desired profits going to Vietnamese or Chinese producers, or because the colonial state needed more efficient means of tax collection, but because monopolization was based on Pastorian technologies that eliminated "impurities" and delivered a healthier product. Social hygienist forms of tuberculosis prevention were called unthinkable in

Pasteur's Empire. Aro Velmet, Oxford University Press (2020). © Oxford University Press.
DOI: 10.1093/oso/9780190072827.001.0001

Indochina not because of French fears that enabling associational life would lead to seditious activity, or because the state was unwilling to commit funds to large-scale infrastructure projects, but because Pastorians argued that appropriately modern public health measures would focus on destroying the pathogenic microbe and leave social and ecological considerations aside. Vaccinators and colonial officials focused on Africans as yellow fever test subjects not because European human trials created high-profile ethical controversies but because bacteriological expertise rendered Africans as "disease reservoirs."

Displacing politics onto biotechnology turned microbes and scientific knowledge into political forces of their own, outside the control of scientists and experts. In Indochina, the higher alcohol content and unfamiliar taste of wine produced using Calmette's Amyloprocess enabled political critiques of the alcohol monopoly, the brutality of the Douanes et Régies, reorganization of Vietnamese village life, and ultimately French rule in general. The Lübeck catastrophe bolstered the claims of European social hygienists who were uncomfortable with Calmette's assertion of expertise. Across the empire, Pastorians and administrators found that bacteriology was a double-edged sword, one that colonial subjects, rival experts, and international oversight organizations could often wield against them.

The very fact that the French had to rely on such a fragile and unpredictable form of microbial technopolitics reveals the manifold limits of imperial rule. In the case of plague outbreaks, the French were constrained by businessmen lobbying to keep the ports open, on the one hand, and the need to demonstrate scientific and administrative superiority over the British, on the other hand. With the Indochinese monopolies, orders from the Ministry of the Colonies, Chinese business interests, French entrepreneurs left out of monopoly contracts, and Vietnamese elites who lost their distilleries all pushed against administrators' and Pastorians' technopolitical plans. Indeed, the alliance between Pastorians and administrators itself was unstable and conflictual. The Pastorians learned during the plague pandemic that in order to thrive they had to make themselves indispensable to colonial officials. Still, the bacteriologists had their own interests, which did not always fit with the plans of administrators. Recall how Calmette's tuberculosis epidemiology revealed patterns of contagion that made Europeans appear as carriers of TB into virgin African soils, embarrassing the defenders of the civilizing mission and empowering the critiques of anticolonial activists.

During the 1890s plague pandemic, the Pastorians developed a specific style of technopolitics, which was premised in equal parts on techno-optimism and limited engagement—"pastorization." In contrast to social hygiene, which gained in popularity in Europe, and was dressed in equally bacteriological—indeed, Pastorian—language in the same period, pastorization in the empire meant a focus on the technical manipulation of disease-generating microbes and disrupting their effects on an abstract, generalized human body. Imperial Pastorians considered social, political, and ecological contexts essentially passive and unimportant. This stance was techno-optimistic: the Pastorians genuinely believed that their inventions would transform the empire and enable the development of colonial territories. It was also, conveniently, highly limited. Pastorization circumscribed public health actions to the domain of microbiological technologies—vaccination, industrial fermentation, serotherapy, and disinfection. It integrated conveniently well with older methods such as quarantine and sanitary cordons. This discourse permitted French officials to refrain from more expansive and costly interventions, which were being undertaken in France and ranged from mass education campaigns inspired by the Rockefeller Foundation to the improvement of living and labor conditions through infrastructure development and legislation. Overwork, malnutrition, and unsanitary housing remained unaddressed in the colonies, while in the metropole these issues were becoming increasingly intertwined with questions of public health.

Pastorization also reframed the scale of public health intervention. It imagined universal solutions, applicable across the globe, while in reality remaining grounded in the far-reaching yet uneven and patchy network of overseas Pasteur Institutes. The Pastorian network extended from Saigon to Dakar and spread well beyond the empire. Even as they competed, Pastorians had connections to both British microbiologists and research at the Rockefeller Foundation. They could borrow from as far as Denmark or bring vaccination programs from Dakar to Paris or from Tunis to Dakar. The creation of this mobile space took a lot of work. It required the construction of laboratories, supply chains, and intellectual networks. Equally important, it required imagining the empire as a single, bounded space, a space that was comparable, essentially uniform, and easily traveled—at least by Pastorians. Some of this work was cultural: over time colonial Pastorians came to see themselves as a single unit within the Pasteur Institute, with an ethos that joined them to the metropolitan Pastorians through their connection to

Louis Pasteur but that was also differentiated by their ambitious, expansive, and quasi-militarist attitude to research and public engagement. Other work was scientific: epidemiological work that encompassed the entire empire, rather than focusing on a single colony, made previously unseen patterns of disease distribution visible. We can see the importance of the connective threads of the Pastorian network in the history of BCG trials. There, Pastorian infrastructure that extended from France to Africa and Indochina, a common colonial ethos, and epidemiological studies that reframe TB as a pan-imperial problem were all central to the success of the project. A net, however, is made up of both threads and gaps. In many instances, the importance of the gaps within the Pastorian network might have been greater still.

The Pastorian world map was patchy and unequal. Not everyone there traveled at the same speed. Epidemics were made visible once they disrupted imperial governance, but otherwise they could go unnoticed. Yellow fever only became a concern once it brought about a political crisis in 1928. Indigenous actors became important once they were seen as disease reservoirs, and they faded from view once they left the hospital or, more likely, the mobile vaccination unit. These inequalities allowed Pastorians to maneuver around ethical, political, and material obstacles, conducting human trials in Africa, where observations were less precise and results magically appeared to support the Pastorians' position, while doing laboratory research in Paris, where high degrees of control were required. The world as seen by Pastorians enabled them to manage uncertainty and avoid many of the costs of medical research. All too often, those costs were instead borne by the colonized.

And yet, contours of other networks and other worlds kept seeping in through the seams. Time and again, Africans and Vietnamese turned out to be more mobile, more visible, and more adept at learning the language of Pastorian hygiene than either bacteriologists or administrators could imagine. Opponents of the Indochinese alcohol monopoly talked about the effects of factory alcohol on heredity and complained about headaches, noting that the product was neither as pure nor as hygienic as Pastorians had promised. Controversies around the management of the 1928 yellow fever epidemic made it all the way to the National Assembly. Pastorian rhetoric about the European origins of colonial tuberculosis echoed at the Anticolonial Exposition of 1931. Though the Pastorian network structurally privileged French scientists and colonial officials, technological, ecological, and scientific factors created spaces where pastorization could be pushed to work in other directions. African and Vietnamese doctors, politicians, and activists were more than up to the task.

Pasteur's empire was technopolitical, limited, pan-imperial, and highly dependent on biomaterial circumstances. This analysis has both conceptual and historiographical implications. Scholars generally agree that imperial ideologies were animated by a fervent belief in the utopian power of technology and medicine, "machines as the measure of men," and "the doctor who would be king."[2] Projects of biomedical development, in particular, have been seen as forms of deepening governmentality that produced colonial subjects, as well as the colonizers themselves. In treaty port China, Chinese elites debated what they saw as their own underdevelopment and translated biomedical concepts of public health into a reforged version of *weisheng*, which looked at Western examples for constructing "hygienic modernity" in China.[3] In the Philippines, American doctors categorized, described, and reshaped Filipino bodies from practices of defecation to mental hygiene, all the while reaffirming their inability to adapt to proper, American norms of hygiene. The inability to achieve "biomedical citizenship," Warwick Anderson has argued, also deferred political citizenship.[4] Other scholars have used Michel Foucault's notions of "biopolitics" or "power/knowledge" to describe how biomedicine and colonialism "used or attempted to use the body as a site for the construction of its own authority, legitimacy, and control" in British India, through legislation and discourse surrounding tropical epidemics, or how representations of Puerto Rican reproductive practices were used to render the inhabitants of the American territory as deviant, undisciplined, and in need of American tutelage.[5]

It is certainly true that colonial doctors had lofty ambitions. Pastorians saw themselves as the equals of "soldiers and administrators," bringing "the benefits of French civilization in their most touching and pure form to our immense colonial empire."[6] Yet there was much disagreement about how the transformation of colonial domains should be achieved. Much of the historiography has focused on domains or times when a developmentalist public health logic prevailed, and the policing of bodies, behavior, and the physical environment was indeed a priority. The overrepresentation of American colonies and territories (the Philippines, Puerto Rico, preindependence Cuba) has particularly shaped this view. In the pre–World War II era French empire, however, medical development was largely dominated by Pastorians, and while they did share the dominant idea about the potential of biomedicine, they were unique in how they defined its limits.

The Pastorian civilizing mission was a limited one, excluding or marginalizing many of the "social" aspects of Western hygiene. The Pastorians paid lip service to the importance of education and the shaping of indigenous morality, completely ignored reorganizations of urban spaces, and scoffed at much of the environmentalist work (the clearing of undergrowth and destruction of mosquito habitats) pioneered by the Rockefeller Foundation. When such efforts were conducted, Pastorians and administrators took care to note that they were outmoded, perhaps even uncivilized—only stopgap measures until a proper vaccine could be developed and deployed. This approach worked well with the goals of colonial officials, who held shoestring budgets and ruled largely through intermediaries. Colonial infrastructure could hardly sustain larger development programs prior to 1945. This approach worked well to foreclose avenues for investment that Vietnamese and African elites increasingly demanded, but it also opened up avenues for technopolitical action in limited spheres: from industry and agriculture to trade and symbolic performances of state power. The Pastorian notion of hygiene was a flexible one, limiting itself to the management of microbial life, but expansive in imagining the technological ways in which that management could be accomplished.

The biopolitical role of Pastorian hygiene, therefore, appears quite different from the conventional story. For all the talk about their responsibility for "the indigenous populations," Pastorians and administrators cared little about the behavior and bodily practices of Africans or Vietnamese.[7] Most of the time, indigenous populations disappeared quickly from the view of the Pastorians, whose attention largely focused on the metropole and on various scientific competitors. Indigenous bodies were important as carriers of microbes, as data points on epidemiological charts, and as subjects of seroprotection tests. Once the presence or absence of the *Yersinia pestis* or the *Mycobacterium tuberculosis* had been determined, the carrier no longer mattered. The conviction that the social and physical environment was of secondary importance in disease etiology, and that, regardless, Africans and Vietnamese were hopelessly unhygienic to begin with, only reinforced this focus on the disease agent. The Pastorians managed microbes, not people or spaces.

The Pastorian perspective forces us to rethink the role of "technological superiority" in the history of imperialist thought. French, British, American, German, and Belgian colonizers all believed that their superior capacity for reason and their high level of technological development gave them the right, even the duty, to civilize less-developed lands. While the evolution of this idea has been charted with considerable nuance across time, scholars working on empire often write about the idea of "European" superiority as if the idea was more or less uniformly articulated across the continent.[8] Recently, historians have highlighted different kinds of "technological styles" that emerged from different imperialist projects.[9] Take, for instance, the British preference for colony-wide, gargantuan hydrostations in Mandate Palestine, even though these stations provided far more electricity than the country needed in the 1920s. So understood, the construction of hydro dams was not simply producing electricity but also producing a specific kind of future for Palestine— a Jewish, industrialized national space with an integrated market.[10]

The French empire certainly pursued its share of gargantuan, centralized engineering projects. The most infamous of those was surely the Congo-Ocean railway, which claimed an estimated seventeen thousand lives and drew the attention of emerging international organizations to the violence of colonial rule.[11] The flagship technological marvel of the empire, however, the network of Pasteur Institutes, was a different beast. Rather than relying on massive engineering feats, it leaned largely on existing infrastructure, using the labor of administrators, soldiers, and local intermediaries to extend the reach of its laboratories, which were largely located in colonial hubs. It did seek to impress with scale, but rather than going big, the Pastorians went small, revealing entire worlds within the colonial empire that Frenchmen could explore and, of course, conquer. While infrastructure projects like the Palestine hydroenergy system or the thousands of kilometers of railways constructed across Africa focused on linking colonies to metropoles, or creating unified spaces within the confines of a single territory, the Pasteur Institute was consciously pan-imperial. It sought to link the various colonies to each other, to imagine a single space of empire that could, if necessary, bypass Paris altogether. This project, too, was producing a particular kind of future, but one that looked very different from the one brought into being by hydroelectric dams or railways. A view from the Pasteur Institutes alters quite dramatically our understanding of the French technological mission civilisatrice.

The history of Pastorian bacteriology also bears on the longer chronology of public health regimes in the Global South. Historians and anthropologists distinguish between the pre–World War II era of colonial public health and the subsequent, developmentalist period, which built on the colonial experience.[12] "International health" policies after 1945, the story goes, largely echoed the prewar colonial logic of *mise-en-valeur*, where investment in infrastructure and health care was designed for the purpose of accelerating economic development and integrating the (former) colonies into the capitalist market. At the same time, these efforts differed, by taking a broader view of the changes necessary to achieve this integration, and by focusing on raising overall living standards, tackling malnutrition, and other questions of social hygiene.[13] As international organizations, most notably the United Nations and the World Health Organization, competed with old metropoles for power over the colonies, they put in place new programs for malaria eradication, family planning, and nutritional support.[14] For a brief period in the 1960s and 1970s, as critiques of development gained ground in the West, health policies focused more on primary care and basic infrastructure, although these efforts, too, remained limited and blinkered by the belief that real expertise lay solely with the West.[15]

From the late 1970s to the early 1990s, coinciding with the rise of neoliberalism in the West and structural adjustment policies in developing countries, "a new *era* in the history of public health" emerged.[16] This regime of "global health" had a dual focus on security—the protection of the West from a variety of emerging diseases—and humanitarianism, the offering of care seemingly out of compassion rather than a profit or development motive.[17] The fight against AIDS, particularly in the new millennium, the global Ebola scare, the fight against malaria, and trials of new wonder drugs—these recent examples all demonstrate how "global health" is accompanied by a rhetoric of acute danger requiring immediate action, and an ethos of heroic triumphalism promising the eradication of this or some other disease in the very near future (but never today).[18] These interventions are often led by Western universities, transnational NGOs, or corporations and come part and parcel with structural adjustment and neoliberal economic policies that have privatized health systems and other public services in the Global South. Such health policies have—thus far—been able to mitigate some of the worst problems of the tropical world but have done little to address, and indeed, have often exacerbated, health inequalities when it comes to access to basic services and medications or the construction of fundamental infrastructure. Dying of malaria or AIDS may have become rarer in twenty-first-century Africa. Dying of malnutrition or untreated infections has become all the more common. While the era of developmentalism was hardly a panacea, it did expand services well beyond what was expected during the years of high colonialism. Pasteur Institutes conducted mobile vaccination and prevention campaigns deep into the hinterlands in Cameroon and elsewhere. It was a time many observers in Africa now regard with a sense of longing and nostalgia.[19] Most of the infrastructure constructed during the age of "international health" has been left to ruination in the age of "global health."

The ruins left to us by the age of development still eerily resemble the palaces of the age of empire. This is not just because the system of sparsely located outposts of Western research institutions, which conduct trials ostensibly for the benefit of the local population, without caring much for their input or, really, interests, echoes the pre–World War II era of high colonialism. Many of the distinctive features of the "new" age of global health can be traced directly back to infrastructures and political relations put into place in the early twentieth century. Scholars have described the world of global health as one of "de-territorialization" and "networks" and one that is "pluralist in its rhetoric," "integrative" with global markets, centered around a future-oriented "economy of promise," filled with "irregular landscape[s]," and generative of its own contradictions (an "autoimmunitary logic").[20] Colonial health unfolded in territories-turned-laboratories, international health was constrained by developmentalist empires hanging on to their power, while global health unfolds in a globalized world—or so the story goes.[21] Yet as the history of Pastorian bacteriology shows, the infrastructure for tightly yet unevenly networked pan-imperial research laboratories that global health programs exploit today was first laid in the late nineteenth century. The logic of projecting the victories of bacteriological research into an ever-deferred future, while using the promise of future benefit as an excuse for inaction in the present was worked out during the plague epidemics of the nineteenth century and the yellow fever epidemics of the twentieth century. The use of technopolitical power to maneuver on a dense landscape of competing human, technological, and microbial actors was brought into the standard arsenal of French bacteriologists with the drug industries in Indochina. Knowledge regimes for apprehending the empire as a unified space were produced through epidemiological studies in the 1920s and 1930s. The mass vaccination campaigns of the postwar era, the trials of the anti–sleeping sickness drug Lomidine, and the pharmaceutical work of the late twentieth and twenty-first centuries all echo the dynamics of early Pastorians and, indeed, often borrow what remains of their infrastructure. Global health experts, as Lachenal has noted, "far from ignorant of or indifferent to the past," evoke colonial health campaigns as precedents to their work, while conveniently forgetting about their failures.[22] In an age in which constraints imposed by economic arbiters like the International Monetary

Fund prevent states from expanding their public infrastructure, one of the few alternatives involves looking to the past for usable alternatives. And the past, in this case, is Pastorian.

History rarely offers lessons directly applicable to the present, but it does teach us where to look. Pastorian power was made and broken in encounters between microbes, technology, and men, which often interacted across great distances with unequal force. All three components mattered. French officials had confidence in their ability to manage people, and the Pastorians believed themselves experts at constructing new technologies for managing microbes. In reality, the interactions between the three were more complex than they could have possibly imagined. Frictions generated by the collisions of these three sets of actors reverberated across the empire, generating new forms of opposition as well as new forms of power. Local improvisation mattered: the ability to turn an unexpected microbial interaction, a troubling "side effect" of a vaccine or a malfunctioning piece of equipment to one's advantage could determine the outcome of a struggle between administrators, scientists, businessmen, and local elites. So did extraversion: the Pastorians consciously built networks through and across empires, and so did their rivals, from Africans sending letters of complaint to the National Assembly to TB activists spreading social hygiene to the colonies. Analyses of globalization generally tend to eschew one perspective to highlight another; the microbiological and the geopolitical are not easily combined. Yet this is precisely the challenge if we are to remedy the inequalities of the global health regime that dominate the tropical world today.

Notes

Introduction

1. G. Bruno, *Le tour de la France par deux enfants* (Paris: Belin Frères, 1922), 303, 314. By 1901, the book had sold more than six million copies and was the single most popular volume in French libraries. Jacques Ozouf and Mona Ozouf, "Le tour de la France par deux enfants: The Little Red Book of the Republic," in *Realms of Memory: The Construction of the French Past*, vol. 2, *Traditions*, ed. Pierre Nora (New York: Columbia University Press, 1997), 125–150. My thanks to Gilles Pécout for pointing me to the epilogue.
2. Bruno, *Le tour de la France*, 305.
3. Representative examples of the "no revolution" thesis include, for instance, Michael Worboys, "Was There a Bacteriological Revolution in Late Nineteenth-Century Medicine?," *Studies in History and Philosophy of Biological and Biomedical Sciences* 38, no. 1 (March 2008) 20–42; David S. Barnes, *The Great Stink of Paris and the Nineteenth-Century Struggle against Filth and Germs* (Baltimore: Johns Hopkins University Press, 2006); for a contrary reading, see K. Codell Carter, *The Rise of Causal Concepts of Disease* (Burlington, VT: Ashgate, 2003), who sees the revolution in concepts of disease causation; J. Andrew Mendelsohn, "'Like All That Lives': Biology, Medicine and Bacteria in the Age of Pasteur and Koch," *History and Philosophy of the Life Sciences* 24, no. 1 (November 1996): 3–36, for whom it lay in the reorganization of diverse scientific theories and practices around the category of "virulence," but also Bruno Latour, *The Pasteurization of France*, trans. Alan Sheridan and John Law (Cambridge, MA: Harvard University Press, 1988), whose revolution was in the creation of actor-networks between hygienists, legislators, and microbes in which the microbiological laboratory was the central node.
4. Ruth Rogaski, *Hygienic Modernity: Meanings of Health and Disease in Treaty-Port China* (Berkeley: University of California Press, 2004), 6–7; Warwick Anderson prefers "biomedical citizenship"; see *Colonial Pathologies: American Tropical Medicine, Race, and Hygiene in the Philippines* (Durham, NC: Duke University Press, 2006), 3.
5. Bruno, *Le tour de la France*, 315, 307.
6. The rise of Pasteur in France has a rich historiography. Classic studies of the "microbiological revolution" in France include Latour, *The Pasteurization of France*; Patrice Debré, *Louis Pasteur*, trans. Elborg Forster (Baltimore: Johns Hopkins University Press, 1998); Gerald L. Geison, *The Private Science of Louis Pasteur* (Princeton, NJ: Princeton University Press, 1995); Barnes, *The Great Stink of Paris*; Alain Corbin, *Le miasme et la jonquille: L'odorat et l'imaginaire social, XVIIIe–XIXe siècles* (Paris: Aubier-Montaigne, 1982).

7. For two such examples, see Pratik Chakrabarti, *Bacteriology and British India: Laboratory Medicine in the Tropics* (Rochester, NY: University of Rochester Press, 2012); Peter Soppelsa is in the early stages of a study of Pasteur Institutes outside the French imperial world.

8. The classic term is from Georges Balandier, "La situation coloniale: Approche théorique," *Cahiers Internationaux de Sociologie* 11 (1954): 44–79.

9. This is the definition most commonly used in international relations. Robert Dahl, "The Concept of Power," *Behavioral Science* 2, no. 3: (1957): 201–215. We might also think of the definition used by Max Weber, which places "interests in the distribution, maintenance, or transfer of power" at the heart of political matters. Weber, "Politics as a Vocation," in *From Max Weber: Essays in Sociology*, ed. and trans. H. H. Gerth and C. Wright Mills (New York: New York University Press, 1948).

10. Gabrielle Hecht, *The Radiance of France: Nuclear Power and National Identity after World War II* (Cambridge, MA: MIT Press, 1998), 15–16. The concept has been also used and developed in Timothy Mitchell, *Rule of Experts: Egypt, Techno-Politics, Modernity* (Berkeley: University of California Press, 2002); Sara Pritchard, *Confluence: The Nature of Technology and the Remaking of the Rhône* (Cambridge, MA: Harvard University Press, 2011); and Fredrik Meiton, *Electrical Palestine: Capital and Technology from Empire to Nation* (Berkeley: University of California Press, 2019).

11. Some examples include Ilana Löwy, *Virus, moustiques et modernité: La fièvre jaune au Brésil entre science et politique* (Paris: Éditions des Archives Contemporaines, 2001); Mariola Espinosa, *Epidemic Invasions: Yellow Fever and the Limits of Cuban Independence, 1878–1930* (Chicago: University of Chicago Press, 2009). For an example of a distinctly different approach to imperial public health, see Helen Tilley, *Africa as a Living Laboratory: Empire, Development, and the Problem of Scientific Knowledge* (Chicago: University of Chicago Press, 2011).

12. This argument runs counter to the understanding that a defining feature of "modernity" is the assumption of a stark divide between human activity and the natural world (including the microbiological world). The actors surveyed in this book certainly did not share a fixed notion of this division, but rather deployed different models of human-microbial interactions depending on their political goals. For some articulations of this divide, see Bruno Latour, *We Have Never Been Modern* (Cambridge, MA: Harvard University Press, 1991); Zygmunt Bauman, *Liquid Modernity* (New York: Wiley, 2000); Martin Heidegger, *The Question Concerning Technology, and Other Essays*, trans. William Lovitt (New York: Harper, 1977).

13. The critical role of technology and nonhuman actors in shaping sociocultural processes is the key insight of science and technology studies (STS). The point here is that technology and the nonhuman environment are not independent of society—they are not *nature* standing apart from *culture*—but neither are they wholly subservient to culture. They are variables that turn ideas and beliefs into reality and facts, but in so doing, technology and the environment also reshape the contours of those ideas and beliefs. This scholarship is usually traced back to Ludwik Fleck, *The Genesis and Development of a Scientific Fact*, trans. F. Bradley and T. J. Trenn (1935; Chicago: University of Chicago Press, 1979). Actor-network theory is perhaps the

best-known strand of this tradition: Bruno Latour, *Science in Action: How to Follow Scientists and Engineers through Society* (Cambridge, MA: Harvard University Press, 1987); Latour, *Reassembling the Social: An Introduction to Actor-Network-Theory* (Oxford: Oxford University Press, 2005); for other approaches, see John Law, "Technology and Heterogeneous Engineering: The Case of Portuguese Expansion," in *The Social Construction of Technological Systems: New Directions in the Sociology and History of Technology*, ed. Wiebe E. Bijker, Trevor P. Hughes, and Trevor J. Pinch (Cambridge, MA: MIT Press, 1987), 111–134. For a more skeptical stance on theories that meld social constructionism and materialism, see Ian Hacking, *The Social Construction of What?* (Cambridge, MA: Harvard University Press, 2000).

14. I owe this phrase to Guy Ortolano.

15. Jacques Revel, ed., *Jeux d'échelles: La micro-analyse à l'expérience* (Paris: Gallimard, 1996).

16. Frederick Cooper and Ann Stoler, eds., *Tensions of Empire: Colonial Cultures in a Bourgeois World* (Berkeley: University of California Press, 1997).

17. Latour, *Science in Action*, 233–257.

18. Noémi Tousignant, *Edges of Exposure: Toxicology and the Problem of Capacity in Postcolonial Senegal* (Durham, NC: Duke University Press, 2018); Guy Ortolano, *Thatcher's Progress: From Social Democracy to Market Liberalism through an English New Town* (Cambridge: Cambridge University Press, 2019).

19. This approach is inspired by a number of ethnographies of "global frictions": Anna Tsing, *Friction: An Ethnography of Global Connection* (Princeton, NJ: Princeton University Press, 2005); for a different, but related approach, see Kapil Raj, "Beyond Postcolonialism . . . and Postpositivism: Circulation and the Global History of Science," *Isis* 104, no. 2 (June 2013): 337–347; Adriana Petryna, *When Experiments Travel: Clinical Trials and the Global Search for Human Subject* (Princeton, NJ: Princeton University Press, 2009).

20. This insight is drawing from an extensive STS literature on circulation, scale, and modeling. See, for instance, Manu Goswami, *Producing India: From Colonial Economy to National Space* (Chicago: University of Chicago Press, 2004); Sheila Jasanoff, "Image and Imagination: The Formation of Global Environmental Consciousness," in *Changing the Atmosphere: Expert Knowledge and Environmental Governance*, ed. C. Miller and P. N. Edwards (Cambridge, MA: MIT Press, 2001), 309–338; Paul N. Edwards, *A Vast Machine: Computer Models, Climate Data and the Politics of Global Warming* (Cambridge, MA: MIT Press, 2010).

21. For an account of microbiology's "golden age," see Paul de Kruif, *Microbe Hunters*, trans. Harry Greenwood Grover (New York: Harcourt, 1926). See also Ann F. La Berge, "Edwin Chadwick and the French Connection," *Bulletin of the History of Medicine* 62 (1988): 23–41; Nancy J. Tomes and John Harley Warner, eds., "Rethinking the Reception of the Germ Theory of Disease: Comparative Perspectives," special issue, *Journal of the History of Medicine and Allied Sciences* 51, no. 1 (January 1997).

22. On Koch, see Christoph Gradmann, *Laboratory Disease: Robert Koch's Medical Bacteriology*, trans. Elborg Forster (Baltimore: Johns Hopkins University Press,

2009); on Japanese bacteriologists, see Victoria Lee, *The Arts of the Microbial World: A History of Japanese Fermentation Science* (forthcoming).

23. The literature on late nineteenth-century imperialism is too long to enumerate, but a good starting point is Frederick Cooper and Jane Burbank, *Empires in World History: Power and the Politics of Difference* (Princeton, NJ: Princeton University Press, 2011).

24. Two comprehensive statements on this are C. A. Bayly, *The Birth of the Modern World, 1780–1914: Global Connections and Comparisons* (Maiden, MA: Blackwell, 2004), and Jürgen Osterhammel, *The Transformation of the World: A Global History of the Nineteenth Century* (Princeton, NJ: Princeton University Press, 2014), esp. 710–743.

25. Barnes, *The Great Stink of Paris*; Michael Worboys, *Spreading Germs: Disease Theories and Medical Practice in Britain, 1865–1900* (Cambridge: Cambridge University Press, 2000); Nancy Tomes, *The Gospel of Germs: Men, Women, and the Microbe in American Life* (Cambridge, MA: Harvard University Press, 1998); Dorothy Porter, *Health, Civilization and the State: A History of Public Health from Ancient to Modern Times* (London: Routledge, 1999), 77–109.

26. For example, see Christopher Hamlin, *Public Health and Social Justice in the Age of Chadwick: Britain, 1800–1854* (Cambridge: Cambridge University Press, 1998); George Rosen, *A History of Public Health* (New York: MD Publications, 1954), 106–160.

27. Judith Walzer Leavitt, *Typhoid Mary: Captive to the Public's Health* (Boston: Beacon Press, 1996).

28. Erwin Ackerknecht, *Rudolf Virchow: Doctor, Statesman, Anthropologist* (Madison: University of Wisconsin Press, 1953); Byron A. Boyd, *Rudolf Virchow: The Scientist as Citizen* (New York: Garland, 1991).

29. Rogaski, *Hygienic Modernity*.

30. Claire Salomon-Bayet et al., *Pasteur et la révolution Pastorienne* (Paris: Payot, 1986), 72–91; Ann F. La Berge, *Mission and Method: The Early-Nineteenth Century French Public Health Movement* (Cambridge: Cambridge University Press, 1992), 207–239.

31. Alain Corbin, *The Foul and the Fragrant: Odor and the French Social Imagination*, trans. Miriam Kochan Berg (Cambridge, MA: Harvard University Press, 1986); David S. Barnes, *The Making of a Social Disease: Tuberculosis in Nineteenth-Century France* (Berkeley: University of California Press, 1995); François Delaporte, *Disease and Civilization: The Cholera in Paris, 1832*, trans. Arthur Goldhammer (Cambridge, MA: MIT Press, 1986).

32. Debré, *Louis Pasteur*.

33. Barnes, *The Great Stink of Paris*, 3–9

34. A notable exception here is Andrew Cunningham, "Transforming Plague: The Laboratory and the Identity of Infectious Disease," in *The Laboratory Revolution in Medicine*, ed. Andrew Cunningham and Perry Williams (Cambridge: Cambridge University Press, 1992), 209–243. Christoph Gradmann has emphasized the imperial dimension of Robert Koch's research, seeing bacteriology as essentially a "traveling discipline"; Gradmann, *Laboratory Disease*, chap. 5.

35. Kim Pelis, *Charles Nicolle, Pasteur's Imperial Missionary: Typhus and Tunisia* (Rochester, NY: Rochester University Press, 2006), xvii.

36. Anne-Marie Moulin, "Patriarchal Science: The Network of the Overseas Pasteur Institutes," in *Science and Empires: Historical Studies about Scientific Development and European Expansion*, ed. Anne-Marie Moulin, Patrick Petitjean, and Catherine Jami (Berlin: Springer, 1992), 307–322, quotations on 308 and 307

37. Latour, *The Pasteurization of France.*

38. Laurence Monnais-Rousselot, *Medecine et colonisation: L'aventure indochinoise, 1860–1939* (Paris: CNRS Editions, 1999); Anne-Marie Moulin, "The Pasteur Institutes between the Two World Wars: The Transformation of the International Sanitary Order," in *International Health Organisations and Movements 1918–1939*, ed. Paul Weindling (Cambridge: Cambridge University Press, 1995), 244–265.

39. Ann Laura Stoler, *Carnal Knowledge and Imperial Power: Race and the Intimate in Colonial Rule* (Berkeley: University of California Press, 2002); see also Emmanuelle Saada, *Empire's Children: Race, Filiation, and Citizenship in the French Colonies* (Chicago: University of Chicago Press, 2012); for technology, see Michael Adas, *Machines as the Measure of Men: Science, Technology, and Ideologies of Western Dominance* (Ithaca, NY: Cornell University Press, 1989); for the materialist side of this argument, see Daniel Headrick, *Tentacles of Progress: Technology Transfer in the Age of Imperialism 1850–1950* (Oxford: Oxford University Press, 1988); for hygiene, see Anderson, *Colonial Pathologies.*

40. Alice Conklin, *A Mission to Civilize: The Republican Idea of Empire in France and West Africa, 1895–1930* (Stanford, CA: Stanford University Press, 1997).

41. Frederick Cooper, *Decolonization and African Society: The Labor Question in French and British Africa* (Cambridge: Cambridge University Press, 1996), esp. 21–108; Conklin, *A Mission to Civilize*; J. P. Daughton, *An Empire Divided: Religion, Republicanism, and the Making of French Colonialism, 1880–1914* (Oxford: Oxford University Press, 2006).

42. Anderson, *Colonial Pathologies*, 3; Megan Vaughan, *Curing Their Ills: Colonial Power and African Illness* (Stanford, CA: Stanford University Press, 1991); Julie Livingston, *Debility and the Moral Imagination in Botswana* (Bloomington: Indiana University Press, 2005); for medical hybridity, see Ellen Amster, *Medicine and the Saints: Science, Islam and the Colonial Encounter in Morocco, 1877–1956* (Austin: University of Texas Press, 2013); Nancy Rose Hunt, *A Colonial Lexicon: Of Birth Work, Medicalization, and Mobility in the Congo* (Durham, NC: Duke University Press, 1999); for scientific critiques of the colonial state, see Alice Conklin, *In the Museum of Man: Race, Anthropology, and Empire in France, 1850–1950* (Stanford, CA: Stanford University Press, 2014); Tilley, *Africa as a Living Laboratory.*

43. For instance, see continuities with contemporary philanthrocapitalism: Linsey McGoey, *No Such Thing as a Free Gift* (New York: Verso, 2015); with AIDS research: Vinh-Kim Nguyen, *The Republic of Therapy: Triage and Sovereignty in West Africa's Time of AIDS* (Durham, NC: Duke University Press, 2010).

44. Susan Pedersen, *The Guardians: The League of Nations and the Crisis of Empire* (Oxford: Oxford University Press, 2015).

45. Deborah Neill, *Networks in Tropical Medicine: Internationalism, Colonialism, and the Rise of a Medical Specialty, 1890–1930* (Stanford, CA: Stanford University Press, 2012).

46. Paul Weindling, ed., *International Health Organisations and Movements, 1918–1939* (Cambridge: Cambridge University Press, 1995); Iris Borowy, *Coming to Terms with World Health: The League of Nations Health Organization, 1921–1946* (Frankfurt am Main: Peter Lang, 2009); for a similar argument regarding the Rockefeller Foundation, see John Farley, *To Cast Out Disease: A History of the International Health Division of the Rockefeller Foundation, 1913–1951* (Oxford: Oxford University Press, 2004).

47. For the postcolonial life of global health, see Richard C. Keller, "Geographies of Power, Legacies of Mistrust: Colonial Medicine in the Global Present," *Historical Geography* 34 (2006): 26–48; Warwick Anderson, "Where is the Post-colonial History of Medicine?," *Bulletin of the History of Medicine* 72 (1998): 522–530; P. Wenzel Geissler, ed., *Para-states and Medical Science: Making African Global Health* (Durham, NC: Duke University Press, 2015); Jessica Lynne Pearson, *The Colonial Politics of Global Health: France and the United Nations in Postwar Africa, 1945–1960* (Cambridge, MA: Harvard University Press, 2018).

48. Noémi Tousignant, *Edges of Exposure: Toxicology and the Problem of Capacity in Postcolonial Senegal* (Durham, NC: Duke University Press, 2018), chap. 2; P. Wenzel Geissler, Guillaume Lachénal, John Manton, and Noémi Tousignant, eds., *Traces of the Future: An Archaeology of Medical Science in Africa* (Chicago: Intellect, 2016).

Chapter 1

1. Photocopy of Yersin's diary, document 11,630, 3, YER.6, AIP.

2. de Kruif, *Microbe Hunters*, 245. The vision of a "heroic age" of Pastorism has survived remarkably well in biographies of famous Pastorians: Noël Bernard, *La vie et l'oeuvre de Albert Calmette, 1863–1933* (Paris: Éditions Albin Michel, 1961); Noël Bernard, *Yersin: Pionnier—Savant—Explorateur 1863–1943* (Paris: La Colombe, 1955); Jean-Pierre Dedet, *Les Instituts Pasteur d'outre-mer: Cent vingt ans de microbiologie française dans le monde* (Paris: L'Harmattan, 2001), 40, and the website of the Association Amicale Santé Navale et d'Outre-Mer, http://www.asnom.org/ (accessed December 16, 2014).

3. The classic triumphalist work on plague and bacteriology is L. Fabian Hirst, *The Conquest of Plague: A Study of the Evolution of Epidemiology* (Oxford: Clarendon Press, 1953). See also Cunningham, "Transforming Plague," 209; Latour, *The Pasteurization of France*, 94–103.

4. Mary P. Sutphen, "Not What, but Where: Bubonic Plague and the Reception of Germ Theories in Hong Kong and Calcutta, 1894–1897," *Journal of the History of Medicine and the Allied Sciences* 52, no. 1 (January 1997): 112; see also similar claims in Worboys, *Spreading Germs*, 8–9; Barnes, *The Great Stink of Paris*, 6–7. Myron Echenberg offers a more measured account of new policies generated by

bacteriology in *Plague Ports: The Global Urban Impact of the Bubonic Plague, 1894–1901* (New York: New York University Press, 2010).

5. For overviews of other imperial powers' plague containment measures, see in particular Rajnarayan Chandavarkar, "Plague Panic and Epidemic Politics in India, 1896–1914," in *Epidemics and Ideas: Essays on the Historical Perception of Pestilence*, ed. Terence Ranger and Paul Slack (Cambridge: Cambridge University Press, 1992), 203–240; David Arnold, *Colonizing the Body: State Medicine and Epidemic Disease in Nineteenth-Century India* (Berkeley: University of California Press, 1999); Mark Harrison, *Public Health in British India: Anglo-Indian Preventive Medicine, 1858–1914* (Cambridge: Cambridge University Press, 2014).

6. Geison, *The Private Science of Louis Pasteur*, 121–125.

7. Barnes, *The Great Stink of Paris*, 194–223. For a different spin on this argument, see Latour, *The Pasteurization of France*.

8. George Weisz, *The Medical Mandarins: The French Academy of Medicine in the Nineteenth and Early Twentieth Centuries* (Oxford: Oxford University Press, 1995); Barnes, *The Making of a Social Disease*, 41–47.

9. Debré, *Louis Pasteur*, 488–490.

10. Jack D. Ellis, *The Physician-Legislators of France: Medicine and Politics in the Early Third Republic* (Cambridge: Cambridge University Press, 1990), 180–189.

11. Pasteur to comte de Laubespin, 12 January 1888, cited in Debré, *Louis Pasteur*, 490.

12. Pasteur to Duclaux, January 1887, cited in Debré, *Louis Pasteur*, 493; Statuts du 20 Mai 1887, document 18450, DR.FND.1, AIP.

13. "L'Institut Pasteur," *La République Française*, November 14 1888, document 16384, DR.FND.2, AIP.

14. The longer history of naval and tropical medicine is recounted in Michael A. Osborne, *The Emergence of Tropical Medicine in France* (Chicago: University of Chicago Press, 2014).

15. Georges Treille, *Organisation sanitaire des colonies: Progrès réalisés—Progrès à faire* (Marseille: Barlatier, 1906), 23.

16. Treille, *Organisation sanitaire des colonies*, 23.

17. Georges Treille, *De l'acclimatisation des Européens dans les pays chauds* (Paris: Octave Doin, 1888), 3; for a history of the founding of the SdS, see B. Brisou, "Naissance du Service de Santé des Colonies: Dix ans de drames," *Médecine et Armées* 24, no. 5 (1996): 423–432; for a longer analysis of Treille's views, see Osborne, *The Emergence of Tropical Medicine in France*, 137–138.

18. Treille, *De l'acclimatisation*, 16–17.

19. Treille, *Organisation sanitaire des colonies*, 84.

20. Treille, *Organisation sanitaire des colonies*, 71.

21. Treille, *Organisation sanitaire des colonies*, 74.

22. Albert Calmette, autobiographical notes, 8–9, document 28,431, CAL.A1, AIP.

23. Georges Treille, *Besoins et organisation de l'enseignement de la médecine et de l'hygiène coloniales* (Paris: Jean Gainche, 1903), 9–10.

24. Yersin to his mother, 28 February 1891, NUM.YERSIN, AIP.

25. Yersin to his mother, 23 January, 1892, NUM.YERSIN, AIP.

26. Pierre Brocheux and Daniel Héméry, *Indochina: An Ambiguous Colonization 1858–1954*, trans. Ly-Lan Dill Klein (Berkeley: University of California Press, 2011), 48–64.

27. Michael P. M. Finch, *A Progressive Occupation? The Gallieni-Lyautey Method and Colonial Pacification in Tonkin and Madagascar, 1885--1900* (Oxford: Oxford University Press, 2013), 120–135.

28. "Création à Saigon d'un Institut microbiologique et de vaccination de la rage après morsure," *L'Avenir du Tonkin*, 18 February 1892.

29. Calmette's letters to his parents, April–November 1892; quotations from Calmette to his parents, 7 November 1891, CAL.A3, AIP; see also Calmette to lt. gov. of Cochinchina, 19 March 1891, GGI 23882, ANOM.

30. Photocopy of Yersin's diary, document 11,630, 4, YER.6, AIP.

31. Grall to governor-general, 12 May 1894, no. 215, GGI 23916, ANOM; Arrêté du 12 June 1894, no. 414, *Bulletin Officiel de l'Indochine Française*, June 1894, 554–556.

32. Chambre du Commerce de Saigon, Extrait du procès-verbal de la séance de 4 April 1898, copy, GGI 6679; Chambre de Commerce, procès-verbal de la séance du 21 May 1894, GGI 23916; Grall to governor-general, 21 June 1894, no. 8, GGI 23916, ANOM.

33. Handwritten note on projet de l'arrêté, 6 May 1894, GGI 23916, ANOM. De Lanessan's ex post facto assessment of his administration of the colony has been recounted in his autobiographical apologia, *La colonisation Française en Indochine* (Évreux: Imprimerie de Charles Hérissey, 1895).

34. Yersin's letter to his mother, 8–9 June 1894, NUM.YERSIN, AIP; Telegrams no. 13289, 13572 (no dates) to governor-general, GGI 23863, ANOM.

35. Latour, *The Pasteurization of France*, 96–100; Cunningham, "Transforming Plague," 209–244.

36. Christos Lynteris, *Ethnographic Plague: Configuring Disease on the Chinese-Russian Frontier* (London: Palgrave Macmillan, 2016), 15–17; Robert Peckham, "Matshed Laboratory: Colonies, Cultures, and Bacteriology," in *Imperial Contagions: Medicine, Hygiene, and Cultures of Planning in Asia*, ed. Robert Peckham and David M. Pomfret (Hong Kong: Hong Kong University Press, 2013), 124–125.

37. Steve Tsang, *A Modern History of Hong Kong* (London: Palgrave Macmillan, 2007), 56–72; Echenberg, *Plague Ports*, 18–20.

38. Photocopy of Yersin's diary, document 11,630, 9–13, YER.6, AIP.

39. Letter of the French consul to minister of the colonies, 26 June 1894, GGI 23863, ANOM.

40. Sutphen, "Not What, but Where," 87–89.

41. Letter of the French consul to minister of the colonies, 26 June 1894, GGI 23863, ANOM.

42. Yersin's report to the governor-general, 18 June 1894, GGI 23863, ANOM.

43. Yersin's report to the governor-general, 18 June 1894, GGI 23863, ANOM.

44. Lowson, cited in Sutphen, "Not What, but Where," 87.

45. Tom Solomon, "Hong Kong, 1894: The Role of James A. Lowson in the Controversial Discovery of the Plague Bacillus," *Lancet*, 5 July 1997, 60.

46. Yersin's report to the governor-general, 17 July 1894, GGI 23863, ANOM.

47. For a history of medical geography and naval medicine, see Osborne, *The Emergence of Tropical Medicine in France*, 47–75; for British views on plague etiology, see Solomon, "Hong Kong, 1894," 60; Sutphen, "Not What, but Where," 87.

48. Commission d'études dite des Odeurs de Paris, cited in Barnes, *The Great Stink of Paris*, 235.

49. For the importance of the Koch-Pasteur controversy in understanding the development of Pasteur's career, see the discussion in Simon Schaffer, "The Eighteenth Brumaire of Bruno Latour," *Studies in the History and Philosophy of Science 22, no. 1* (March 1991): 187–189.

50. For a while Kitasato and Yersin shared credit for the discovery of the plague microbe. French scientists and Pastorians tended to emphasize Yersin's contributions. For a technical analysis of the difference between Yersin's and Kitasato's cultures, see David J. Bibel and T. H. Chen, "Diagnosis of Plague: An Analysis of the Yersin-Kitasato Controversy," *Bacteriological Reviews*, September 1976, 633–651. For reports of Yersin's poor English skills and socializing problems, see the report of the French consul to the governor-general of Indochina, 19 June 1894, GGI 23863, ANOM; Solomon, "Hong Kong, 1894," 61.

51. Yersin's personal diary, "Mon voyage à Hong-Kong au sujet de la peste," 4 September 1894, YER.6, AIP.

52. Yersin's notes for the fourth report, undated, YER.6, AIP.

53. Lei from Xiamen to Yersin, 10 September 1896, YER.6, AIP. My thanks to Albert Wu for translating this letter.

54. For the spread of the plague from 1894 to 1901, see Myron Echenberg, "Pestis Redux: The Initial Years of the Third Bubonic Plague Pandemic, 1894–1901," *Journal of World History 13, no. 2* (Fall 2002): 429–449.

55. Émile Roux to Paul-Louis Simond, personal letter, 21 August 1898, SIM.4; Félix Mesnil to Paul-Louis Simond, personal letter, 10 January 1898, SIM.4, AIP.

56. Paul-Louis Simond, "La propagation de la peste," *Annales de l'Institut Pasteur*, October 1898, 684.

57. Simond, "Propagation de la peste," 625–685.

58. Ernest Hankin, "La propagation de la peste," *Annales de l'Institut Pasteur*, November 1898, 761.

59. Hankin, "La propagation de la peste," 761.

60. Hankin, "La propagation de la peste," 762.

61. Echenberg, *Plague Ports*, 307.

62. Mark Harrison, *Contagion: How Commerce Has Spread Disease* (New Haven: Yale University Press, 2013), 180–183.

63. Mark Harrison, "Disease, Diplomacy and International Commerce: The Origins of International Sanitary Regulation in the Nineteenth Century," *Journal of Global History* 1 (2006): 197–217.

64. W. F. Bynum, "Policing the Hearts of Darkness: Aspects of the International Sanitary Conferences," *History and Philosophy of the Life Sciences* 15, no. 3 (1993): 421–434; Norman Howard-Jones, *The Scientific Background of the International Sanitary Conferences, 1851–1938* (Geneva: World Health Organization, 1975).

65. *Procès-verbaux de la Conférence sanitaire internationale ouverte à Constantinople le 13 février 1866* (Constantinople: Imprimerie Centrale, 1866), 10, cited in Valeska Huber, "The Unification of the Globe by Disease? The International Sanitary Conferences on Cholera, 1851–1894," *Historical Journal* 42, no. 2 (Spring 2006): 462.

66. Huber, "The Unification of the Globe by Disease?," 466–468.

67. *Conference sanitaire internationale de Venise, 16 février–19 mars 1897: Procès-verbaux* (Rome: Forzani, et cie, imprimeurs du Sénat 1897), 23–24.

68. *Conférence sanitaire internationale de Venise*, 225–261.

69. M. le Commandeur Santoliquido, *Conférence sanitaire internationale de Paris, 10 octobre–3 décembre 1903: Procès-verbaux* (Paris: Imprimerie Nationale, 1904), 29.

70. *Conférence sanitaire international de Paris*, 34; see also 48–49.

71. Première séance plenière, *Conférence sanitaire internationale de Paris*, 18.

72. Santoliquido, *Conférence sanitaire international de Paris*, 34

73. See, for instance, the discussion over the potential of cargo to transmit the plague; *Conférence sanitaire international*, 357–360.

74. Lettre de Yersin sur Hong Kong, undated (ca. 1896), RSTNF 03803, ANOM.

75. Albert Calmette, "Médecine coloniale: Le rôle des sciences médicales dans la colonisation," *Revue Scientifique*, 8 April 1905, 420.

76. *Conférence sanitaire internationale de Paris*, 18–19.

77. Howard-Jones, *The Scientific Background of the International Sanitary Conferences*, 81–85.

78. Alexandre Yersin, "Sur la peste bubonique (séro-thérapie)," *Annales de l'Institut Pasteur*, January 1897, 81–93

79. C. Huart (Consul de France à Canton), "Le sérum anti-pesteux du Dr. Yersin," *Revue Générale des Sciences Pures et Appliquées 17*, 15 September 1896; Jean Hess, "Le Docteur Yersin et le vaccin de la peste," *Le Monde Illustré*, 9 January 1897; "Le Docteur Yersin," *Écho de la Semaine*, 14 February 1897.

80. Yersin's notes, "Mission sur la peste aux Indes," YER.6, AIP.

81. Calmette's lecture notes, "Moyens de défense contre la peste," 21 November 1900, CAL.D12, AIP.

82. *Conférence sanitaire internationale de Paris*, 233–234. See also Albert Calmette and Dr. Hautefeuille, *Rapport sur la désinfection par le procédé Clayton à bord des navires* (Paris: Masson et Cie, 1902).

83. *Conférence sanitaire internationale de Paris*, 156–159.

84. Harrison, *Contagion*, 197.

85. Emil Zuschlag and Harald Goldschmitt, *Rotterne samt deres Forhold til det moderne Samfundsliv: Et Agitationsskrift for Rottesagen* (Copenhagen: Fr. Bagge, 1900); Emil Zuschlag, *Le rat migratoire et sa destruction rationnelle* (Copenhagen: Fr. Bagge, 1903).

86. Zuschlag, *Le rat migratoire*, 29–35, 20–21.

87. Zuschlag, *Le rat migratoire*, 46

88. Zuschlag, *Le rat migratoire*, 139.

89. Karin Johannisson, "Public Health Policies in Sweden," in *The History of Public Health and the State*, ed. Dorothy Porter (London: Routledge, 1996), 165–182; Andreas Vilhelmsson, "Folkhälsoarbetets historia i socialmedicinsk belysning," *Socialmedicisnk Tidskrift* 89, no. 1 (2012): 44–53; Signe Mellemgaard, "Bourgeois Ideals in Nineteenth-Century Hygiene: The Evidence of a Danish Medical Topography," *Ethnologia Scandinavica: A Journal for Nordic Ethnology* 22 (1992): 27–35.

90. For a history of the Danish "social question" and the role different strategies of hygiene played within this, see Anne Løkke, "Creating the Social Question: Imagining Society in Statistics and Political Economy in Late Nineteenth-Century Denmark," *Histoire Sociale/Social History* 35, no. 70 (2002): 393–422; Lars-Henrik Schmidt and Jens Erik Kristensen, *Lys, luft og renlighed: Den moderne socialhygiejnes fødsel* (Copenhagen: Akademisk Forlag, 1986).

91. Zuschlag and Goldschmitt, *Rotterne samt deres Forhold*, 122–124.

92. Zuschlag and Goldschmitt, *Rotterne samt deres Forhold*; the original petition to the Folketing is reprinted in Zuschlag, *Le rat migratoire*, 104–106.

93. Adrien Loir, "Prophylaxie sanitaire internationale: La question des quarantaines et mesures sanitaires contre la peste," in *Congrès maritime international de Copenhague, 1902* (Paris: Assocation Internationale de la Marine, 1902), 751; Alexandre Kermorgant, *Instructions à nos colonies au sujet de mesures à prendre en cas de peste* (Paris: Imprimerie Nationale, 1900); Albert Calmette, "Les missions scientifiques de l'Institut Pasteur et l'expansion coloniale de la France," *Revue Scientifique* 3 (February 1912): 418.

94. Yersin to Kermorgant, 22 July 1897, no. 24.230, IND.A2, AIP.

95. Yersin to the governor-general, report on the plague outbreak, 16 July 1898, GGI 6676, ANOM.

96. Yersin to governor-general, report on the plague outbreak, 22 July 1898, GGI 6676, ANOM.

97. Yersin to Kermorgant, 22 July 1897, no. 24.230,; IND.A2, AIP, Alexandre Yersin, "L'épidémie de peste à Nha Trang de juin à octobre, 1898," *Annales d'Hygiène et de Médecine Coloniales* 2 (1899): 381–390.

98. Yersin to Roux, 22 July 1897, no. 24.230, IND.A2, AIP.

99. Yersin to Kermorgant, 22 July 1897, no. 24.230, IND.A2, AIP.

100. Yersin to the governor-general, report on the plague outbreak, 16 July 1898, GGI 6676, ANOM.

101. Marchoux to Simond, personal letter, 21 July 1898, "Institut Pasteur et Pastoriens," SIM.6.2, AIP.

102. Monnais-Rousselot, *Médecine et colonisation*, 22.

103. Monnais-Rousselot, *Médecine et colonisation*, 57–63.

104. Clavel to the governor-general, "Instructions relatives à l'hygiène des populations et à l'assainissement du pays," 23 January 1907, GGI 6722, ANOM.

105. Governor-general circular, "Instructions relatives au developpement des mesures d'hygiène et de protection de la santé publique," 31 January 1907, GGI 6722; governor-general to minister of the colonies, 19 September 1908, doc. No 2,906, GGI 6722, ANOM.

106. Inspecteur des services civils de Nanh-Tinh to resident-superior of Tonkin, 17 February 1904, GGI 6726; see also administrateur de Chai-Nguyen to resident-superior of Tonkin, 31 January 1904, GGI 6726, ANOM.

107. Administrateur Resident of Phu Lien to resident-superior of Tonkin, 3 February 1904, GGI 6726, ANOM.

108. Governor-general to the minister of the colonies, report, 19 September 1908, GGI 6724, ANOM.

109. Roy des Barrès, "Ville de Hanoi, Rapport sur l'épidémie de peste de 1903," handwritten report, GGI 6738, ANOM.

110. Prefect of Van Bu to resident-general of Tonkin, 27 January 1904, GGI 6725; see also prefect of Backan to resident-general of Tonkin, 26 January 1904, GGI 6725, ANOM.

111. Prefect of Phu Lien to resident-general of Tonkin, 8 February 1904, GGI 6725, ANOM.

112. Medical officer of Phu Lien to resident-general of Tonkin, 4 February 1904, GGI 6725, ANOM.

113. The difficulties in implementing deratization measures in Hanoi are the subject of a splendid analysis by Michael Vann: "Of Rats, Rice, and Race: The Great Hanoi Rat Massacre, an Episode in French Colonial History," *French Colonial History* 4 (2003): 191–203. My discussion here generally follows his argument.

114. Dr. Serez to governor-general, 7 July 1907, GGI 6675, ANOM.

115. Resident-superior of Tonkin to the governor-general, 26 February 1904, GGI 6724, ANOM.

116. Vann, "Of Rice, Rats, and Race," 198.

117. Vann, "Of Rice, Rats, and Race," 199.

118. Resident-superior of Tonkin to the governor-general, 15 January 1904, GGI 6725, ANOM; for later epidemics, see Laurent Joseph Gaide and Henri Bodet, *La peste en Indochine* (Hanoi: Imprimerie d'Extrême-Orient, 1930).

119. For Hanoi, see "A. S. des mesures sanitaires imposées aux habitants dans l'épidémie de peste, et des formalités dans la déclaration des décès, 1908–1909," GGI 23867, and Roy des Barrès, "Ville de Hanoi, Rapport sur l'épidémie de peste de 1903," handwritten report, GGI 6738, ANOM. For Phnom Penh, see resident superior to governor-general, report, 19 September 1909, GGI 17068, ANOM.

120. The story of this outbreak has been analyzed by Myron Echenberg, *Black Death, White Medicine: Bubonic Plague and the Politics of Public Health in Senegal, 1914–1945* (Portsmouth, NH: Heinemann, 2002).

121. In Indochina, "Rapport sur les mesures prises et les résultats obtenus au point de vue de l'hygiène et de la santé publique pendant l'année 1915, province de Mytho," GouCoch. IA.8/232, VNA-II. In Senegal, see Comité local de l'hygiène, Séance de 20 Mai 1914, Senegal H-70, ANS.

122. Secretary-general of Indochina to governor-general, report, 12 September 1904, IND.B, AIP.

123. Institut Pasteur, convention, 1904, IND.B, AIP.

124. Circular of the governor-general, 31 January 1907, GGI 6722, ANOM.

125. "Épidémie de peste et de choléra. État sanitaire en Indochine et dans les pays voisins—1889–1905," GGI 66345, ANOM.
126. Citizens of Hanoi to governor-general, 31 March 1906, GGI 6739, ANOM.
127. Governor-general par interim circular, no. 83, 1 June 1908, GGI 2526, ANOM.
128. Resident superior to governor-general, 19 June 1908, GGI 2526, ANOM.
129. Albert Calmette, "Médecine coloniale—le rôle des sciences médicales dans la colonization," *Revue Scientifique*, 8 April 1905, 416–421.
130. Calmette, "Les missions scientifiques," 419.
131. Calmette, "Les missions scientifiques," 420.
132. Calmette, "Les missions scientifiques," 418.
133. Calmette, "Les missions scientifiques," 420.
134. Calmette, "Les missions scientifiques," 421.
135. Calmette, "Les missions scientifiques," 421.
136. Monnais-Rousselot, *Médecine et colonisation*, in particular 78–95, 139–173.
137. Ferdinand Heckenroth, "Traitement de la peste dans les colonies," in *Congres de la santé publique et de la prévoyance sociale, Marseille, 11–17 septembre 1922* (Paris, 1922), 307.

Chapter 2

1. "Société française des distilleries de l'Indo-Chine," *Les Annales Coloniales*, August 15, 1922, 4; for other similar advertisements, see "Société française des distilleries de l'Indo-Chine," *Le Courrier Colonial Illustré*, December 15, 1928; *L'industrie de l'alcool en Indochine* (Hanoi: SFDIC, 1938).
2. "Société française des distilleries de l'Indo-Chine," *Les Annales Coloniales*, 15 August 1922, 4.
3. *L'industrie de l'alcool*, 4.
4. Session of 27 April 1907, *Procès-verbal du Conseil colonial de la Cochinchine française* (Saigon: Imprimerie Nationale, 1907), 17–18. Vietnamese responses to the alcohol regime are analyzed in detail in Erica J. Peters, "Taste, Taxes, and Technologies: Industrializing Rice Alcohol in Northern Vietnam, 1902–1913," *French Historical Studies* 27, no. 3 (Summer 2003): 569–600. A similarly insightful analysis can be found in Gerard H. Sasges, "Contraband, Capital, and the Colonial State: The Alcohol Monopoly in Northern Viet Nam, 1897–1933" (PhD diss., University of California, Berkeley, 2006). Both scholars have shaped my analysis here in key respects.
5. Albert Sarraut, confidential letter to the minister of the colonies, 31 October 1912, FP 9 PA 16, ANOM.
6. Chantal Descours-Gatin, *Quand l'opium finançait la colonisation en Indochine: L'élaboration de la régie générale de l'opium (1860 à 1914)* (Paris: L'Harmattan, 1992), 95–97.
7. Report of the governor-general of Indochina to the minister of the colonies, 4 April 1908, FM 1 AFF-POL 2417/4, ANOM.

8. Calmette, letter to family, dated 21 May 1892, CAL.A3, AIP.
9. On alcohol, see Sasges, "Contraband, Capital, and the Colonial State"; Charles van Onselen, "Randlords and Rotgut 1886–1903: An Essay on the Role of Alcohol in the Development of European Imperialism and Southern African Capitalism," *History Workshop Journal* 1, no. 2 (Autumn 1976): 33–89; Charles Ambler and Jonathan Crush, eds., *Liquor and Labor in Southern Africa* (Athens: Ohio University Press, 1992); on opium, see Descours-Gatin, *Quand l'opium finançait la colonisation en Indochine*; Philippe le Failler, *Monopole et prohibition de l'opium en Indochine: Le pilori des chimères* (Paris: L'Harmattan, 2001); Yvette Bision, "Le monopole des stupéfiants" (PhD diss., Université de Paris X-Nanterre, 1993); Diana Kim, *Empires of Vice: The Rise of Opium Prohibition in Colonial Southeast Asia* (forthcoming).
10. An exception here is Peters, "Taste, Taxes, and Technologies," 569–600; Erica J. Peters, "What the Taste Test Showed: Alcohol and Politics in French Vietnam," *Social History of Alcohol and Drugs* 19 (2004): 94–110. I build significantly on her analysis.
11. Bernard-Marcel Peyrouton, *Étude sur les monopoles en Indo-Chine. Thèse pour le doctorat* (Paris: Émile Larose, 1913), 62–65.
12. Sasges, "Contraband, Capital and the Colonial State," 26–27.
13. Brocheux and Hémery, *Indochina*, 93.
14. Peyrouton, *Étude sur les monopoles en Indo-Cine*, 140–144; Le Thanh Khoi, *Le Viet-Nam: Histoire et civilisation* (Paris: Les Éditions de Minuit, 1955), 369.
15. Paul Bert quoted in René Monier, *La question du monopole de l'alcool au Tonkin et dans le Nord-Annam* (Paris: Émile Larose, 1914), 20.
16. Sasges, "Contraband, Capital and the Colonial State," 14–17. The original Vietnamese phrasing reads: "Cơm no rượu say rồi." See also Albert Sarraut's report on the alcohol regime, and the saying "fête sans alcool, fête incomplete et sans efficacité" and the following description of Vietnamese drinking customs; confidential letter from Albert Sarraut to the minister of the colonies, 31 October 1912, FP 9 PA 16, ANOM.
17. Calmette, "De quelques industries de Cochinchine," 655; Descours-Gatin, *Quand l'opium finançait la colonisation en Indochine*, 144–147.
18. Lauret, "Monopoles de l'Indochine et leur remplacement," 8–11, INDO GGI 8456, ANOM.
19. Lauret, "Monopoles de l'Indochine et leur remplacement," 12, INDO GGI 8456, ANOM; *Rapports et procès-verbaux du Comité International de l'Opium* (Shanghai, 1909), 124 INDO GGI 8769, ANOM; G. Geoffray, *Règlementation des régies Indochinoises. Tome premier. Opium, alcools, sels* (Paris: Édition, 1936).
20. "Étude sur la consommation de l'opium en Cochinchine," INDO GGI 42996, ANOM.
21. Brocheux and Hémery, *Indochina*, 80.
22. Brocheux and Hémery, *Indochina*, 78–80, 91–92.
23. Governor of Cochinchina, letter reproduced in F. des Tournelles, *Procédés de de préparation de l'alcool de riz de Cochinchine: Rapport de mission* (Paris: Challamel et Cie, 1888), 5–6.
24. Peyrouton, *Étude sur les monopoles en Indo-Cine*, 76–77; Lauret, Report to the governor-general, "Monopoles en Indo-Chine et leur remplacements" published in 1909, 75, INDO GGI 8456, ANOM.

25. Jacob M. Price, "Tobacco Use and Tobacco Taxation: A Battle of Interests in Early Modern Europe," in *Consuming Habits: Drugs in History and Anthropology*, ed. Jordan Goodman, Paul Lovejoy, and Andrew Sherratt (London: Routledge, 1995), 167–168.

26. David T. Courtwright, *Forces of Habit: Drugs and the Making of the Modern World* (Cambridge, MA: Harvard University Press, 2001), 152–155.

27. For a biographical sketch of Doumer, who went from being a provincial working-class mathematics teacher to being a member of the Chamber of Deputies, and from there to the governor-generalof Indochina, and eventually the president of France, see Amaury Lorin, *Paul Doumer, governeur general de l'Indochine* (Paris: L'Harmattan, 2004).

28. Monier, *La question du monopole*, 22.

29. Monier, *La question du monopole*, 32. See also de Lanessan, "Arrêté de 3 avril 1893," *Journal Officiel*, 3 April 1893, 498,and the debate particularly in "Séance du 19 décembre, Commission des affaires diverses. Régime des alcools—rapport au conseil colonial," *Journal Officiel*, 19 December 1891, 121–125. For an overview of the budgets of Annam-Tonkin, see *Le Tonkin en 1893* (Hanoi, 1893), 56–59.

30. Peyrouton, *Étude sur les monopoles en Indo Chine*, 6–7.

31. The Administration des douanes et régies, translated roughly as "Department of Customs and State-Owned Companies," which I will from here on abbreviate as Douanes et Régies, was the muscle of French commerce in Indochina. It was in charge of maintaining ports and borders, collecting tariffs and excise taxes, administering state-owned companies (especially the alcohol, opium, and salt monopolies), and fighting contraband with an army of customs agents. Gerard Sasges has translated the name as "Department of Customs and Excise," but I have opted for the French original, since it better conveys the breadth of the department's jurisdiction—it handled questions ranging from the setting of tax policy to shopping for the raw opium required for the Saigon factory. Monier, *La question du monopole*, 33–35. In contrast to de Lanessan's "ultraliberalism," Monier dubs Doumer's politics "ultrafiscalism," which puts budgetary balance before all other ideological concerns, including those of trade liberalization.

32. "Dossier contentieux de Nguyen Thai Xuan, Vo Van Tri au sujet de fabrication et de vente d'alcool sans permissions des années," dated 1890, GouGoch 1719, VNA-II; Brocheux and Hémery, *Indochina*, 165–166, Peters, "Taste, Taxes, and Technologies," 579–580.

33. Descours-Gatin, *Quand l'opium financait la colonisation en Indochine*, 174–177; Lauret, "Monopoles de l'Indochine et leur remplacement," INDO GGI 8456, ANOM; René De Saint-Mathurin, *La ferme de l'opium au Tonkin: Mémoire présenté a la Commission extraparlementaire* (Paris: L. Woestendieck, 1896).

34. Louis Pasteur, "Mémoire sur la fermentation appelée lactique," *Annales de Chimie et de Physique*, 3rd ser., 52 (1858): 404–418. For a brilliant semiotic analysis of this text, see Bruno Latour, "Pasteur on Lactic Acid Yeast: A Partial Semiotic Analysis," *Configurations* 1, no. 1 (1993): 126–146.

35. Gerald Geison, "Louis Pasteur," in *The Dictionary of Scientific Biography*, vol. 10 (New York: Charles Scribner's Sons, 1974), 362.

36. Louis Pasteur, *Études sur la bière: Ses maladies, causes qui les provoquent, procédé pour la rendre inaltérable; avec une théorie nouvelle de la fermentation* (Paris: Gauthier-Villars, 1876), vii–viii.

37. For the standard version of the Bigo story, see René Vallery-Radot, *La vie de Pasteur* (Paris: Hachette, 1911), 91–97. Gerald Geison has persuasively argued that this is most likely a fabrication and certainly did not have the determining effect on Pasteur's research as biographers have often claimed—rather, Pasteur's interest in fermentation should be seen as almost entirely theoretical and growing out of his study of optical isomers in soluble substances; Geison, *The Private Science of Louis Pasteur*, 91–94.

38. Albert Calmette, letter to family, 12 September 1891; Calmette, letter to family, 23 October 1891, CAL.A3, AIP.

39. Calmette, personal notes titled "Plantes aromatiques entrant dans la composition de la levure chinoise", n.d.; *Journal l'Indochinois*, 22 January 1887, CAL.D7, AIP. He also drew on prior work by a French civil engineer named Lezé. Des Tournelles, *Procédés de de préparation de l'alcool de riz de Cochinchine*, 6; Calmette's letter to his family, dated 21 May 1892, CAL.A3, AIP.

40. Calmette, personal notes titled "Plantes aromatiques entrant dans la composition de la levure chinoise," n.d., and "Préparation de l'alcool de riz à la distillerie de Thu-Tienh, en face de Saigon," n.d., CAL.D7, AIP; Albert Calmette, "Contribution à l'étude des ferments de l'amidon: La levure chinoise," *Annales de l'Institut Pasteur*, October 1892, 605.

41. Calmette, "La levure chinoise," 612.

42. Calmette, "La levure chinoise," 612.

43. Calmette, "La levure chinoise," 616–618.

44. Calmette, "La levure chinoise," 620.

45. For the "beasts of burden" argument, see Peyrouton, *Étude sur les monopoles en Indo-Chine*, 79–81.

46. Letter of minister of the colonies to the governor-general, 14 August 1896, INDO GGI 8280; Report by A. Frézoul, inspector of the colonies, to the governor-general, 30 November 1898, INDO GGI 8280, ANOM.

47. "Arrêté règlementant la fabrication de l'alcool indigène au Nord-Annam et Tonkin," *Bulletin Officiel de l'Indochine Française*, June 1897, 802–810.

48. "Arrêté portant règlementation de l'exercice dans les distilleries et fabriques de liquers de l'Indo-Chine du 9 mars, 1900," *Bulletin Officiel de l'Indochine Française*, March 1900, 357–364.

49. Monier, *La question du monopole*, 45.

50. "Arrêté relatif au régimes des alcools en Indo-chine du 20 décembre 1902," *Bulletin Officiel de l'Indochine Française*, December 1902, 956–992; "Arrêté réglementant la vente des alcools en Indo-Chine du 22 décembre 1902," *Bulletin Officiel de l'Indochine Française*, December 1902, 1004–1011. See also draft legislation in INDO GGI 1319, ANOM.

51. Monier, *La question du monopole*, 54–61; this process is also discussed at length in Sasges, "Contraband, Capital and the Colonial State," 106–137.

52. Lauret, report to the governor-general, "Monopoles en Indo-Chine et leur remplacements" published in 1909, 96–97, INDO GGI 8456, ANOM.

53. Calmette, "De quelques industries de Cochinchine," 659.

54. Draft letter from Albert Sarraut to Ministry of the Colonies, undated, FP 9PA-15, ANOM.

55. Monier, *La question du monopole*, 10.

56. Pham Quynh, "Van de rirou a dai hoi nghi," *Nam Phong* 168 (January 1932): 11, cited in Sasges, "Contraband, Capital, and the Colonial State," 54.

57. Société des Distillateurs Français de l'Indo-Chine, *Industrie de l'alcool en Indochine*, 4, BIB Br 9581 C, ANOM.

58. Société des Distillateurs Français de l'Indo-Chine, *Industrie de l'alcool en Indochine*, 4, BIB Br 9581 C, ANOM.

59. "Rapport au gouverneur général au sujet du régime des alcools indigènes en Cochinchine," 22 May 1912, 15, FP 9 PA 16, ANOM.

60. J. Sanguinetti, "Contribution à l'étude de l'amylomyces Rouxii, de la levure chinoise et de moisissures ferments de l'amidon," *Annales de l'Institut Pasteur*, December 1897, 264–276; A. Boidin and E. Rolants, "Contribution a l'étude de l'utilisation de l'*Amylomyces Rouxii* de la levure chinoise," *La Biere et les Boissons Fermentées*, March 1897, CAL.D7, AIP.

61. "Institut Pasteur de Lille," *Le Nord-Économiste*, 8 September 1898.

62. Jean-Louis de Lanessan, *L'expansion coloniale de la France* (Paris: F. Alcan, 1886), 581. Saint-Mathurin, owner of the opium monopoly, regularly compared opium to tobacco use in France. de Saint-Mathurin, *Ferme de l'opium au Tonkin*, 1.

63. Report of the lt. gov of Cochinchina to minister of the colonies, 7 February 1908, INDO GGI 42996, ANOM.

64. Paul Gide, *L'opium—Thèse de doctorat* (Paris: Recueil Sirey, 1910), 11; see also 8–14.

65. Letter of F. Drouhet, secretary-general of the colonies, to lt. gov of Cochinchina, 13 November 1911, GouGoch IB.29/013, VNA-II.

66. Calmette, "De quelques industries de Cochinchine," 655; "Au sujet de la qualité de l'opium et des moyens à employer pour la fabrication de cette drogue," *Journal Officiel de L'Indochine Française*, 20 January 1896, extract in GouGoch IB.29/017, VNA-II.

67. Saint-Mathurin's side of the story is recounted in *La ferme de l'opium à Tonkin*; for the administration's side, see INDO GGI 10102, ANOM. For a later summary, see Peyrouton, *Étude sur les monopoles de l'Indo-Chine*, 146–149.

68. E. Lalande, "Opium des fumeurs," *Archives de Médecine Navale et Coloniale 54* (1890): 33–76.

69. Gide, *L'opium*, 50–54; Descours-Gatin, *Quand l'opium finançait la colonisation en Indochine*, 12–14.

70. Albert Calmette's manuscript, "Le ferment de l'opium des fumeurs et la fermentation artificielle des chandoos," 16 October 1891, CAL.C, AIP. For the composition of Raulin's medium, see Alexandre Guilliermond, *Yeasts: Culture, Identification, and Microbiology* (Boston: Stanhope Press, 1920), 149.

71. Official telegram from the lt. gov of Cochinchina to the Gov. Gen, 25 September 1892, INDO GGI 23882, ANOM.

72. Translation of a Chinese *affiche, Courrier de Saigon,* July 18, 1894.

73. "Au sujet de la qualité de l'opium et des moyens à employer pour la fabrication de cette drogue," *Journal Officiel de l'Indochine Française,* 20 January 1896, 159, GouGoch IB.29/017, VNA-II.

74. Bérenguier cited in "Au sujet de la qualité de l'opium et des moyens à employer pour la fabrication de cette drogue," *Journal Officiel de l'Indochine Française,* 20 January 1896, 159, GouGoch IB.29/017, VNA-II.

75. "Des diverses préparations de l'opium à la bouillerie de Saigon," GouGoch IB.29/017, VNA-II.

76. *Courrier de Saigon,* July 18, 1894.

77. Dir. of the Douanes et Régies cited in "Au sujet de la qualité de l'opium et des moyens à employer pour la fabrication de cette drogue," *Journal Officiel de l'Indochine Française,* 20 January 1896, 158, GouGoch IB.29/017, VNA-II.

78. Calmette, "Industries de Cochinchine," 657.

79. "Des diverses préparations de l'opium à la Bouillerie de Saigon," GouGoch IB.29/017, VNA-II; "Rapport no 2 sur l'étude des opiums des fumeurs," 30 May 1902, INDO GGI 8686, ANOM; "Organisation de la manufacture de l'opium à Saigon, fonctionnement en 1910," 3, INDO GGI 43,025, ANOM.

80. "Rapport no 2 sur l'étude des opiums des fumeurs," 30 May 1902, INDO GGI 8686, ANOM.

81. "Rapport no 2 sur l'étude des opiums des fumeurs," 30 May 1902, INDO GGI 8686, ANOM; Gide, *L'opium,* 44.

82. Monier, *La question du monopole,* 34; Paul Doumer, *Situation de l'Indochine française de 1897 à 1901* (Hanoi: F. H. Schneider, 1902), 157.

83. Doumer, *Situation de l'Indochine,* 553.

84. Sasges, "Contraband, Capital, and the Colonial State," 71–83; Le Conte, "Rapport sur la Régie des alcools en Indochine," 24 June 1930, Fonds Ministeriels INDO NF 2481, ANOM;

85. For price adjustments and licensing fees, see arrêté du Governor-general, 16 April 1906, GouCoch IB.29/027, VNA-II; "Arrêté du 29 juin 1905 fixant le prix de l'hectolitre d'alcool en 1905," INDO GGI 1320, ANOM.

86. "Arrêté du 7 janvier 1907," *Journal Officiel de l'Indo-Chine Française,* GouCoch IB.29/032, VNA-II.

87. lý trưởng Trinh-ca Giang to le chef Debeaux, undated; lý trưởng Tran-van-Chu to Quan Huyen of Vuban, undated, INDO GGI 1360, ANOM.

88. Compagnie Générale du Tonkin et du Nord-Annam to the governor-general, 11 April 1910; resident superior p.i. to the governor-general, 29 April 1910, INDO GGI 1360, ANOM.

89. Sasges, "Contraband, Capital, and the Colonial State," 142; Dominique Niollet, *L'épopée des douaniers en Indochine 1874–1954* (Paris: Éditions Kailash, 1998), 232, 242.

90. *Reglements concernant la procedure,* INDO GGI 8267, ANOM.

91. *Meurtre de M. Beaussar agent de la ferme des alcools 1899,* INDO GGI 8774; Lauret, "Monopoles de l'Indo-Chine et leur remplacement," 91–96, INDO GGI 8456,

ANOM; Circular of the lt. gov. of Cochinchina to administrators and provincial chiefs, 30 May 1906, GouCoch IB.29/032, VNA-II.

92. Jules Morel to the lt. gov. of Cochinchina, 8 May, 1906, GouCoch IB.29/032, VNA-II; "De la répression de la contrebande d'alcool dans les provinces du Nord-Annam 1908," INDO GGI 1344, ANOM.

93. For the repeal, see "Arrêté du 11 December 1908," and the following procés-verbal, INDO GGI 8457, ANOM; Berges, "Note sur l'arrêté des 20 et 22 decembre 1902, sur le régime des alcools," GouCoch 12473, VNA-II; Circular of lt. gov of Cochinchina to administrators and provincial chiefs, March 1906, GouCoch 12473, VNA-II.

94. lt. gov. of Cochinchina to the governor-general., 3 October 1903, GouCoch, 12473 VNA-II

95. Report of M. Doceul to the lt. gov. of Cochinchina, 3 February 1904, GouCoch 12473, VNA-II

96. See the circular of the lt. gov. of Cochinchina from 25 August 1904 showing nineteen cases invoking Article 96 in 1904 alone, 12473, VNA-II; administrator of Bien-Hoa to lt. gov. of Cochinchina, 11 September 1903, GouCoch12473, VNA-II; extracts from political reports, 1903, INDO GGI 8457, ANOM.

97. Lauret, "Monopoles de l'Indo-Chine et leur remplacement," 95, INDO GGI 8456, ANOM; Le Thuan Phu to M. Le Rés. De France a Vinh Yen, 10 January 1912, RST 20.513, VNA-I.

98. This was a central argument for enforcing Article 96; Crayssac, dir. of the Douanes et Régies, to lt. gov. of Cochinchina, 15 September 1903 and 9 October 1903, GouCoch 12473, VNA-II; Dir. of the Douanes et Régies to the governor-general, 24 May 1906, INDO GGI 8280, ANOM.

99. "Opinions Annamites," Le Pionnier Indochinois, 28 November 1907, INDO GGI 1357, ANOM.

100. "Enquête sur la régie de l'alcool à Chuong My, Ha Dong, 1904," Résidence de Hadong, 4218, VNA-I; Letter of Le Thuan Phu to Rés. de France a Vinh Yen, 10 January 1912, RST 20.513, VNA-I.

101. Letter of Le Thuan Phu to Rés. de France a Vinh Yen, 10 January 1912, RST 20.513, VNA-I.

102. Letter of M. Maspero, administrator of Bien-Hoa, to the lt. gov. of Cochinchina, 1 June 1906, IB.29/032, VNA-II; letter of Le Thuan Phu to Rés. de France à Vinh Yen, 10 January 1912, RST 20.513, VNA-I.

103. Lauret, "Monopoles de l'Indochine et leur remplacement," 94, INDO GGI 8456, ANOM.

104. Report of governor-general Albert Sarraut to the minister of the colonies, 34, FP 9 PA 16, ANOM.

105. "A. S. De diverses propositions présentées par M. De Monpezat, 1908," INDO GGI 1333; Report to governor-general Albert Sarraut, 2, no date, FP 9 PA 15, ANOM.

106. Letter of Sanguinetti to Calmette, reproduced in a report to the governor-general, 26 September 1905, INDO GGI 1326, ANOM.

107. Governor-general to the Ministry of the Colonies, 18 October 1905.

108. For instance, see "Gros scandale imminent: Le monopole de l'alcool en Indochine," *Le Petit Bleu Illustré*, 12–19 June 1913, FP 9 PA 15, ANOM.

109. "Alcool et attentat à Hanoi," FP 9 PA 16, ANOM. For a history of Vietnamese resistance to colonial rule, see Charles Fournieau, *Vietnam: Domination coloniale et résistance nationale 1858–1914* (Paris: Les Indes Savantes, 2002), esp. 775–782.

110. Letter of the governor-general to the resident superior of Tonkin, 14 January 1913, RST 20.978, VNA-I; Malan's report to the minister of the colonies, 23 February 1912, 33–38, FP 9 PA 16, ANOM.

111. Letter of Le quan An to the resident of France at Kien-An, 10 January 1912, RST 20.972, VNA-I; Letter of Le tri-phu of Nghoa Hung to resident of Namdinh, 27 December 1911, VNA-I. "Rapport du Résident de Hung Yen sur le régime des alcools au Tonkin 1912," RST 20.799, VNA-I.

112. Malan's report to the minister of the colonies, 23 February 1912, 55–86, FP 9 PA 16, ANOM.

113. Note of the director of Douanes et Régies to the governor-general, undated (ca. 1912), esp. "II—Liberté de fabrication et de vente," FP 9 PA 15, ANOM.

114. Malan's report to the minister of the colonies, 23 February 1912, 74–75, FP 9 PA 16, ANOM.

115. Malan's report to the minister of the colonies, 23 February 1912, 57–64, FP 9 PA 16, ANOM.

116. See the discussion and draft legislation at the meeting of the Conseil Colonial, *Supplement du Journal Officiel de l'Indochine Française*, VIII–XXII, FP 9 PA 16, ANOM.

117. See Peters, "Taste, Taxes, and Technologies," 595; Dossier 192, unsigned note, December 1922, AgEcFOM 208, ANOM.

118. In 1934, when the existing system of awarded contracts and production quotas was abolished, this turned out to be exactly the case: although nominally under a system of free trade, the SFDI continued to dominate the Indochinese market. Sasges, "Contraband, Capital, and the Colonial State," 346–350.

119. Doumer, *Situation en Indochine*, 157.

120. "Arrêté concernant le régime des opiums en Indo-Chine du 7 février 1899," *Journal Officiel de l'Indochine Française*, February 1899, 182; see also "Contrôle et surveillance de la ferme de l'opium au Tonkin 1890–1899," Résidence de Hadong, 4366, VNA-I.

121. Sasges, Contraband, Capital, and the Colonial State," 5–6. For the importance of rượu byproducts for pig feed, see letter of Le Quan An to the resident of France at Kien-An, 10 January 1912, RST 20982, VNA-I.

122. "Rapport: Mission de M. Gigaux de Grandpré Commis de 4e Classe entre Yen Bay et Van Bu pour visiter les cultures de pavot et rechercher des terrains propices à cette culture," 13 December 1901; "Rapport de M. Lussan sur la culture du pavot au Haut-Laos," 8 July 1898, INDO GGI 41878, ANOM.

123. Letter of Kérébel, pharmacist 1st class to lt. gov. of Cochinchina, 20 December 1895, GouCoch IB.29/064, VNA-II; "Mission Bertrand-Spéder relatif à l'étude des procédés et fabrication de l'opium à fumer," 10 April 1901, FM 1AFF-POL 2417/

5, ANOM; letter of M. Frézoul, director of the Douanes et Régies to the governor-general, 18 January 1901, INDO GGI 8686, ANOM.

124. For the background of the International Opium Conventions, see David F. Musto, *The American Disease: Origins of Narcotics Control* (New Haven, CT: Yale University Press, 1973), 24–53; Joy Mott and Philip Bean, "The Development of Drug Control in Britain," in *The Control of Drugs and Drug Users: Reason or Reaction?*, ed. Ross Coomber (Amsterdam: Harwood Academic Publishers, 1998), 31–48; Gregory Blue, "Opium for China: The British Connection," in *Opium Regimes: China, Britain, and Japan, 1839–1952*, ed. Timothy Brook and Bob Tadashi (Berkeley: University of California Press, 2000), 31–54.

125. *Rapports et procés-verbaux du Comité International de l'Opium* (Shanghai, 1909), 84, INDO GGI 8679, ANOM.

126. *Convention International de l'Opium à la Haye, 1911–1912*, INDO GGI 43064, ANOM.

127. Report of Klobukowski, governor-general of Indochina, to the minister of the colonies, 27 December 1910; Letter of Lebrun, minister of the colonies, to the governor-general of Indochina, 17 May 1912, INDO GGI 43064, ANOM.

128. *Le Matin*, 22 April 1913; *Le Petit Journal*, 24 April 1913; *La Bataille Syndicaliste*, 4 May 1913, FP 9 PA 10, ANOM.

129. "Les ravages de l'opium dans la marine," *Le Petit Journal*, 24 April 1913, FP 9 PA 10, ANOM.

130. "Contre l'opium," *La France*, 30 April 1913, FP 9 PA 10, ANOM.

131. Report of the governor-general of Indochina to the minister of the colonies, 4 April 1908, FM 1 AFF-POL 2417/4, ANOM.

132. For instance, the letter of the resident of Than Hoa to the resident superior of Annam, 20 August 1907, INDO GGI 42994, ANOM; letter of the administrator of Cholon to the lt. gov. of Cochinchina, 16 December 1907; letter of the Inspecteur des Services Civils to the lt. gov. of Cochinchina, 14 December 1907; administrator of Gocong to the lt. gov. of Cochinchina, 14 December 1907, INDO GGI 42996, ANOM.

133. For instance, the discussion in the Chamber of Deputies, session of Wednesday, 23 July 1913, *Journal Officiel*, 24 July 1913, 2009–2011; see also telegram of Ernest Roume, governor-general of Indochina, to the minister of the colonies, 22 March 1916; Report of Ernest Roume, governor-general of Indochina, to the minister of the colonies, 16 May 1916, INDO GGI 43005, ANOM.

134. Letter of the governor-general to the resident-superior of Tonkin highlighting the "once again vigorously surging . . . movement against opiomania in the metropole thanks to the ravages the drug is causing in France, in some maritime or colonial milieux." 3 October 1913, INDO GGI 43007, ANOM.

135. Letter of the Inspecteur des Services Civils to the lt. gov. of Cochinchina, 14 December 1907, INDO GGI 42996; "Politique indochinoise de l'opium," Director of the Douanes et Régies to the governor-general, July 1922, INDO GGI 43070, ANOM.

136. Letter of the governor-general to the resident superior of Tonkin, 3 October 1913, INDO GGI 43007, ANOM.

137. "Des mesures prises depuis 1907 en Indo-Chine pour diminuer la consommation de l'opium et de leur effet pratique," in *Rapports et procés-verbaux du Comité International de l'Opium* (Shanghai, 1909), 124–125, INDO GGI 8679.

138. M. F. Drouhet, mayor of the City of Cholon, to the lt. gov. of Cochinchina, 13 November 1911, GouCoch IB.29/013, VNA-II; Director of the Douanes et Régies to the governor of Cochinchina, 10 August 1918, GouCoch IB.29/057, VNA-II.

139. Contrast, for instance, the discussion of the two monopolies in "Monopoles de l'Indo-Chine et leur remplacement," INDO GGI 8456, ANOM. The alcohol monopoly was said to have caused "discontent that at certain points translated into an outright revolt against our authority."

140. Letter of Albert Calmette to M. Leybold, 15 March 1892, CAL.B2.

141. For example, Albert Calmette, "L'oeuvre de Pasteur et les progrès de l'hygiène," *Bulletin de l'Académie Nationale de Medecine*, 26 December 1922; Albert Calmette, "Influence de l'oeuvre de Pasteur sur l'expansion colonisatrice des peuples," n.d., CAL.F, AIP. For the establishment of Pasteur Institutes in the Maghreb, see Kmar Annabi-Ben Nefissa, "L'Organisation Sanitaire en Tunisie à la veille de la création de l'Institut Pasteur de Tunis," *Archives de l'Institut Pasteur de Tunis* 71 (1994): 345–349.

Chapter 3

1. de Kruif, *Microbe Hunters*. For the language of "heroics" and "intrepid" adventuring, see description of Pasteur on p. 81; Yersin and Roux on p. 182, and throughout.

2. Céline, *Journey to the End of the Night*, trans. Ralph Manheim (New York: New Directions, 2009 [1932]), 239–240.

3. de Kruif, *Microbe Hunters*, 181–182; Céline, *Journey*, 239.

4. Céline, *Journey*, 243, 245.

5. Céline, *Journey*, 241.

6. Edward Berenson, *Heroes of Empire: Five Charismatic Men and the Conquest of Africa* (Berkeley: University of California Press, 2011).

7. Céline, *Voyage au bout de la nuit* (Paris: Gallimard, 2014), 316. I am using my own translation from the original French here: "Dans les fossés de la grande déroute," where the more accurate translation of "ditch" or "trench" conveys both the reference to the war and the inescapable sorriness of interwar society, while Manheim's translation of "mass grave" emphasizes the context of the war.

8. Robert Nye, "Medicine and Science as Masculine 'Fields of Honor,'" *Osiris* 12 (1996): 60–79; Erika Lorraine Milam and Robert Nye, "An Introduction to Scientific Masculinities," *Osiris* 30 (2015): 1–12; Andrew Warwick, *Masters of Theory: Cambridge and the Rise of Mathematical Physics* (Chicago: University of Chicago Press, 2003); Robert Kohler, *Lords of the Fly: Drosophila Genetics and the Experimental Life* (Chicago: University of Chicago Press, 1993).

9. Heather Ellis, *Masculinity and Science in Britain, 1831–1918* (Basingstoke: Palgrave Macmillan, 2018).

10. See Milam and Nye, "An Introduction to Scientific Masculinities," 3–4; Ellis, *Masculinity and Science in Britain*, 2, 5–6, for calls for further research.

11. There is a wide body of scholarship on the crisis of degeneration and manhood in fin-de-siècle France. Key works include Robert Nye, *Masculinity and Male Codes of Honor in Modern France* (Berkeley: University of California Press, 1998); Daniel Pick, *Faces of Degeneration: A European Disorder, c. 1848–1918* (Cambridge: Cambridge University Press, 1993); André Rauch, *Le premier sexe: Mutations et crise de l'identité masculine* (Paris: Hachette, 2000); Christopher Forth and Bertrand Taithe, eds., *French Masculinities: History, Culture and Politics* (Basingstoke: Palgrave Macmillan, 2007); Christopher Forth and Elinor Accampo, eds., *Confronting Modernity in Fin-de-Siècle France: Bodies, Minds and Gender* (New York: Palgrave Macmillan, 2009); Joan Tumblety, *Remaking the Male Body: Masculinity and the Uses of Physical Culture in Interwar and Vichy France* (Oxford: Oxford University Press, 2012).

12. Margaret Cook Andersen, *Regeneration through Empire: French Pronatalists and Colonial Settlement in the Third Republic* (Lincoln: University of Nebraska Press, 2015); Elizabeth Ezra, *The Colonial Unconscious: Race and Culture in Interwar France* (Ithaca, NY: Cornell University Press, 2000), 21–47; Aro Velmet, "Beauty and Big Business: Race and Civilizational Decline in French Beauty Pageants, 1920–37," *French History* 28, no. 1 (March 2014): 66–91. Others have highlighted how the empire could pose a threat to the French race. Eliza Camiscioli, *Reproducing the French Race: Immigration, Intimacy, and Embodiment in the Early Twentieth Century* (Durham, NC: Duke University Press, 2009).

13. On science and the mission civilisatrice, see Conklin, *A Mission to Civilize*, 38–70; Patrick Petitjean, "Science and the 'Civilizing Mission': France and the Colonial Enterprise," in *Science across the European Empires—1800–1950*, ed. Benediky Stutchey (Oxford: Oxford University Press, 2005), 107–128; Berenson, *Heroes of Empire*.

14. For a theorization of the scientific "persona," see Lorraine Daston and H. Otto Sibum, "Introduction: Scientific Personae and Their Histories," *Science in Context* 16, nos. 1/2 (2003): 1–8, as well as other essays in the special issue, in particular Janet Browne, "Charles Darwin as a Celebrity," 175–194, and Cathryn Carson, "Objectivity and the Scientist: Heisenberg Rethinks," 243–269.

15. Steven Shapin's argument on how truth-telling depended on possessing and publicly demonstrating honorable qualities is made in the context of early modern England in *A Social History of Truth: Civility and Science in Seventeenth-Century England* (Chicago: University of Chicago Press, 1994). Robert Nye argues that honor (though transformed from an aristocratic into a bourgeois quality) remained an important indicator of credibility in nineteenth-century France; see Nye, "Medicine and Science as Masculine 'Fields of Honor,'" 65–69.

16. The notion of a "moral economy" of scientific exchange is from Kohler, *Lords of the Fly*. Warwick Anderson makes a similar argument in *The Collectors of Lost Souls: Turning Kuru Scientists into Whitemen* (Baltimore: Johns Hopkins University Press, 2006).

17. Latour, *The Pasteurization of France*, 69; Barnes, *The Great Stink of Paris*; Geison, *The Private Science of Louis Pasteur*.

18. Louis Pasteur cited in René Doumic, "Une biographie de savant," *Revue des Deux Mondes* 162 (1900): 465.

19. Geison, *The Private Science of Louis Pasteur*, 269.

20. Lorraine Daston, "Objectivity and the Escape from Perspective," *Social Studies of Science* 22, no. 4 (November 1992): 597–618; see also Lorraine Daston and Peter Galison, *Objectivity* (Cambridge, MA: MIT Press, 2007).

21. Peter Galison, "Objectivity Is Romantic," in *The Humanities and the Sciences*, ed. P. Galison, S. Haack, and J. Friedman, ACLS Occasional Papers 14 (1999), 17–18.

22. Galison, "Objectivity Is Romantic," 25–26.

23. Steven Shapin makes a similar argument in the Anglo-American context in *The Scientific Life: A Moral History of a Late Modern Vocation* (Chicago: University of Chicago Press, 2008), 21–46; Philip Mirowski has critiqued his argument in *Science-Mart: Privatizing American Science* (Cambridge, MA: Harvard University Press, 2011), 87–89.

24. Claude Bernard, *An Introduction to the Study of Experimental Medicine*, trans. Henry Copley Greene (New York: Henry Schuman, 1949 [1865]), 18–23. Contrast this, for instance, to Ernest Renan's conception of science as unity in human self-development toward perfection in *The Future of Science: Ideas of 1848*, trans. Albert D. Vandam and C. B. Pitman (London: Chapman and Hill, 1891 [1890]). Even Renan, however, noted that the key quality of the best scientists was their "courage to abstain" (235).

25. Bernard, *An Introduction to the Study of Experimental Medicine*, 35.

26. Bernard, *An Introduction to the Study of Experimental Medicine*, 39.

27. Nye, *Masculinity and Male Codes of Honor*, 31–32.

28. Bernard cited in Patrice Debré, "Louis Pasteur et Claude Bernard: autour d'un conflit posthume," *Biologie aujourd'hui* 211, no. 2 (2017), 161.

29. Pasteur cited in Geison, *The Private Science of Louis Pasteur*, 20.

30. *L'inauguration de l'Institut Pasteur, compte-rendu* (Paris: Scéaux, 1888); "L'Institut Pasteur," *La République Française*, 14 November 1888, DR.FND.2, AIP.

31. Alexis Lemaistre, *L'Institut de France et nos grands établissements scientifiques* (Paris: Hachette, 1896), 197.

32. Lemaistre, *L'Institut de France*, 208.

33. "Le Palais de la rage," *Le Gaulois*, 15 November 1888; "L'Institut Pasteur," *Le Temps*, 14 November 1888, DR.FND.2, AIP.

34. "L'Institut Pasteur," *Le Matin*, 14 November 1888, DR.FND.2, AIP.

35. "Le Palais de la rage," *Le Gaulois*, 15 November 1888.

36. On staff living arrangements before the inauguration of the Pasteur Institute, see Yersin's letters to his mother, 26 December. 1886, 13 March 1887; after the institute's inauguration, see 20 January 1889, NUM.YERSIN, AIP.

37. Geison, *The Private Science of Louis Pasteur*, 51.

38. "Le palais de la rage," *Le Gaulois*, 15 November 1888.

39. "Le palais de la rage," *Le Gaulois*, 15 November 1888; "Au jour le jour: l'Institut Pasteur," *La Liberté*, 14 November 1888, DR.FND.2, AIP.

40. "L'Institut Pasteur," *Le Monde Illustrée*, 15 November 1888; Gustave Fischbach, "Souscription pour l'Institut Pasteur," *Strasbourg*, 11 March 1886.

41. Discours de M. Christophe, "Inauguration de l'Institut Pasteur," 14 November 1888 (Paris: Sceaux, 1888), 23, DR.FND.2, AIP.

42. Yersin's letter to his mother, 7 November 1885, NUM.YERSIN, AIP.

43. Yersin's letter to his mother, 3 April 1886, NUM.YERSIN, AIP.

44. Yersin's letter to his mother, 8 May 1886, NUM.YERSIN, AIP.

45. Yersin's letter to his mother, 20 November. 1886, NUM.YERSIN, AIP.

46. Yersin's letters to his mother, 30 December 1888; 13 January 1889; 3 February 1889, NUM.YERSIN, AIP;

47. Yersin's letter to his mother, 3 January 1886, NUM.YERSIN, AIP.

48. Henri H. Mollaret and Jacqueline Brossollet, *Alexandre Yersin, 1863–1943: Un Pasteurien en Indochine* (Paris: Bellin, 1993), 55; Yersin's letter to his mother, 16 December 1888, NUM.YERSIN, AIP.

49. Discours de M. Pasteur, "Inauguration de l'Institut Pasteur," 14 November 1888 (Paris: Sceaux, 1888), 28, DR.FND.2, AIP.

50. Discours de M. Pasteur, 29, DR.FND.2, AIP.

51. Discours de M. Pasteur, 29, DR.FND.2, AIP.

52. Discours de M. Pasteur, 27, DR.FND.2, AIP.

53. Ed Cohen, *A Body Worth Defending: Immunity, Biopolitics, and the Apotheosis of the Modern Body* (Durham, NC: Duke University Press, 2009).

54. "Le Palais de la rage," *Le Gaulois*, 15 November 1888, DR.FND.2, AIP.

55. On diphtheria, see Jonathan Simon, *Diphtheria Serum as a Technological Object: A Philosophical Analysis of Serotherapy in France 1894–1900* (Lanham, MD: Lexington Books, 2016), 72, 91–92, 107–113. Other examples include BCG and rabies; Geison, *The Private Science of Louis Pasteur*, 263.

56. Simon, *Diphtheria Serum as a Technological Object*, 113, 105.

57. Nye, "Medicine and Science as Masculine 'Fields of Honor,'" 61–63; Kohler, *Lords of the Fly*, 93–112; see also Ellis, *Masculinity and Science in Britain*, 133–141.

58. E. Roux, "À propos d'une observation de MM. Moizard et Bouchard," *Journal de Clinique et de Thérapeutique Infantiles*, 1 August 1895, 601–604. There are many other examples of Pastorians dissociating themselves from their products, when these are embroiled in controversies; see, for example, Albert Calmette's responses to the Lübeck controversy in the 1920s, where a contaminated batch of the Pastorian BCG vaccine caused the death of dozens of infants. Calmette's letter to the lawyer of Alstaed, July 1931; Calmette's letter to Kolle, 6 October 1931, BCG.16, AIP.

59. G. Variot, "Une querelle médicale," *Journal de Clinique et de Thérapeutique Infantiles*, August 1, 1895, 605.

60. Yersin's letter to his mother, 13 October 1889; Yersin's letter to his mother, 20 October 1889, NUM.YERSIN, AIP.

61. Yersin's letter to his mother, 1 December 1889, NUM.YERSIN, AIP.

62. Yersin's letter to his mother, 1 December 1889, NUM.YERSIN, AIP.

63. Berenson, *Heroes of Empire*.

64. Edward Berenson, *The Trial of Madame Caillaux* (Berkeley: University of California Press, 1992), 209; Berenson, *Heroes of Empire*, 25–26.

65. Yersin's letter to his mother, 20 October 1889, NUM.YERSIN, AIP.

66. Yersin's letter to his mother, 3 December 1890, NUM.YERSIN, AIP.

67. Yersin's letters to his mother, 20 March 1892, 2 Nov. 1892, NUM.YERSIN, AIP.

68. Yersin's letter to his mother, 20 March 1892, NUM.YERSIN, AIP.

69. Raoul Jully, "Le Docteur Yersin chez les mois," *Le Journal des Voyages*, 26 May 1895 and onward, YER.6, AIP.

70. Raoul Jully, "Le Docteur Yersin chez les mois VII," *Le Journal des Voyages*, YER.6, AIP.

71. "Le retour du Dr. Yersin," *Le Journal de Morges*, 5 December 1895.

72. Hess, "Le Docteur Yersin et le vaccin de la peste"; ; see also "Le Docteur Yersin," *Écho de la Semaine*, 17 February 1897.

73. Yersin's letter to his mother, 11 December 1897, NUM.YERSIN, AIP; see also Eric Jennings, *Imperial Heights: Dalat and the Making and Undoing of French Indochina* (Berkeley: University of California Press, 2011), 21–34.

74. Mitchitake Aso, "Forests without Birds: Science, Environment, and Health in French Colonial Vietnam" (PhD diss., University of Wisconsin–Madison, 2011), 55–57.

75. Yersin's letters to his sister, 28 September 1908; 27 January 1911, NUM. YERSIN, AIP.

76. Yersin's letters to his sister, 6 April 1910; 7 May 1910; 2 June 1910; 27 August 1910, NUM.YERSIN, AIP.

77. For the economic arguments around the Nha Trang laboratory, see, for example, Yersin to the governor-general of Indochina, 1 September 1896, GGI 2510, ANOM.

78. Here I am drawing from Robert Kohler's *Lords of the Fly*; the notion of a "moral economy," of course, comes originally from E. P. Thompson, "The Moral Economy of the English Crowd in the Eighteenth Century," *Past and Present* 50 (February 1971): 76–136.

79. Calmette to Simond, 19 May 1898, SIM.4.1, AIP.

80. Calmette to Simond, 28 September 1897; 18 July 1898; 19 May 1898, SIM.4.1, AIP.

81. Calmette to Simond, 9 January 1899, SIM.4.1, AIP.

82. Calmette to Simond, 14 January 1899, SIM.4.1, AIP.

83. Calmette to Simond, 14 January 1899, SIM.4.1, AIP.

84. Calmette to Simond, 5 October 1898, SIM.4.1, AIP.

85. Calmette to Simond, 5 October 1898, SIM.4.1, AIP.

86. On self-restraint and managing of passions as masculine ideals, see George L. Mosse, *The Image of Man: The Creation of Modern Masculinity* (New York: Oxford University Press, 1996), 94–98.

87. Christopher E. Forth, *The Dreyfus Affair and the Crisis of French Manhood* (Baltimore: Johns Hopkins University Press, 2006), 12.

88. Calmette to Simond, 14 January 1899, SIM.4.1, AIP.

89. Nicolle to Félix Mesnil, 21 October 1931, NCP.11, AIP.

90. Annabi-Ben Nefissa, "L'Organisation Sanitaire en Tunisie à la veille de la création de l'Institut Pasteur de Tunis," *Archives de l'Institut Pasteur de Tunis* 71 (July 1994): 345–349; Anne-Marie Moulin, "Les Instituts Pasteur de la Méditerranée

Arabe: Une religion scientifique en pays d'Islam," in *Santé, Médecine et Société dans le Monde Arabe*, ed. Elisabeth Longuenesse (Paris: L'Harmattan, 1995), 136.

91. Charles Nicolle, "L'Institut Pasteur de Tunis," *Archives de l'Institut Pasteur de Tunis* 1 (1906): 4–34.

92. Paul Rabinow, *French Modern: Norms and Forms of the Social Environment* (Chicago: University of Chicago Press, 1989), 282–288.

93. Nicolle, "L'Institut Pasteur de Tunis," 6; Charles Nicolle, cited in Pierre Nicolle, "Un événement historique dans la vie de Charles NICOLLE: l'inauguration officielle, il y aura 70 ans cette année, de l'Institut Pasteur de Tunis (d'après des lettres de Charles Nicolle, retrouvées et commentées par Pierre Nicolle)," *Archives de l'Institut Pasteur de Tunis* 69 (1975), 197.

94. Nicolle, "Un événement historique," 198; Nicolle, "L'Institut Pasteur de Tunis," 8.

95. Nicolle, "L'Institut Pasteur de Tunis," 8.

96. Nicolle, "Un événement historique," 202.

97. Nicolle, "Un événement historique," 199.

98. Nicolle, "Un événement historique," 197.

99. Pelis, *Charles Nicolle*, 59–64.

100. Pelis, *Charles Nicolle*, 72–73.

101. Charles Nicolle to Ludovic Blaizot, 25 October 1918, 146 J 36; Marthe Conor to Charles Nicolle, 9 April 1914, 146 J 25, ADSM. This episode is described in detail in Pelis, *Charles Nicolle*; I largely follow Pelis's discussion in the following paragraphs.

102. Annick Guénel and Anne-Marie Moulin, "L'Institut Pasteur et la naissance de l'industrie de la santé," in *La philosophie du remède*, ed. Jean-Claude Beaune (Paris: Éditions Champs-Vallon, 1993), 100–104.

103. Ludovic Blaizot to Charles Nicolle, 27 February 1914, 146.J.23, ADSM.

104. John Strachan, "The Pasteurization of Algeria?," *French History* 20, no. 3 (August 2006): 274.

105. Strachan, "The Pasteurization of Algeria?," 273–275.

106. Francisco Javier Martinez, "Double Trouble: French Colonialism in Morocco and the Early History of the Pasteur Institutes of Tangier and Casablanca (1895–1932)," *Dynamis* 36, no. 2 (2016) 317–339; for Morocco, see Amster, *Medicine and the Saints*.

107. Albert Calmette, *Association pour l'extension des études Pastoriennes, rapport du Dr. Calmette* (Paris: R. Tancrède, 1921), 5, CAL.F, AIP.

108. Albert Calmette, *Association pour l'extension des études Pastoriennes, Rapport du Dr. Calmette* (Paris: R. Tancrède, 1921), 5, CAL.F, AIP.

109. Albert Calmette, *Association pour l'extension des études Pastoriennes, Rapport du Dr. Calmette* (Paris: R. Tancrède, 1921), 8–14, CAL.F, AIP.

110. Albert Calmette, *Association pour l'extension des études Pastoriennes, Rapport du Dr. Calmette* (Paris: R. Tancrède, 1921), 21, CAL.F, AIP.

111. Calmette to Nicolle, 2 January 1919, NIC.3, AIP.

112. Roger Kervran, *Albert Calmette et le B.C.G.* (Paris: Librairie Hachette, 1962), 143–144.

113. Yersin to his sister, 14 December 1919, NUM.YERSIN; Calmette to Yersin, 20 June 1920, NIC.3, AIP.

114. For Tunis, see Pelis, *Charles Nicolle*, 92; for Indochina, see Yersin to his sister, 2 February 1917; 1 May 1917; 3 August. 1917, NUM.YERSIN; for Dakar, see Constant Mathis, *Oeuvre des Pastoriens en Afrique Noire, Afrique Occidentale Française* (Paris: Presses Universitaires de France, 1946), 52–56.

115. Mathis, *Oeuvre des Pastoriens*, 53; Albert Calmette, *Association pour l'extension des études Pastoriennes, Rapport du Dr. Calmette* (Paris: R. Tancrède, 1921), 15–16, CAL.F, AIP; Pelis, *Charles Nicolle*, 94–95.

116. Yersin to his sister, 12 October 1914, NUM.YERSIN, AIP.

117. Yersin to his sister, 2 February 1917; 1 May 1917, NUM.YERSIN, AIP.

118. Pelis, *Charles Nicolle*, 94.

119. Mosse, *The Image of Man*, 108–114.

120. Peter J. Bloom, *French Colonial Documentary: Mythologies of Humanitarianism* (Minneapolis: University of Minnesota Press, 2008), ix.

121. *La Maladie du Sommeil*, directed by Alfred Chaumel (1930; Gaumont-Pathé, 1930), DVD, CNC.

122. *Promenade en Afrique Équatoriale Française*, directed by J. K. Raymond-Millet (Comité du Propagande Colonial par le Film, 1931), DVD, CNC.

123. Leredde to Nicolle, 26 December 1916, NIC.3, AIP.

124. Burnet to Nicolle, 24 June 1922; 1 July 1925; 7 July 1925; 18 July 1925, NIC.3, AIP.

125. Leredde to Nicolle, 29 March 1920, NIC.3, AIP.

126. Leredde to Nicolle, 29 March 1920, NIC.3, AIP.

127. Leredde to Nicolle, 29 March 1920, NIC.3, AIP.

128. Burnet to Nicolle, 24 June 1922, NIC.3 AIP.

129. Nicolle to Vallery-Radot, 5 August 1920, NCP.12, AIP.

130. Calmette to Nicolle, 24 January 1920, NIC.3 AIP.

131. Calmette to Nicolle, 31 May 1919, NIC.3 AIP

132. "La cérémonie de l'Institut Pasteur," *Le Temps*, 28 December 1922.

133. "La cérémonie de l'Institut Pasteur."

134. Discours de M. le Dr. É. Roux, 26 December 1922, DIR.CR1, AIP.

135. "La cérémonie de l'Institut Pasteur."

136. "Pasteur," review, undated, DIR.CR2, AIP.

137. "Comment fut tourné le film: Pasteur," review, undated, DIR.CR2, AIP.

138. *Pasteur*, directed by J. Epstein and J. Benoit-Lévy (Ministère d'Agriculture, 1922), DVD, CNC.

139. "Discours de M. Édmond Sergent," 16 June 1923; "Discours de M. le Gouverneur-Général," 16 June 1923, DIR.C3, AIP.

140. "Discours de M. le Gouverneur-Général," 16 June 1923, DIR.C3, AIP.

141. "Discours de M. Édmond Sergent," 16 June 1923, DIR.C3, AIP.

142. "Souvenir offert aux écoliers de Tunisie," 27 December 1922, DIR.CR3, AIP.

143. "La semaine de Pasteur à l'école (cinq brèves causeries)," undated, DIR. CR3, AIP.

144. "Discours de M. Édmond Sergent," 16 June 1923, DIR.C3, AIP.

145. Nicolle to Vallery-Radot, 4 February 1921, NCP.12, AIP.

146. Charles Nicolle, "Le péril des études microbiennes en France," *Le Temps*, 8 October 1920.

147. Nicolle, "Le péril des études microbiennes en France."

148. Charles Nicolle, "Une heure avec le Docteur Charles Nicolle. La grande misère de l'Institut Pasteur: Un cri d'alarme," *Les Nouvelles Litteraires*, 3 February 1934.

149. Roux to Nicolle, 18 October 1920, 146 J 33, ADSM.

150. Calmette to Nicolle, 23 March 1918, NIC.3; Mathis to Mesnil, 9 January 1927, MES.6, AIP.

151. Maurice Barrès, "Les fils spirituels de Pasteur," *Les Échos*, n.d. (most likely around 1919–1920), CAL.F, AIP.

152. Maurice Barrès, "Les fils spirituels de Pasteur," *Les Échos*, n.d. (most likely around 1919–1920), CAL.F, AIP.

153. Maurice Barrès, "Les fils spirituels de Pasteur," *Les Échos*, n.d. (most likely around 1919–1920), CAL.F, AIP.

154. *Association pour l'extension des études Pastoriennes* (Paris: R. Tancrède, 1921).

155. Calmette, *Association pour l'Extension des études Pastoriennes*.

156. Georges Duhamel, "Le docteur Nicolle expliqué par Georges Duhamel," *Le Jour*, 25 November 1933.

157. Pasteur Vallery-Radot, "Rapport sur l'organisation des Instituts Pasteur d'Outre-mer," 12 January 1938, IPOM, AIP.

158. Pasteur Vallery-Radot, "Les Instituts Pasteur d'Outre-Mer," *Institut Pasteur, Cérémonie du 15 Mars 1939*, 39, DIR.CR.6 AIP.

159. Pasteur Vallery-Radot, "Les Instituts Pasteur d'Outre-Mer," *Institut Pasteur, cérémonie du 15 Mars 1939*, 40, DIR.CR.6 AIP.

160. Pasteur Vallery-Radot, "Le bilan de l'effort français: l'Institut Pasteur," *Revue des Deux Mondes*, 1 April 1939, 609–610.

161. Pierre Mauriac, "Pasteur en marge des discours officiels," *Le Bulletin Médical*, no date (1923), DIR.CR3, AIP.

162. Pierre Mauriac, "Pasteur en marge des discours officiels," *Le Bulletin Médical*, no date (1923), DIR.CR3, AIP.

163. de Kruif, *Microbe Hunters*.

164. For instance, see the periodization into a "heroic era" and a "mature era" in Dedet, *Les Instituts Pasteur d'Outre-Mer*, 16; Mollaret and Jacqueline Brossollet, *Alexandre Yersin*; Bernard, *La vie et l'oeuvre de Albert Calmette*.

Chapter 4

1. Tuberculosis epidemiology in Algeria is the subject of an upcoming study by Clifford Rosenberg, *Infection, Inequality, and the Colonial State: The Spread of TB from France to Algeria and Back, 1830–c. 1970* (forthcoming).

2. Albert Calmette, "La tuberculose des indigènes en Afrique occidentale française," *La Presse Médicale 72*, 7 September 1929, 1178; Pasteur Vallery-Radot and Noël

Bernard, "Les missionnaires de Pasteur," *Patrie: Revue Mensuelle Illustrée de l'Empire* 6 (1942): 44.

3. "Scale-making" is a term developed by Anna Tsing; see Tsing, *Friction*, 56–60.

4. This process might be compared to how objects previously thought of as "natural" or as belonging to the commons are transformed into commodities through the production of market devices; or how the study of retroviruses in Cameroon reframed the country from being a locus of a multiplicity of serious yet easily treatable diseases to one that posed a threat to global "biosecurity" by potentially harboring a new, deadly, but completely hypothetical (and ultimately nonexistent) HIV strain. In all of these cases, ecological objects and processes such as the discovery of uranium or the spread of HIV are politically (re)constructed in order to privilege certain actors over others. Gabrielle Hecht, *Being Nuclear: Africans and the Global Uranium Trade* (Cambridge, MA: MIT Press, 2012), esp. 49–78; Michel Callon, *Laws of the Markets* (London: Wiley-Blackwell, 1998); Donald MacKenzie, Fabian Muniesa, and Lucia Siu, eds., *Do Economists Make Markets?* (Princeton, NJ: Princeton University Press, 2007); Guillaume Lachenal, "Lessons in Medical Nihilism: Virus Hunters, Neoliberalism, and the AIDS Pandemic in Cameroon," in Geissler, *Para-states and Medical Science*, 103–141.

5. See Gouvernement général de l'Afrique Occidentale Française, *Exposition coloniale internationale de 1931*, vol. 3 (Paris: Société d'éditions géographiques, maritimes et coloniales, 1931), 214–216, for discussion of the spread of TB; the citation is from S. Rosso, "Alors que l'Exposition se ferme," *Le Cri des Nègres*, November 1931.

6. Randall M. Packard, *White Plague, Black Labor: Tuberculosis and the Political Economy of Health and Disease in South Africa* (Berkeley: University of California Press, 1989).

7. Barnes, *The Making of a Social Disease*, 5.

8. Contemporary statisticians in the League of Nations also drew attention to the unreliability of epidemiological data drawn from mortality and morbidity statistics, due to irregularities in data collection, disease ontologies that changed over time and space, and changes in statistical classifications. Finally, critics noted that even if the statistical data were correct, it would be difficult to draw conclusions about changing etiology based on changing mortality statistics alone. S. Rosenfeld, *Tuberculosis Statistics: Summary of the Report* (Geneva, 1926), R.881, and "Some observations on method of statistical research and upon the interpretation of statistical data with particular reference to the programme of the TB commission," undated (ca. 1927), R.882 LNA.

9. William W. Stead and Joseph H. Bates, "Epidemiology and Prevention of Tuberculosis," in *Pulmonary Diseases and Disorders*, 2nd ed., ed. Alfred P. Fishman (New York: McGraw-Hill, 1988), vol. 3, 1795.

10. Barnes, *The Making of a Social Disease*, 6–8.

11. Barnes, *The Making of a Social Disease*; for the connection between social, moral, and political anxieties and TB, see also Isabelle Grellet and Caroline Kruse, *Histoires de la tuberculose: Les fièvres de l'âme, 1800–1940* (Paris: Ramsay, 1983); Dominique Dessertine and Olivier Faure, *Combattre la tuberculose* (Lyon: Presse Universitaire de Lyon, 1988); Corbin, *Le miasme et la jonquille*.

12. Barnes, *The Making of a Social Disease*, 76.

13. Barnes, *The Making of a Social Disease*, 112–174.

14. For instance, a 1922 Health Congress presentation lamented that TB had only been the subject of a "restrained number of systematic studies"; Kérandel, "La tuberculose chez les indigènes dans les colonies françaises," in *Congrès de la santé publique et de la prévoyance sociale, Marseille, 11–17 septembre 1922* (Paris: Imprimerie Nationale, 1923).

15. *Rapport d'ensemble annuel: Gouvernement général de l'Afrique occidentale française* (Paris: Émile Larose, 1909), 14; *Rapport d'ensemble annuel: Gouvernement général de l'Afrique occidentale française* (Paris: Émile Larose, 1910), 42; *Rapport d'ensemble annuel: Gouvernement général de l'Afrique occidentale française* (Paris: Émile Larose, 1911), 212.

16. For example, *Indochine: Situation générale de la colonie pendant l'année 1912* (Hanoi: Imprimerie d'Êxtreme-Orient, 1913), 8–10, 18–19, 47–49; tuberculosis is only mentioned as an "occasional disease" in a report from Koang-Tchéou-Wan, 70; *Rapports au Conseil Supérieur, Session ordinaire de 1910* (Hanoi: Imprimerie d'Êxtreme-Orient, 1913), 162.

17. Marcel Leger discusses these dissertations in his overview of tuberculosis studies in West Africa, "La tubérculose au Sénégal, étude historique," *Bulletin du Comité d'études historiques et scientifiques de l'Afrique occidentale française, 1922*, 534–536.

18. Alexandre Kermorgant, *La tuberculose dans les colonies Françaises et plus particulièrement chez les indigènes* (Paris: Imprimerie Nationale, 1906).

19. Packard, *White Plague, Black Labor*, 22–32, 194–210. For the discursive uses of the virgin soil theory with other diseases, specifically in the conquest of the Americas, see David S. Jones, "Virgin Soils Revisited," *William and Mary Quarterly* 60, no. 4 (October 2003): 703–742.

20. Kermorgant, *La tuberculose dans les colonies Françaises*, 6–8.

21. Kermorgant, *La tuberculose dans les colonies Françaises*.

22. M. le dr. Hénaff, "La tuberculose chez les indigènes de Cochinchine," *Annales d'Hygiène et de Médecine Coloniales* 6 (1903): 51–52.

23. Hénaff, "La tuberculose chez les indigènes de Cochinchine," 50; M. le dr. Angier, "La tuberculose au Cambodge," *Annales d'Hygiène et de Médecine Coloniales* 6 (1903): 65.

24. Kermorgant, *La tuberculose dans les colonies Françaises*, 22.

25. J. P. F. Thévenot, *Traité des maladies des Européens dans les pays chauds et spécialement au Sénégal* (Paris: J-B Bailliére, 1840), 252; for claims to a consensus, see Louis-Joseph Janvier, *Phtisie pulmonaire: Causes, traitement préventif* (Paris: Impr. A Parent, 1884), 24–26. According to Marcel Leger, this consensus began to fracture in the late 1880s with the first hospital statistics in Saint-Louis and Dakar on tuberculosis patients; "La tubérculose au Sénégal, étude historique," 534–536.

26. J. Crambs, *Contribution à la géographie médicale du Soudan occidental (région aurifère entre le haut Sénégal et le haut Niger)* (Bordeaux: Thèse de doctorat, 1887); Alphonse Voillot, *Contribution à l'étude de la tuberculose aux colonies* (Paris: Thèses médicales, 1898), 45.

27. Kermorgant, *La tuberculose dans les colonies Françaises*, 13.

28. Voillot, *Contribution à l'étude de la tuberculose aux colonies*, 21. See also Dr. Crespin, "Paludisme et tuberculose," in *Congrès International de la Tuberculose tenu à Paris du 2 au 7 octobre 1905* (Paris: Masson et Cie, 1906), 540.

29. Hénaff, "La tuberculose chez les indigènes de Cochinchine," 59.

30. E. Jeanselme, "La tuberculose dans la presqu'île Indo-Chinoise et dans le Yunnan," in *Congrès International de la Tuberculose tenu à Paris du 2 au 7 octobre 1905* (Paris: Masson et Cie, 1906), 546–547.

31. J. Mahé, "Programme de séméiotique et d'étiologie pour l'étude des maladies exotiques et principalement des maladies des pays chauds," *Archives de Médecine Navale* 32 (1879): 47.

32. Kermorgant, *La tuberculose dans les colonies Françaises*, 14. See also Voillot, *Contribution à l'étude de la tuberculose aux colonies*, 43.

33. Voillot, *Contribution à l'étude de la tuberculose aux colonies*, 43.

34. Kermorgant, *La tuberculose dans les colonies Françaises*, 13.

35. Dr. Feuillet cited in Dr. Gillot, "Progression de la tuberculose en Algérie," in *Congrès International de la Tuberculose tenu à Paris du 2 au 7 octobre 1905* (Paris: Masson et Cie, 1906), 549.

36. J. C. M. Boudin, *Traite de geographie et de statistique médicales et des maladies endemiques* (London: J. B. Bailliere et fils, 1857), 96.

37. Dr. Crespin, "Paludisme et tuberculose," in *Congrès International de la Tuberculose tenu à Paris du 2 au 7 octobre 1905* (Paris: Masson et Cie, 1906), 541.

38. Georges Darenberg, *La Phtisie Pulmonaire*, vol. 2 (Paris: J. Rueff, 1892), 115; H. Hérard, V. Cornil, and V. Hanot, *La phtisie pulmonaire*, 2nd ed. (Paris: Felix Alsan, 1888), 364–365.

39. Hénaff, "La tuberculose chez les indigènes de Cochinchine," 54–55.

40. For an overview of reports emphasizing the spread of TB in Senegal, see Marcel Leger, "La tubérculose au Sénégal, étude historique," *Bulletin du Comité d'études historiques et scientifiques de l'Afrique occidentale française, 1922*, 535–537. By contrast, see Kermorgant's argument about the relative lack of tuberculosis compared with metropolitan France, *La tuberculose dans les colonies Françaises*.

41. Kermorgant, *La tuberculose dans les colonies Françaises*, 23–24.

42. Circular of the governor-general of the AOF to govs. gen. of AOF, Indochina and Madagascar and to the comissaire general of the Congo, *Bulletin Administratif du Gouvernement général de l'Afrique occidentale française*, 2 March 1900; Circular of the governor-general of the AOF to govs. gen. of AOF, Indochina and Madagascar and to the comissaire general of the Congo, *Bulletin Administratif du Gouvernement général de l'Afrique occidentale française*, 19 February 1904.

43. Abbatucci and Gravellat, *Prophylaxie de la tuberculose parmi les troupes indigènes coloniales* (Paris: Masson et Cie, 1923), 3.

44. Albert Calmette, autobiographical notes, 17, CAL.A1, AIP.

45. Bernard, *La vie et oeuvre de Albert Calmette*, 137–145; A. Calmette and M. Breton, *L'ankylostomasie. Anémie des mineurs* (Paris: Masson et Cie, 1905).

46. Albert Calmette, "Dispensaires pour tuberculeux," in *Moyens pratiques de combattre la propagation de la tuberculose*, ed. Commission de la Tuberculose (Paris: Masson et Cie, 1900), 331.

47. Louis Bernard, cited in L. Martin and G. Brouardel, *Traité d'hygiène*, vol. 23 (Paris: Baillière, 1929), 149.

48. Lion Murard and Patrick Zilberman, "L'autre guerre (1914–1918): La santé publique en France sous l'œil de l'Amérique," *Revue Historique* 276, no. 2 (October–December 1986): 372.

49. Charles Nordmann, "La croisade des américains contre la tuberculose," *Revue des Deux Mondes*, 15 September 1919, 458, Folder 266, Box 28, Series 500 T, RG 1.1, RAC.

50. Murard and Zilberman, "L'autre guerre (1914–1918)," 378; Vincent Viet, *La santé en guerre, 1914–1918: Une politique pionnière en univers incertain* (Paris: Presses de Sciences Po, 2015).

51. Dessertine and Faure, *Combattre la tuberculose*, 36–43.

52. Lion Murard and Patrick Zilberman, "Les fondations indestructibles: La santé publique en France et la Fondation Rockefeller," *Médicine/Sciences* 18, no. 5 (2002): 625–632.

53. Farley, *To Cast Out Disease*, 48–50; school assignment cited on p. 50.

54. Farley, *To Cast Out Disease*, 51–54.

55. Examples from the collection of TB stamp campaigns, CNDT.A1, AIP

56. Étienne Bernard, *Tuberculose et médecine sociale* (Paris: Masson et Cie, 1938), 147–149.

57. Auguste Lumière, *Tuberculose: Contagion, hérédité* (Lyon: Joannès Desvigne et Cie, 1931).

58. "International Health Board, Work in France, Summary of Report Activities 1922," Folder 276, Box 32, Series 500 T, RG 1.1, RAC.

59. Commission for the Prevention of Tuberculosis in France, final report vol. 1, Folder 260, Box 28, Series 500 T, RG 1.1, RAC.

60. Albert Calmette, *L'effort nationale de défense contre la tuberculose* (Paris: Comité Nationale de Défense contre la Tuberculose, 1920), 2.

61. Calmette, *L'effort nationale*, 6.

62. Albert Calmette, *Infection bacillaire et la tuberculose chez l'homme et chez les animaux* (Paris: Masson et Cie, 1920), 600.

63. Calmette, *Infection bacillaire et la tuberculose*, 604.

64. The term "epidemiological devices" is inspired by Michel Callon's concept of market devices, technical instruments that intervene in the construction and reshaping of markets. Michel Callon, *Market Devices* (New York: Wiley, 2007). See also Gerald Oppenheimer, "Causes, Cases and Cohorts: The Role of Epidemiology in the Historical Construction of AIDS," in *AIDS: The Making of a Chronic Disease*, ed. Elizabeth Fee and Daniel Fox (Berkeley: University of California Press, 1992).

65. René Collignon and Charles Becker, *Santé et population en Sénégambie des origines à 1960 Bibliographie annotée* (Paris: Institut National d'Études Démographiques, 1989), 237–247.

66. Carol A. Dyer, *Tuberculosis* (Santa Barbara, CA: Greenwood, 2010), 17–18; Lee B. Reichman and Earl S. Hershfield, *Tuberculosis: A Comprehensive International Approach*, 2nd ed. (New York: Marcel Dekker, 2005), 29–31.
67. Albert Calmette, "Enquête sur l'épidémiologie de la tuberculose dans les colonies françaises," *Annales de l'Institut Pasteur* 26 (July 1912): 499.
68. For instance, Kérandel, "La tuberculose chez les indigènes dans les colonies françaises."; Mathis, *Oeuvre des Pastoriens*, 333.
69. Leger, "La tuberculose au Sénégal," 537–538.
70. Leger, "La tuberculose au Sénégal," 533–534.
71. Calmette, "Enquête sur l'épidémiologie de la tuberculose dans les colonies françaises," 498. For other instances of the rhetorical claims to precision, see Mathis, *Oeuvre des Pastoriens*, 333.
72. Calmette, "Enquête sur l'épidémiologie de la tuberculose dans les colonies françaises," 499.
73. Calmette, "Enquête sur l'épidémiologie de la tuberculose dans les colonies françaises," 499.
74. Kermorgant, *La tuberculose dans les colonies Françaises et plus particulièrement chez les indignèes*, 9, 11–12.
75. Calmette, "Enquête sur l'épidémiologie de la tuberculose dans les colonies françaises," 507–510; for previous studies, see Hénaff, "La tuberculose chez les indigènes de Cochinchine," 52–55; Angier, "La tuberculose au Cambodge," 61–66 Kermorgant, "La tuberculose dans les colonies Françaises et plus particulièrement chez les indigènes," 6.
76. Calmette, "Enquête sur l'épidémiologie de la tuberculose dans les colonies françaises," 500–501; Kermorgant, "La tuberculose dans les colonies Françaises et plus particulièrement chez les indigènes," 6–7.
77. Calmette, "Enquête sur l'épidémiologie de la tuberculose dans les colonies françaises," 542.
78. Calmette, "Enquête sur l'épidémiologie de la tuberculose dans les colonies françaises," 542.
79. Calmette, "Enquête sur l'épidémiologie de la tuberculose dans les colonies françaises," 543.
80. Calmette, "Enquête sur l'épidémiologie de la tuberculose dans les colonies françaises," 497.
81. Calmette, "Enquête sur l'épidémiologie de la tuberculose dans les colonies françaises," 498.
82. "La tuberculose des indigènes en Afrique Occidentale Française," *La Presse Médicale*, 7 September 1929, 1176–1177, BCG.37, AIP.
83. F. Noc and H. Huchard, "La tuberculose à Dakar," *Bulletin de la Société Médico-Chirurgicale l'Ouest-Africain*, 1920, 168–170; M. Léger and G. Huchard, "Contribution à l'étude de la tuberculose au Sénégal: Cuti-réaction chez les enfants de Dakar," *Bulletin de la Société de la Pathologie Exotique*, 1922, 344–347; Mathis, *Oeuvre des Pastoriens*, 334–335; Lasnet, "Infection tuberculeuse et vaccination BCG dans les colonies françaises et pays de protectorat," manuscript notes, BCG.37, AIP.

84. Abbatucci and Gravellat, *Prophylaxie de la tuberculose*, 2–3; Louis Bui, *La tuberculose en Indochine. Étude épidémiologique, clinique, prophylactique. Projet d'armement antituberculeux* (Paris: Vigot Frères, 1933).

85. Dr. Gaide and Dr. Dorolle, *La tuberculose et sa prophylaxie en Indochine Française* (Hanoi: Imprimerie Nationale, 1930), 8.

86. Overviews of the Colonial Exposition can be found in Patricia Morton, *Hybrid Modernities: Architecture and Representation at the 1931 Colonial Exhibition, Paris* (Cambridge, MA: MIT Press, 2000), esp. chap. 1; Catherine Hodeir and Michelle Pierre, *1931: L'Exposition Coloniale* (Paris: Éditions Complexe, 1991); *Exposition Coloniale Internationale á Paris en 1931: Guide officiel* (Paris: Imprimerie Nationale 1931), 17–18.

87. Minister of the colonies circular to governors-general of the colonies, 31 May 1928, GGI 66725, ANOM.

88. Délégué Général du Commissaire de l'Indochine to the Colonial Exposition in Paris, 8 August 1930, GGI 66725, ANOM; see also *L'assistance médicale indigène en AOF. Exposition Coloniale Internationale de Paris. Commissariat de l'AOF* (Rochefort: Impr. Thoyon-Theze, 1931), ANS.

89. Société d'éditions géographiques, maritimes et coloniales, *Exposition coloniale internationale de Paris. Commissariat général* (Paris: Exposition Coloniale, 1931), 162; Le Conseil des recherches scientifiques de l'Indochine, *Exposition coloniale internationale, Paris, 1931, Indochine française, Section des sciences* (Paris: Exposition Coloniale, 1931), 36.

90. Société d'éditions géographiques, maritimes et coloniales, *Exposition coloniale internationale de 1931. Volume 3. Sénégal. Gouvernement général de l'Afrique Occidentale Française* (Paris: Exposition Coloniale, 1931), 214; see also Société d'éditions géographiques, maritimes et coloniales, *Exposition coloniale internationale de 1931. Volume 2. Dakar et Dépendences. Gouvernement général de l'Afrique Occidentale Française* (Paris: Exposition Coloniale, 1931), 102; Société d'éditions géographiques, maritimes et coloniales, *Exposition coloniale internationale de 1931. Volume 10. La Guinée Française. Gouvernement général de l'Afrique Occidentale Française* (Paris: Exposition Coloniale, 1931), 110.

91. Société d'éditions géographiques, maritimes et coloniales, *Exposition coloniale internationale de 1931. Volume 3. Sénégal. Gouvernement général de l'Afrique Occidentale Française*, 216.

92. Société d'éditions géographiques, maritimes et coloniales, *Exposition coloniale internationale de 1931. Volume 3. Sénégal. Gouvernement général de l'Afrique Occidentale Française*, 216.

93. Albert Calmette, undated manuscript notes (around 1931), "La lutte antituberculeuse dans les colonies françaises, principalement en Afrique Occidentale," 2–3, BCG.37, AIP; see also "La tuberculose des indigènes en Afrique occidentale française," *La Presse Médicale* 7 (September 1928), BCG.37, AIP.

94. Albert Calmette, undated manuscript notes (around 1931), "La lutte antituberculeuse dans les colonies françaises, principalement en Afrique Occidentale," 4, BCG.37; Noël Bernard, "Le rôle des Instituts de microbiologie et d'hygiène aux colonies," 13

April 1931, BRN.2, AIP; Société d'éditions géographiques, maritimes et coloniales, *Exposition coloniale internationale de 1931. Volume 2. Dakar et Dépendences. Gouvernement général de l'Afrique Occidentale Française*, 191.

95. Michael Goebel, *Anti-imperial Metropolis: Interwar Paris and the Seeds of Third World Nationalism* (Cambridge: Cambridge University Press, 2015); Jennifer Boittin, *Colonial Metropolis: The Urban Grounds of Anti-imperialism and Feminism in Interwar Paris* (Lincoln & London: University of Nebraska Press, 2010); Claude Liauzu, *Aux origines des Tiers-Mondismes: Colonisés et anti-colonialistes en France (1919–1939)* (Paris: L'Harmattan, 1981).

96. Rosso, "Alors que l'Exposition se ferme."

97. Saumane, "L'Exposition Coloniale Internationale," *La Race Nègre*, April 1931.

98. S. Rosso, "L'impérialisme aux abois," *Le Cri des Nègres*, September 1931.

99. Modris Eksteins, *Rites of Spring: The Great War and the Birth of the Modern Age* (Toronto: Vintage Canada, 2012);

100. *Le Cri des Nègres*, October 1931, 4; André Thirion, *Revolutionaries without Revolution*, trans. Joachim Neugroschel (New York: Macmillan, 1975), 289. For an overview of the Anti-colonial Exposition, see Jody Blake, "The Truth about the Colonies, 1931: *Art indigàne* in the Service of the Revolution," *Oxford Art Journal* 25, no. 1 (January 2002): 38.

101. José Pierre, ed., *Tracts Surréalistes et déclarations collectives, 1922–1969*, vol. 1 (Paris: La Terrain Vague, 1980), 197, 199.

102. "Encore un exemple du colonialisme: Choses du Laos!," *L'Ère Nouvelle*, 1 May 1928; "Saigon sous la poussière," *L'Écho Annamite*, 22 November 1921; Nguyen The Truyen, *La Nation Annamite*, June 1927. See also Daniel Héméry, "Du patriotisme au marxisme: L'immigration vietnamienne en France de 1926 à 1930," *Le Mouvement Social* 90 (January–March 1970): 3–54.

103. Tranh Phu, "The Political Theses of the Indochinese Communist Party (October 1930)," in *Colonialism Experienced: Vietnamese Writings on Colonialism, 1900–1930*, ed. and trans. Truong Buu Lâm (Ann Arbor: University of Michigan Press, 2000), 283.

104. Tranh Huy Lieu, "A Bag Full of Confidences (1927)," in Lâm, *Colonialism Experienced*, 256

105. Maurice Blanchard to Albert Calmette, 23 May 1932, BCG.37, AIP.

106. Dr. Biraud, "Tuberculosis Mortality in France," April 1926, League of Nations Health Organization Tuberculosis Sub-Committee second meeting, 9 October 1926, 21–22, R.881, LNA.

107. Tilley, *Africa as a Living Laboratory*.

Chapter 5

1. We can think of this process as co-production; Sheila Jasanoff, ed., *States of Knowledge: The Co-production of Science and the Social Order* (London: Routledge, 2004).

2. Pedersen, *The Guardians*, 4.

3. Pedersen, *The Guardians*, 9. A sampling of scholarship that highlights the League of Nations technical institutions as ushering in an age of international experts includes Barbara H. M. Metzger, "Towards an International Human Rights Regime during the Interwar Years: The League of Nations' Combat of Traffic in Women and Children," and Kevin Grant, "Human Rights and Sovereign Abolitions of Slavery, c. 1885–1950," in *Beyond Sovereignty: Britain, Empire and Transnationalism, c. 1880–1950*, ed. Kevin Grant, Philippa Levine, and Frank Trentmann (London: Palgrave Macmillan, 2007), 54–79 and 80–102; Claudena M. Skran, *Refugees in Interwar Europe: The Emergence of a Regime* (Oxford: Clarendon Press, 1995).

4. Contrast, for instance, Weindling, *International Health Organisations and Movements, 1918–1939*, as well as Keller, "Geographies of Power, Legacies of Mistrust," 26–48; Anderson, "Where Is the Post-colonial History of Medicine?," 522–530.

5. Clifford Rosenberg, "The International Politics of Vaccine Testing in Interwar Algiers," *American Historical Review* 117, no. 3 (June 2012): 671–697.

6. Historians are increasingly paying attention to how groups ostensibly critical of globalization used the international stage for building alliances and making claims that critiqued new, supranational forms of sovereignty. See, for example, the international history of anti-BCG movements, Albert Wu, "Re-considering the Lübeck Disaster: Towards a Global History of Anti-vaccination" (paper presented at the Sovereignty, Economy and the Global Histories of Natural Resources symposium, University of Cambridge, Cambridge, UK, 18–19 December 2017).

7. The historiography of the outsourcing of clinical trials and medical experimentation is growing. Some examples include Petryna, *When Experiments Travel*; João Biehl and Adriana Petryna, eds., *When People Come First: Critical Studies in Global Health* (Princeton, NJ: Princeton University Press, 2013); Geissler, *Para-states and Medical Science*; Kaushik Sunder Rajan, "Pharmaceutical Crises and Questions of Value: Terrains and Logics of Global Therapeutic Politics," *South Atlantic Quarterly* 111, no. 2 (Spring 2012): 321–346; Kaushik Sunder Rajan, *Lively Capital: Biotechnologies, Ethics and Governance in Global Markets* (Durham, NC: Duke University Press, 2012); Melissa Graboyes, *The Experiment Must Continue: Medical Research and Ethics in East Africa* (Athens: Ohio University Press, 2015); see also the special issue of the *International Journal of African Historical Studies* 47, no. 3 (September 2014): 379–506.

8. For other histories of the BCG vaccine, which have generally contextualized BCG development within national or imperial politics, without interrogating the impact of BCG *on* politics, see Christian Bonah, "'As Safe as Milk or Sugar Water': Perceptions of the Risks and Benefits of the BCG Vaccine in the 1920s and 30s in France and Germany," in *The Risks of Medical Innovation: Risk Perception and Assessment in Historical Context*, ed. Thomas Schich and Ulrich Thöler (London: Routledge, 2006); Laurence Monnais, "Uses of the BCG Vaccine in French Colonial Vietnam between the Two World Wars," *International Journal of Asia-Pacific Studies* 2, no. 1 (May 2006): 40–66.

9. Dorothy Porter and Roy Porter, "What Was Social Medicine? An Historiographical Essay," *Journal of Historical Sociology* 1 (January 1989): 90–106.

10. Murard and Zilberman, "L'autre guerre (1914–1918)," 367–398; Dessertine and Faure, *Combattre la tuberculose.*

11. History Source Material vol. 8, 1900–1901, Series 900, Box 9, RG 3, RAC.

12. Overview of the Rockefeller mission to France, summary, Folder 266, Series 500 T, Box 28, RG 1.1, RAC; "La croisade des Américains contre la tuberculose en France," *Revue des Deux Mondes*, 15 September 1919, 459.

13. For example, Bernard, *Tuberculose et médecine sociale*, 2–3 (statistics on p. 7).

14. "La croisade des américains contre la tuberculose en France," *Revue des Deux Mondes*, 15 September 1919, 461, Box 28, Series 500 T, RG 1.1, RAC.

15. Cohen, *A Body Worth Defending*, 206–267.

16. Cohen, *A Body Worth Defending*, 254–267.

17. Calmette, *Infection bacillaire et la tuberculose*, 595–597; see also Edmond Sergent, "Calmette et la prémunition contre la tuberculose par le vaccin B.C.G." (no date), BCG.37, AIP.

18. Albert Calmette, Camille Guérin, and Benjamin Weill-Hallé, "Essais d'immunisation contre l'infection tuberculeuse," *La Presse Médicale* 2 (1924): 553–555.

19. Albert Calmette, Camille Guérin, and Benjamin Weill-Hallé, "Essai d'immunisation contre l'infection tuberculeuse," *Bulletin de l'Académie Nationale de Médecine* 91 (1924): 787–796; Albert Calmette and Camille Guérin, "Vaccination des bovidés contre la tuberculose et méthode nouvelle de prophylaxie de la tuberculose bovine," *Annales de l'Institut Pasteur* 38 (May 1924): 371–398.

20. Calmette, Guérin and Weill-Hallé, "Essais d'immunisation contre l'infection tuberculeuse," *La Presse Médicale* 2 (1924): 555.

21. Christian Bonah, *Histoire de l'expérimentation humaine en France: Discours et pratiques, 1900–1940* (Paris: Belles Lettres, 2007), 52–75; Rosenberg, "The International Politics of Vaccine Testing in Interwar Algiers," 676–678; Nye, "Honor Codes and Medical Ethics in Modern France," 91–111; Giovanni Maio, "Medical Ethics and Human Experimentation in France after 1945," in *Twentieth Century Ethics on Human Subjects Research: Historical Perspectives on Values, Practices and Regulations* ed. V. Roelcker and M. Giovanni (Stuttgart: Steiner, 2004), 235–252.

22. Bonah, *Histoire de l'expérimentation humaine en France*, 112–138.

23. Albert Calmette, "La Conférence Internationale du BCG," 2, "Réponse à M. Lignières," *Bulletin de l'Académie de Médecine*, 23 October 1928, 1042, BCG.14, AIP.

24. L. Roueche, "À propos de la vaccination antituberculeuse par le B.C.G.," *L'Oeuvre Médicale*, n.d.; A. Calmette, "À propos du BCG. Réponse à M. Taillens (de Lausanne)," *Revue Médicale de la Suisse Romande*, 25 September 1931, 684–689; Calmette's response to L. Tixier, 8 March, 1929, BCG.15, AIP.

25. J. Lignières, "Le vaccin BCG, bien que tres atténué et sans action tuberculigène, reste encore trop pathogène pour l'espèce humaine," *Académie de Médecine*, Séance du 24 juillet 1928, 877; J. Lignières, "Nouvelle contribution à l'étude des propriétés pathogène du vaccin BCG et son application à la prophylaxie de la tuberculose," *Académie de Médecine*, Séance du 15 mai, 1928, 513, BCG.14, AIP.

26. J. Lignières, "Quelques réflexions sur les mesures d'hygiène appliquées a la prophylaxie de la tuberculose humaine et sur l'emploi du BCG," *Académie de Médecine*, Séance du 2 octobre, 1928, 931, BCG.14, AIP.

27. J. Lignières, "Quelques réflexions sur les mesures d'hygiène appliquées a la prophylaxie de la tuberculose humaine et sur l'emploi du BCG," *Académie de Médecine*, Séance du 2 octobre, 1928, 932–933, BCG.14, AIP.

28. J. Lignières, "Nouvelle contribution a l'étude des propriétés pathogène du vaccin BCG et son application a la prophylaxie de la tuberculose," *Académie de Médecine*, Séance du 15 mai, 1928, 522, BCG.14, AIP.

29. Léon Bernard, "Le drame de Lübeck et le BCG," *La Presse Médicale*, 26 December 1931, 1900–1903, BCG.17, AIP.

30. Comptes-rendus du procès de Lübeck, 1931, 3ème session, BCG.17, AIP.

31. Comptes-rendus du procès de Lübeck, 1931, 20ème session, BCG.17, AIP.

32. Comptes-rendus du procès de Lübeck, 1931, 49ème session, BCG.17, AIP.

33. Calmette to Norbert Bachrach, 4 January 1932; Calmette to Dr. Cantor, 26 October 1931, BCG.16, AIP

34. Matthew Ramsey, "Public Health in France," in *The History of Public Health and the State*, ed. Dorothy Porter (Amsterdam: Rodopi, 1994), 82–91; for statistical modes of thinking, see Theodore M. Porter, *The Rise of Statistical Thinking, 1820–1900* (Princeton, NJ: Princeton University Press, 1986); Ian Hacking, *The Taming of Chance* (Cambridge, MA: Harvard University Press, 1990).

35. For the elaboration of the Swedish concept of Folkhem, a model of government that brings together all social classes without governing, but through the "paternalistic authority" of the state, see Thomas Etzemüller, *Alva and Gunnar Myrdahl: Social Engineering in the Modern World* (London: Lexington Books, 2014); Marjaana Niemi, *Public Health and Municipal Policy Making: Britain and Sweden, 1900–1940* (London: Routledge, 2016), 144–154.

36. Arvid Wallgren, "Observations critiques sur la vaccination antituberculeuse de Calmette," *Acta Pædiatrica* 12 (1928): 120–137.

37. P. Greenwood, "Professor Calmette's Statistical Study of B.C.G. Vaccination," *British Medical Journal* 3514 (14 May 1928): 793.

38. Greenwood, "Professor Calmette's Statistical Study of B.C.G. Vaccination," 794.

39. Wallgren, "Observations critiques sur la vaccination antituberculeuse de Calmette," 130.

40. Wallgren, "Observations critiques sur la vaccination antituberculeuse de Calmette," 137.

41. Rajchman cited in Martin David Dubin, "The League of Nations Health Organization," in Weindling, *International Health Organisations and Movements, 1918–1939*, 67.

42. Dubin, "The League of Nations Health Organization," 56–80; Borowy, *Coming to Terms with World Health*.

43. Borowy, *Coming to Terms with World Health*, 32–33.

44. Dubin, "The League of Nations Health Organization," 62–63, 72–73.

45. Borowy, *Coming to Terms with World Health*, 14–17.

46. Letters of Yves M. Biraud to Albert Calmette, 1924–1925, R.881, LNA.

47. "Report of the Technical Conference for the Study of Vaccination against Tuberculosis by Means of BCG," 15–18 October 1928, 7, 8, C.H.745, LNA.

48. Albert Calmette, "La vaccination préventive de la tuberculose par le B.C.G.—Objections qui onte été faites a cette méthode," BCG.9; "Réponse a M. S.A. Petroff par Albert Calmette," n.d. (ca. 1930), BCG.14. Calmette's references to the LNHO conference were also picked up by journalists in France and Germany, for instance, translation of *Breslauer Neueste Nachricher*, 28 May 1930, BCG.19; "Le procés de Lubeck: Les débats ne sont pas encore terminés," *Le Matin*, 1 November 1931, BCG.17, AIP.

49. "Report of the President of the Health Committee upon the Results of the Conference on Vaccination by B.C.G.," CH.767, LNA.

50. "Report of the President of the Health Committee upon the Results of the Conference on Vaccination by B.C.G.," 4–5, CH.BCG.34, LNA.

51. Albert Calmette, "Réponse a M. Lignières," *Académie de Médecine*, Séance du 23 octobre, 1928, 1043, BCG.14, AIP

52. For example, Calmette's reply to M. Petroff; Albert Calmette and Harry Plotz, "On the Vaccination against Tuberculosis by the BCG," manuscript notes, BCG.14, AIP.

53. S. A. Petroff and Arnold Branch, "Bacillus Calmette-Guérin (B.C.G.): Animal Experimentation and Prophylactic Immunization of Children," *American Journal of Public Health* 18, no. 7 (July 1928): 860.

54. Petroff and Branch, "Bacillus Calmette-Guérin," 861, 864; League of Nations Health Organization, *Report of the Technical Conference for the Study of Vaccination against Tuberculosis by Means of BCG* (Geneva, 1928), 46, CH.767; Société des Nations Organization d'Hygiene, "Vaccination antituberculeuse par le BCG," 4, CH.BCG34, LNA.

55. Rosenberg, "The International Politics of Vaccine Testing in Interwar Algiers," 676.

56. The tension between statistical and clinical/experimental evidence is also highlighted in Bonah, "'As Safe as Milk or Sugar Water,'" 71–92.

57. Philippe Menut, "The Lübeck Catastrophe and Its Consequences for Anti-tuberculosis BCG Vaccination," in *Singular Selves: Historical Issues and Contemporary Debates in Immunology*, ed. Anne-Marie Moulin and Alberto Cambroisio (New York: Elsevier, 2000), 207.

58. Albert Calmette to Charles Nicolle, 3 June 1930, NIC.3; Calmette to Prof. W. Kolle, 6 October 1931, BCG.16, AIP.

59. Susan Pedersen, *Family, Dependence and the Origins of the Welfare State, Britain and France, 1914–1945* (Cambridge: Cambridge University Press, 1993); Mary Louise Roberts, *Civilization without Sexes: Reconstructing Gender in Postwar France, 1917–1927* (Chicago: University of Chicago Press, 1994).

60. Andres Horacio Reggiani, "Procreating France: The Politics of Demography, 1919–1945," *French Historical Studies* 19, no. 3 (Spring 1996): 725–754; Marie-Monique Huss, "Pronatalism in the Inter-war Period in France," *Journal of Contemporary History* 25, no. 1 (January 1990): 39–68. For a history of French eugenics, see William Schneider, *Quality and Quantity: The Quest for Biological Regeneration in Twentieth-Century France* (Cambridge: Cambridge University Press, 1990)

61. These claims are too numerous to count, but in administrative circles, see, for instance, Édouard Daladier, "Rapport au président de la République Française," 1 November 1924, 2013 ZK 005 223 SHD-Toulon.

62. On imperial regeneration, see Velmet, "Beauty and Big Business," 66–91; Cook Andersen, *Regeneration through Empire*, 25–60. On the overly virile other, see Camiscioli, *Reproducing the French Race*; Ezra, *The Colonial Unconscious*, 21–47; Clifford Rosenberg, "Albert Sarraut and Republican Racial Thought," in *Race in France: Interdisciplinary Perspectives on the Politics of Difference*, ed. Herrick Chapman and Laura Frader (New York: Berghahn Books, 2004), 36–53.

63. Margaret Cook Andersen, "Creating French Settlements Overseas: Colonial Medicine and Familial Reform in Madagascar," *French Historical Studies* 33, no. 3 (Summer 2010): 417–444.

64. "Développement des services sanitaires et des oeuvres d'hygiène et d'assistance aux Territoires d'Outre-mer de 1925 à 1928," 3, 2013 ZK 005 223, Instructions de M. Daladier—ministre des colonies," 30 December 1924, 2, 2013 ZK 005 161, SHD-Toulon.

65. Nogue and Adam, "La mortinatalité et la mortalité infantile dans les colonies françaises," in *Congrès de la santé publique et de la prévoyance sociale, Marseille, 11–17 septembre 1922* (Paris: Hatchel, 1922), 445.

66. Édouard Daladier, "Rapport et projet de décret au président de la République par le ministre des Territoires d'Outre-mer Daladier sur le service de santé (1924)," 2013 ZK 005 223, SHD-Toulon.

67. Édouard Daladier, "Rapport au Président de la République Française," 1 November 1924, 2013 ZK 005 223, SHD-Toulon.

68. C. Chippaux, "L'Institut de Médecine Tropicale du Service de Santé des Armées et l'oeuvre de Santé Publique des Médecins des troupes de Marine dans les Pays d'Outre-Mer," 1988, 22, 2013 ZK 005 449; Report "Développement des services sanitaires et des oeuvres d'hygiène et d'assistance aux Territoires d'Outre-mer de 1925 à 1928," 1928, 2013 ZK 005 223, SHD-Toulon.

69. Conklin, *A Mission to Civilize*, 142–211; Martin Thomas, *The French Empire between the Wars: Imperialism, Politics, and Society* (Manchester: Manchester University Press, 2005), 17–91.

70. Governor-general Jules Carde, circular to the lt. gov.-s and prefects of the AOF, 12 March 1924, 2013 ZK 005 161, SHD-Toulon.

71. Minister of the colonies Daladier, circular to the governors-general of colonies and protectorates, 23 May 1925, 2013 ZK 005 161, SHD-Toulon.

72. "L'Oeuvre Sanitaire de la France en Afrique Occidentale Française, 1940," 013 ZK 005 161, SHD-Toulon.

73. Minister of the colonies Daladier, circular to the governors-general of colonies and protectorates, 30 December 1924, 2013 ZK 005 161, SHD-Toulon.

74. Minister of the colonies Daladier, circular to the governor-generals of Madagascar, AOF and Indochina, 20 September 1924; Daladier's circular to the governors of Togo and Cameroun, 30 August 1929, BCG.37, AIP.

75. Daladier to governor-general of Madagascar, 20 September 1924; Daladier's circular to the governors of Togo and Cameroun, 30 August 1929, BCG.37, AIP.
76. Daladier to governor-general of Madagascar, 20 September 1924, BCG.37, AIP.
77. Calmette to Charles Nicolle, 23 July 1926, NIC.3, AIP.
78. Daladier's circular to the governors of Togo and Cameroun, 30 August 1929, BCG.37, AIP.
79. J. Bablet, "Les vaccinations antituberculeuse des nourrissons par ingestion de BCG en Cochinchine (1924–25)," BCG.37, AIP.
80. Institut Pasteur du Hanoi, "Instruction relative à l'emploi du *vaccin du BCG* dans les essais d'immunisation des nouveau-nés contre l'infection tuberculeuse," undated; Resident superior of Tonkin, circular to local prefects and residents, 1 March 1928, RSTNF 3865, ANOM.
81. Annual report of the Pasteur Institute 1929, 17–19, 2 G 29–33, ANS.
82. For the cold abscesses, see Mathis to Calmette, 10 October 1929; for the efficacy debate, see confidential report, "Rapport de mission d'inspection des Tirailleurs sénégalais vaccinés au B.C.G. Affectués en exécution de l'ordre de Mission no 334-I/B du 17/2/30"; for the three BCG-vaccinated TB victims, see Col. Blanchard to Ministre de la Guerre, 13 November 1930, BCG.37, AIP.
83. C. Mathis and C. Durieux, "Resultats fournis par l'épreuve à la tuberculine effectuée sur un contingent de tirailleurs sénégalais," 4–9, quotation on p. 9, BCG.37, AIP.
84. Annual report of the Pasteur Institute 1929, 17–19, 2 G 29–33, ANS.
85. C. Mathis and C. Durieux, "Resultats fournis par l'épreuve à la tuberculine effectuée sur un contingent de tirailleurs Sénégalais," 21, BCG.37, AIP.
86. "Report of the President of the Health Committee upon the Results of the Conference on Vaccination by B.C.G." 4–5, CH.BCG.34, LNA.
87. Rosenberg, "The International Politics of Vaccine Testing in Interwar Algiers," 686–688.
88. "Infection tuberculeuse et vaccination BCG dans les colonies françaises et pays de protectorat," 1930; "L'état actuel de nos connaissances sur la vaccination antituberculeuse," conference of medical journals, Paris, 19 July 1929; "La vaccination préventive de la tuberculose par le BCG," conference at the Royal Society, 9 June 1931, BCG.37, AIP.
89. Albert Calmette, "La vaccination préventive de la tuberculose par le BCG dans les colonies et pays de protectorat français," BCG.37, AIP.
90. Albert Calmette, "La vaccination préventive de la tuberculose par le BCG," Conference de Bruxelles, 29 November 1929; "La vaccination préventive de la tuberculose par le BCG," conference at the Royal Society, 9 June 1931, BCG.37, AIP.
91. Monnais-Rousselot, *Médecine et colonisation*, 269–299; Aso, "Forests without Birds," 154–208.
92. J. Bablet, "Les vaccinations antituberculeuses des nourrisons par ingestion de BCG en Cochinchine (1924–1925)," BCG.37, AIP; "Comité d'hygiène de la ville de Cholon, procès verbal du Comité d'Études pour la Lutte Contre la Tuberculose," 13 December 1924, IIB.56/094, GouCoch, VNA-II.

93. "Rapport au grand conseil des intêret économiques et financiers et au conseil de gouvernement de l'Indochine sur le fonctionnement des Instituts Pasteur d'Indochine, 1928," 9, IND.C1, AIP; Letter of the governor-general to the Pasteur Institute of Saigon, IIA.53/2415, GouGoch, VNA-II.

94. Monnais, "Uses of the BCG Vaccine in French Colonial Vietnam between the Two World Wars," 40–66.

95. Brocheux and Hémery, *Indochina*, 305–314.

96. Brocheux and Hémery, *Indochina*, 318.

97. Aso, "Forests without birds," 199. For famines in Tonkin, see Van Nguyen-Marshall, "The Moral Economy of Colonialism: Subsistence and Famine Relief in French Indo-China, 1906–1917," *International History Review* 27, no. 2 (June 2005): 237–258.

98. Aso, "Forest without Birds," 204–206.

99. Aso, "Forest without Birds," 200.

100. André Honnorat, sénateur, président de la CNDT, to the resident superior of Tonkin, 30 March 1926, RST 32.090, VNA-I.

101. Directeur local de la santé to resident superior of Tonkin, 18 May 1926 RST 32.090, VNA-I.

102. Ministry of the Colonies to the resident superior of Tonkin, 2 March 1926, RST 32.090, VNA-I.

103. Albert Calmette, "L'effort national de defense contre la tuberculose," RST 32.090, VNA-I.

104. See, for instance, the report of the translation of Guérin's brochure by Dr. Nguyen Van Khai and the demand for further vulgarization by Mr. Huy in "Comité d'hygiène de la ville de Cholon, Procès verbal du Comité d'Études pour la Lutte Contre la Tuberculose," 13 December 1924, IIB.56/094, GouCoch, VNA-II; and "La vie saine," December 1926, 7163, GouCoch, VNA-II.

105. "Organisation de la lutte contre la tuberculose à Tonkin," 8 October 1936, RSTNF 3864; C. Mandel to the Ligue des Droits de l'Homme et de Citoyen, 5 October 1936, RSTNF 1484; Demande de capacité juridique, 1933, RSTNF 660, ANOM.

106. Report by Hoang Mong Luong, 1939, Dossier relatif aux autres épidémies dans les diverses provinces en Annam années 1911–1938, S.125, VNA-IV.

107. Report by Hoang Mong Luong, 1939, Dossier relatif aux autres épidémies dans les diverses provinces en Annam années 1911–1938, S.125, VNA-IV.

108. Le Chef du 1er Bureau du Gouvernement to Le Chef du Service des Affaires Economiques et Administratives, January 1929, 7193, GouCoch, VNA-II.

109. G. Striedter, Inspecteur des Affaires Politiques et Administratives to the governor of the colony, 10 August 1932, 7193, GouCoch, VNA-II.

110. G. Striedter, Inspecteur des Affaires Politiques et Administratives to the governor of the colony, 10 August 1932, 7193, GouCoch, VNA-II.

111. L'Inspecteur Général de l'Hygiène et de la Santé Publiques to le Directeur Local de la Santé en Cochinchine, 24 October 1935, 7193, GouCoch, VNA-II.

112. L'Inspecteur Général de l'Hygiène et de la Santé Publiques to le Directeur Local de la Santé en Cochinchine, 24 October 1935, 7193, GouCoch, VNA-II.

113. G. Striedter, Inspecteur des Affaires Politiques et Administratives, to the governor of the colony, 10 August 1932, 7193, GouCoch, VNA-II.

114. Brocheux and Hémery, *Indochina*, 291–292.

115. L'Inspecteur Général de l'Hygiène et de la Santé Publiques en Indochine to Monsieur le Directeur Local de la Santé, 6 November 1936, RST NF 03864, ANOM.

116. Response of Administrateur Chef du 1er Bureau to the Demande de Capacité Juridique, 24 May 1928, RST NF 660, ANOM.

117. Rapport du Directeur Local de la Santé sur la tuberculose au Tonkin, 26 June 1928, RST NF 660, ANOM.

118. Rapport du Directeur Local de la Santé sur la tuberculose au Tonkin, 26 June 1928, RST NF 660, ANOM.

119. Note du 1er bureau, 24 May 1928, RST NF 660, ANOM.

120. G. Striedter, Inspecteur des Affaires Politiques et Administratives, to the governor of the colony. 10 August 1932, GouCoch, 7193, VNA-II.

121. G. Striedter, Inspecteur des Affaires Politiques et Administratives, to the governor of the colony. 10 August 1932, GouCoch, 7193, VNA-II.

122. Dr. Morin, Commission de BCG à l'Institut Pasteur, Seance of 29 October 1936, BCG.22, AIP.

123. Rosenberg, "The International Politics of Vaccine Testing in Interwar Algiers," 689–692.

Chapter 6

1. We might think of Pastorian technologies as "interscalar vehicles," to use Gabrielle Hecht's term. Hecht, "Interscalar Vehicles for an African Anthropocene: On Waste, Temporality, and Violence," *Cultural Anthropology* 33, no. 1 (January 2018): 109–141. As she notes, citing Carr and Fisher, scalar practices can be both integrative and divisive; they can both highlight interconnectedness and serve to discriminate. Indeed, we have seen how Pastorian technologies have done both; the analyst should make these processes visible, to "connect stories and scales usually kept apart."

2. Echenberg, *Black Death, White Medicine*.

3. Dr. Huot, "Rapport d'ensemble sur l'épidémie de peste 1914–1915," 3 March 1915, Senegal H 55, ANS.

4. Clarac and Mainguy, "Épidémie de peste de Majunga en 1902," *Annales d'Hygiène et de Médecine Coloniales* 7 (1904): 28–47; Charles Nicolle, "La peste en Tunisie pendant 1907," *Bulletin de la Société de Pathologie Exotique* 1 (1908): 165–167.

5. Collomb, Huot, and Lecomte, "Note sur l'épidémie de peste au Senegal en 1914," *Annales de Médecine et de Pharmacie Coloniales* 19 (1921: 39–40.

6. Echenberg, *Black Death, White Medicine*, 99–107.

7. Dr. Huot, "Rapport sur l'épidémie de peste à Dakar," 2 June 1914, 2–3, Senegal H 73, ANS

8. Overview of the AOF medical budget, "L'oeuvre sanitaire de la France en Afrique Occidentale Française, 1940," 2013 ZK 005 161, SHD-Toulon.

9. I am drawing here on Guillaume Lachenal's analysis of "medical nihilism" in the context of late twentieth-century AIDS outbreaks in Cameroon. Lachenal argues that US researchers working in well-funded laboratories affiliated with the University of California system spent the majority of their time on highly theatrical and well-publicized attempts to discover new strains of HIV in order to prevent "the next pandemic." At the same time, these scientists deliberately disengaged themselves from the ongoing public health crisis in Cameroon, which they did not have the resources to remedy. Guillaume Lachenal, "Lessons in Medical Nihilism," 103–135.

10. Dr. Huot, "Rapport sur l'épidémie de peste à Dakar," 2 June 1914, 2–3, Senegal H 73, ANS (my emphasis).

11. Dr. Huot, "Rapport sur l'épidémie de peste à Dakar," 2 June 1914, 4, Senegal H 73, ANS.

12. Governor-general Merlin to minister of the colonies, letter dated 22 December 1919, Senegal H 57, ANS; A. Esquier, "La deuxième épidémie de peste à Dakar," *Archives de Médecine et Pharmacie Navales* 110 (1920): 203. See also Echenberg, *Black Death, White Medicine*, 186–187.

13. Minutes of the sanitary council meeting, dated 6 December 1919, Senegal H 49 (2), ANS.

14. G. Wesley Johnson, *The Emergence of Black Politics in Senegal: The Struggle for Power in the Four Communes, 1900–1920* (Stanford, CA: Stanford University Press, 1971), 147–153.

15. Amady Aly Dieng, *Blaise Diagne, premier député africain* (Paris: Karthala, 1990), 61–72; Johnson, *The Emergence of Black Politics*, 160–173; Hilary Jones, *The Métis of Senegal: Urban Life and Politics in French West Africa* (Bloomington: Indiana University Press, 2013), 156–180.

16. This argument is convincingly made by Echenberg, *Black Death, White Medicine*, 60–68.

17. Johnson, *The Emergence of Black Politics*, 170–171.

18. Echenberg, *Black Death, White Medicine*, 63; *La Démocratie*, 23 May 1914.

19. Echenberg, *Black Death, White Medicine*, 66.

20. Echenberg, *Black Death, White Medicine*, 79–81; Haut-Comissaire de Dakar to lt. gov. of Senegal, 13 November 1914, Senegal H 55, ANS.

21. "Rapport sur l'épidemie de peste qui a sévi dans la Ville de Dakar pendant l'année 1919," undated, Senegal H 49 (1), ANS.

22. William H. Sewell's classic example is the taking of the Bastille, where a population torn between two competing articulations of sovereignty—that of the king and of the National Assembly—invented the concept of a popular revolution in which categories of popular violence and popular sovereignty were fused through a series of rituals (processions through the streets of Paris with the flag captured at the Bastille, to name just one example) enacted in the days following the conquering of the prison. William H. Sewell, "Historical Events as Transformations of Structures: Inventing Revolution at the Bastille," *Theory and Society* 25, no. 6 (December 1996): 841–881.

23. Chef du Service de Santé du Senegal to lt. gov of Senegal, 10 March 1933, report, 24–26, Senegal H 93, ANS.

24. This claim has been uncritically reproduced by many scientists and historians. Mariola Espinosa has convincingly argued that there is almost certainly no empirical basis for claiming that Africans had genetic immunity to the disease, and at best one can speak of acquired immunity in very particular contexts. Mariola Espinosa, "The Question of Racial Immunity to Yellow Fever in History and Historiography," *Social Science History* 38, nos. 3–4 (January 2014): 437–453; see 441, and 443–444 for the West African context in particular.

25. Osborne, *The Emergence of Tropical Medicine in France*, 96; Erwin H. Ackerknecht, "Yellow Fever," in *History and Geography of the Most Important Diseases* (New York: Hafner, 1965), 50–59; J. S. Marr and J. T. Cathey, "The 1802 Saint-Domingue Yellow Fever Epidemic and the Louisiana Purchase," *Journal of Public Health Management and Practice 19*, no. 1 (January–February 2013): 77–82.

26. Government General publication no 105, "Notice sur la fièvre jaune," undated, AOF 1 H 11, ANS.

27. Maurice Mathis, *Contribution à l'étude du virus amaril et à la vaccination de la fièvre jaune* (Paris: Impremierie P. et A. Davy, 1934).

28. For Mathis' own recollections of the Dakar lab, see Mathis, *Oeuvre des Pastoriens*, esp. 22–25.

29. Constant Mathis to Felix Mesnil, personal letter, 15 January 1926, MES.6, AIP.

30. Lasnet, "Fièvre jaune au Senegal en 1927," *Conférence Africaine de la Fièvre Jaune (Dakar, 1928)*, Gouvernement Général de l'Afrique Occidentale Française, ed. (Paris: Imprimerie Militaire Universelle, 1928).

31. Note sur des visites d'inspection à M'Bour, 2 July 1927; Commissaire Spécial to Directeur de la Police, 5 September 1927, AOF 1 H 11, ANS.

32. The people administrators referred to as "Syrian" were most likely migrants from the territory of the French mandate of Lebanon, and members of the diasporic community today refers to themselves as such. The term used by administrators dates from the pre–World War I era, when the Syria-Lebanon region was known as the province of Syria under the Ottoman Empire. In the following text, I have opted to preserve the language of the historical actors. See Mara A. Leichtman, *Shi'i Cosmopolitanisms in Africa: Lebanese Migration and Religious Conversion in Senegal* (Bloomington: Indiana University Press, 2015), 40–42.

33. Chief of Staff report to lt. gov. of Senegal, 1 July 1927, AOF 1 H 11, ANS.

34. Confidential letter to lt. gov of Senegal, 12 July 1927, AOF 1 H 11, ANS.

35. Commissaire Spécial to Directeur de la Police, 5 September 1927, AOF 1 H 11, ANS.

36. Note sur des visites d'inspection à M'Bour, 2 July 1927, AOF 1 H 11, ANS.

37. Circular of the governor-general, 6 May 1927, *Journal Officiel de l'Afrique Occidentale Française*, 21 May 1927, AOF 1 H 11, ANS.

38. Personal letter to Carde, 14 September 1927, AOF 1 H 11, ANS; Mathis to Mesnil, personal letter, 10 August 1927, MES.6, AIP.

39. Mathis to Mesnil, personal letter, 9 November 1927, MES.6, AIP.

40. Comissaire Central to mayor of Dakar, 19 September 1927, AOF 1 H 12, ANS.

41. Chamber of Commerce to governor-general, 7 September 1927, AOF 1 H 12, ANS.

42. Collective letter to governor-general, 22 September 1927, AOF 1 H 12, ANS.

43. Minister of the colonies to governor-general, 14 December 1927, AOF 1 H 11, ANS.

44. *Le Madagascar*, 20 December, 1927.

45. G. F. Gerard, "La science jugulera la fièvre jaune," July 1927, AOF 1 H 12, ANS; "La fièvre jaune," *La Vielle Cocarde*, 7 November 1927.

46. Pierre Vega, "Les épidémies de fièvre jaune au Senegal," *Dépêche de Toulouse*, 1 July 1927.

47. "Lettre ouverte à M. le Président de l'Union Coloniale Française à Paris," 20 August 1927, AOF 1 H 12, ANS; Georges G. Joutel, "Les Syriens sont-ils responsables de la fièvre jaune?," *Presse Coloniale*, 30 November 1927; Francis Mury, "Ceux qui guérissent de la fièvre jaune," *Courrier Colonial*, 11 November 1927.

48. Docteur Orticoni, "La fièvre jaune à Dakar," *Le Matin*, 11 October 1927.

49. "Toujours le typhus amaril," *La France Coloniale*, 14. September 1927.

50. "Le retour offensif de la fièvre jaune au Senegal," *Le Matin*, 13 October 1927.

51. "La fièvre jaune à Dakar," *Le Matin*, 15 October 1927.

52. "La fièvre jaune au Senegal," *La France Militaire*, 10 October 1927; "La fièvre jaune," *Annales Coloniales*, 15 October 1927; "La fièvre jaune," *Écho de Paris*, 17 October 1927; "La fièvre jaune en Afrique Occidentale Française," *Le Journal des Coloniaux*, 22 October 1927.

53. A. W. Sellards, "Nouvelles obligations pour le contrôle de la fièvre jaune," in *Conférence Africaine de la Fièvre Jaune (Dakar, 1928)*, 268.

54. Governor-general Carde, "Circulaire au sujet de l'application des mesures destinées à prévenir ou à faire cesser les épidémies de typhus amaryl en Afrique occidentale française," 22 October 1927, 3–5, AOF 1 H 11, ANS.

55. Communiqué, Conseil de l'hygiène de Dakar, 26 November 1927, AOF 1 H 11, ANS.

56. Lasnet, "Fièvre jaune au Senegal en 1927," 45–49; Decret de 27 September 1927, AOF 1 H 11, ANS.

57. Mathis to Mesnil, personal letter, 9 November 1927, MES.6, AIP.

58. Jean Laigret, "Hommage à Jean Laigret, la petite histoire de la découverte de la vaccination contre la fièvre jaune," *La Presse Médicale*, 5 November 1966, 2441, cited in Hervé Bazin, *Vaccination: A History: From Lady Montagu to Genetic Engineering* (Montrouge: John Libbey Eurotext, 2011), 415–416.

59. "La fièvre jaune doit disparaitre," *Le Matin*, 17 October 1927.

60. "Quelques vérités sur la fièvre jaune en Afrique Occidentale," *Presse Coloniale*, 7 November 1927, AOF 1 H 12, ANS.

61. Governor-general to minister of the colonies, 29 July 1928, LAI, AIP.

62. "La santé de la plus grande France," *Dépêche Coloniale*, 18 October 1927; "La guerre contre la fièvre jaune," *Petite Gironde*, 9 October 1927; "La fièvre jaune à Dakar," *L'Oeuvre*, 26 October 1927.

63. *Presse Coloniale*, 3 November 1927; *Le Bien Public*, 18 October 1927; *Le Temps*, 1 November 1927.

64. "La fièvre jaune à Dakar," *Le Matin*, 14 October 1927.

65. Lasnet, "Fièvre jaune au Senegal en 1927," 24.

66. Laigret, "Hommage a Jean Laigret," cited in Bazin, *Vaccination*, 416.

67. H. Beeuwkes, "Report of the West African Yellow Fever Commission for the Year 1920," Folder 2652, Box 214, Series 3, RG5.3 IHB RG5.3, RAC.
68. H. Beeuwkes, "Report of the West African Yellow Fever Commission for the Year 1925," 5, received with the letter of 24 March 1926, Folder 2652, Box 214, Series 3, RG5.3 IHB RG5.3, RAC.

Chapter 7

1. F. N. MacNamara, "Reactions Following Neurotropic Yellow Fever Vaccine Given by Scarification in Nigeria," *Transactions of the Royal Society of Tropical Medicine and Hygiene* 47, no. 3 (May 1953): 199–208; P. B. Stones and F. N. MacNamara, "Encephalitis Following Neurotropic Yellow Fever Vaccine Administered by Scarification in Nigeria: Epidemiological and Laboratory Studies," *Transactions of the Royal Society of Tropical Medicine and Hygiene* 49, no. 2 (March 1955): 176–186.
2. Laigret, "Hommage à Jean Laigret, 2441.
3. Noémi Tousignant, "Trypanosomes, Toxicity and Resistance: The Politics of Mass Therapy in French Colonial Africa," *Social History of Medicine* 25, no. 3 (August 2012): 625–643; Guillaume Lachenal, *Le médicament qui devait sauver l'Afrique: Un scandale pharmaceutique aux colonies* (Paris: La Découverte, 2015).
4. I use the term "infrastructure" in the broad sense in which it is used in science and technology studies—as material networks that tie together technical, administrative, semiotic, and personal systems. This definition may seem overly capacious, but as Thomas Hughes and others have noted, it highlights the interdependency of material infrastructures and the legal, administrative, financial, and semiotic infrastructures that make the material infrastructures work; what they have in common is an emphasis on routinization and extension. For a theorization of networks and infrastructure, see Thomas Hughes, *Networks of Power: Electrification in Western Society, 1880–1930* (Baltimore: Johns Hopkins University Press, 1993); Brian Larkin, *Signal and Noise: Media, Infrastructure and Urban Culture in Nigeria* (Durham, NC: Duke University Press, 2008), 5–10; Andrew Barry, *Political Machines: Governing a Technological Society* (London: Athlone Press, 2001), 85–103; Andrew Barry, *Material Politics: Disputes along the Pipeline* (West Sussex: Wiley-Blackwell, 2014), 1–30. Historians have engaged with infrastructural politics, particularly in Pritchard, *Confluence*, and in Chandra Mukerji, *Impossible Engineering: Technology and Territoriality on the Canal Du Midi* (Princeton, NJ: Princeton University Press, 2015).
5. Susan Leigh Star and Karen Ruhleder, "Steps toward an Ecology of Infrastructure: Design and Access for Large Information Spaces," *Information Systems Research* 7, no. 1 (March 1996): 113.
6. What can be read from colonial archives has been brilliantly analyzed by Ann Laura Stoler, *Along the Archival Grain: Epistemic Anxieties and Colonial Common Sense* (Princeton, NJ: Princeton University Press, 2009); the limits of the colonial archive have been theorized in Guillaume Lachenal, *Le médicament qui devait sauver*

l'Afrique, esp. chaps. 10 and 11. For an analysis of the limitations of expert networks, see Vanessa Ogle, *The Global Transformation of Time* (Cambridge, MA: Harvard University Press, 2015).

7. For a history of the Oswaldo Cruz Institute, see Nancy Stepan, *Beginnings of Brazilian Science: Oswaldo Cruz, Medical Research and Policy, 1890–1920* (New York: Science History Publications, 1976).

8. Löwy, *Virus, moustique et modernité*, 70–79.

9. The most common reference point for critics was Cuba—where the disease had been effectively eliminated in Santiago and Havana. Brazil was also frequently referenced. "Chronique médicale: La fièvre jaune," *Le Temps*, 1 November 1927; "La fièvre jaune en France," *Paris*, 9 October 1927; for the campaign in Cuba, see Espinosa, *Epidemic Invasions*.

10. Espinosa, *Epidemic Invasions*, 117–124.

11. Farley, *To Cast Out Disease*, 88–92.

12. Robert E. Noble to the general director of the International Health Board, undated report; Juan Guiteras to General R. E. Noble, "Report on the General Situation on the West Coast of Africa, with Respect to *Yellow Fever* with Suggestions as to Subsequent Investigations," October 1920, Folder 328, Box 52, Series 2, RG.5 IHD/D, RAC.

13. "List of Localities in West Africa Where Yellow Fever Has Occurred and Years in Which Reported," 28 March 1924, Folder 329, Box 52, Series 2, RG.5 IHD/D, RAC.

14. Henry Beeuwkes, diary entry, vol. 1, 15 April 1925, Folder 27, Box 4, Series 495, RG.1.1, RAC.

15. Henry Beeuwkes, diary entry, vol. 1, 24 April 1925, Folder 27, Box 4, Series 495, RG.1.1, RAC.

16. *The Rockefeller Foundation Annual Report, 1926* (New York: Rockefeller Foundation, 1927), 40–41.

17. Henry Hanson, diary entry, 9 January 1926, Box 196, F-L (FA392), RG.12, RAC.

18. "West Africa—Yellow Fever—Additional Appropriations," 13 April 1928, Folder 4950, Box 1.1, Series 495, RG 1.1, RAC.

19. Henry Beeuwkes to F. F. Russell, 3 May 1928, Folder 4950, Box 1, Series 495 RG.1.1, RAC.

20. F. F. Russell to Henry Beeuwkes, 10 January 1930, Folder 4950, Box 1, Series 495 RG.1.1, RAC.

21. F. F. Russell to A. W. Sellards, 15 January 1926; A. W. Sellards to F. F. Russell, 25 January 1926, Folder 3487, Box 275, Series 1.2, RG.5 IHB/D, RAC.

22. Constant Mathis, A. Watson Sellards, and Jean Laigret, "Sensibilité du *Macacus rhesus* au virus de la fièvre jaune," *Comptes Rendus des Séances de l'Académie des Sciences* 186 (1928): 604–606.

23. F. F. Russell to W. G. McCallum, 14 October 1927, Folder 1632, Box 120, Series 1.1, RG.5 IHB/D, RAC.

24. Henry Beeuwkes, diary entries, 16–19 September 1927, Folder 4950, Box 5, Series 1.1, RG.5, RAC.

25. "Rapport annuel de l'Institut Pasteur de Dakar," 1928, 2 G 28–27, ANS; A. Watson Sellards and Constant Mathis, "Expériences de transmission du virus amaril au

'Macacus Rhesus,'" in *Conférence Africaine de la Fièvre Jaune* (Paris: Imprimerie Militaire Universelle, 1928), 10–11.

26. Sellards to Émile Roux, personal letter, July 1 1931; Sellards to Roux, 9 February 1932, CAL.B6, AIP; Bazin, *Vaccination*, 429–430.

27. Mathis to Mesnil, personal letter, 13 September 1931, MES.6; see also Sellards to Roux, personal letter, 9 February. 1932, CAL.B6, AIP.

28. Laigret, "La vaccination de la fièvre jaune," *Conférence faite le 22 mars à l'Union Colonial Française*, 10–11, LAI, AIP.

29. "La lutte contre la fièvre jaune," *La Nature* 2944 (January 1, 1935): 26.

30. Georges Stefanopolou, "Rapport de la fièvre jaune en AOF, Mission du Gouvernement Général de l'AOF," October 1931–July 1932, 3–5, 11–13, STF.3, AIP.

31. Georges Stefanopolou, "Rapport de la fièvre jaune en AOF, Mission du Gouvernement Général de l'AOF," October 1931–July 1932, 8–9, STF.3, AIP.

32. Pierre-Émile-Jean Rigollet, *Prophylaxie de la fièvre jaune notamment par la vaccination anti-amarile* (Bordeaux: Imprimerie Delmas, 1939), 50–60.

33. Espinosa, "The Question of Racial Immunity to Yellow Fever in History and Historiography," 441–442.

34. Technically, the Pastorians did not understand the immunity as being conferred by antibodies, which were not discovered until 1937. They talked of "protective substances" and "immunity through sera," although for the reader's convenience, the anachronistic term "antibodies" is used here.

35. Georges Stefanopolou, "Rapport de la fièvre jaune en AOF, Mission du Gouvernement Général de l'AOF," October 1931–July 1932, 102, STF.3, AIP.

36. "L'avenir de la prophylaxie de la fièvre jaune," *Le Temps Colonial*, 18 January. 1931; "Les foyers de fièvre jaune en Afrique," *Le Siècle Médical*, 15 January 1933; "La lutte contre la fièvre jaune en AOF," *Le Matin*, 14 January 1932.

37. "Sur la détermination des foyers de l'endémicité amaril," *Écho de Médecine*, 18 January 1933.

38. Maurice Prax, "Une découverte que les français ne voulaient pas . . . découvrir," *Le Nouveau Cri*, 8 September 1934.

39. Prax, "Une découverte que les français ne voulaient pas . . . découvrir."

40. Jean Laigret, "La vaccination contre la fièvre jaune au IIème Congrès international de microbiologie," *La Presse Médicale*, 23 September 1936.

41. Laigret, "La vaccination contre la fièvre jaune au IIème Congrès international de microbiologie."

42. Rigollet, *Prophylaxie de la fièvre jaune notamment par la vaccination anti-amarile*, 35–37; Laigret to minister of the colonies, official report, 3 August 1935, IP.SER.1, AIP-Dakar.

43. Constant Mathis, Camille Durieux, and Maurice Mathis, "Est-il prudent de se faire vacciner contre la fièvre jaune en Afrique Occidentale Française," *Bulletin de la Société de Pathologie Exotique* 27 (1936): 1042; Letter of Mathis to Mesnil, 23 June 1936, MES.6, AIP.

44. Pierre Mollaret, *Le traitement de la fièvre jaune* (Paris: Librairie J.-B. Baillière et fils, 1936), 113–114.

45. Mollaret, *Le traitement de la fièvre jaune*, 115.
46. Laigret to minister of the colonies, official report, 3 August 1935, IP.SER.1, AIP; Jean Laigret and Charles Nicolle, "La vaccination contre la fièvre jaune par le virus amaril vivant, desséché et enrobé," *Comptes Rendus des Séances de l'Académie des Sciences*, 29 July 1935, 312.
47. Rigollet, *Prophylaxie de la fièvre jaune notamment par la vaccination anti-amarile*, 36.
48. Mathis to Mesnil, personal letter, 14 September 1936, MES.6, AIP.
49. G. M. Findlay, *Immunisation contre la fièvre jaune*, 22 January 1935, 10–11, BPT. Doc.23, AIP.
50. G. M. Findlay, *Immunisation contre la fièvre jaune*, 22 January 1935, 13, BPT. Doc.23, AIP.
51. G. M. Findlay, *Immunisation contre la fièvre jaune*, 22 January 1935, 13, BPT. Doc.23, AIP.
52. H. Darré and P. Mollaret, "Étude clinique d'un cas de méningo-encéphalite au cours de la séro-vaccination anti-amarile," *Bulletin de la Société de Pathologie Exotique*, 12 February 1936, 169–171.
53. P. Mollaret, "Étude étiologique et microbiologique d'un cas de méningo-encéphalite au cours de la séro-vaccination anti-amarile," *Bulletin de la Société de Pathologie Exotique*, 12 February 1936, 184.
54. Medecin Inspecteur-General Sorel, *La vaccination anti-amarile en Afrique occidentale française. Mise en application du procédé du vaccination Sellards-Laigret* (Paris: OIHP, 1936), 1325.
55. J. Laigret, "Au sujet des réactions nerveuses de la vaccination contre la fièvre jaune," *Bulletin de la Société de Pathologie Exotique*, 14 October 1936, 825.
56. J. Laigret, "Immunisation contre la fièvre jaune," *La Presse Médicale*, 27 January 1935, 7.
57. Laigret, "Au sujet des réactions nerveuses de la vaccination contre la fièvre jaune," 825.
58. J. Laigret, "La vaccination contre la fièvre jaune," 22 March 1935, LAI, AIP.
59. J. Laigret, "De l'interprétation des troubles consécutifs aux vaccination par les virus vivants, en particulier à la vaccination de la fièvre jaune," *Bulletin de la société de pathologie exotique et de ses filiales*, 11 March 1936, 230. See also similar claims in Laigret, "Immunisation contre la fièvre jaune," 7.
60. "Les Services d'Hygiène, Santé Publique et Assistance Médicale Aux Colonies Sous le Ministère de M. André Hesse (Mars à Octobre 1925)," 2013 ZK 005 106, SHD-Toulon; "Instructions du Gouverneur général Carde sur le développement de l'Assistance médicale indigène sociale et sur la protection sanitaire des travailleurs en AOF," Paris, 1931, 2013 ZK 005 161, SHD-Toulon.
61. Mathis to Mesnil, personal letter, 20 June 1936, MES.6, AIP.
62. Georges Stefanopolou to Dr. Sawyer, 16 October 1934, Folder 313, Box 28, Series 4 IHB/D, RG 5, RAC.
63. Georges Stefanopolou to Dr. Sawyer, 16 October 1934, Folder 313, Box 28, Series 4 IHB/D, RG 5, RAC.
64. W. A. Sawyer to Georges Stefanopolou, 1 November 1934, Folder 313, Box 28, Series 4 IHB/D, RG 5, RAC.

65. Richard G. Hahn to Dr. Strode, 7 November 1946, Folder 404, Box 36, Series 4 IHB/D, RG5, RAC.
66. M. Peltier, "Vaccination antiamarile, simple ou associée à la vaccination antivariolique . . . ," undated, IP.DIR.5, AIP-Dakar.
67. J. Gordon Frierson, "The Yellow Fever Vaccine: A History," *Yale Journal of Biology and Medicine* 83, no. 2 (June 2010): 77–85.
68. Bazin, *Vaccination*, 437.
69. Bazin, *Vaccination*, 441.
70. Bazin, *Vaccination*, 452.
71. Médecin-colonel Robert, Note de service, "vaccinations antiamariles," 394/SD, 23 June 1939, IP.DIR.5, AIP-Dakar.
72. Médecin Lt. Col Durieux to M. le Médecin Général, report, 30 July 1941, IP.DIR.5, AIP-Dakar.
73. Instruction pour l'application de l'arrêté du 10 september 1941 rendant obligatoire la vaccination anti-amaryle en Afrique Occidentale Française," IP.DIR.5, AIP-Dakar.
74. Governor-general of the AOF to local colonial governors, 23 April 1940, IP.DIR.5, AIP-Dakar.
75. Governor-general of the AOF to local colonial governors, 23 April 1940, IP.DIR.5, AIP-Dakar.
76. Médecin Lt. Col Durieux, to M. le Médecin Général, report, 30 July 1941, IP.DIR.5, AIP-Dakar.
77. Médecin-Capitaine Bergouniou to Chef du Service de Santé à Abidjan, official report, 17 April 1940, IP.SER.3, AIP-Dakar.
78. Circular by Médecin-Colonel Robert, 23 June 1941, IP.DIR.5, AIP-Dakar.
79. For an example of a hagiographical rendition, see Léon Lapeyssonnie, *Moi Jamot, le vainqueur de la maladie du sommeil* (Brussels: Éditions Louis Musin, 1987).
80. Tousignant, "Trypanosomes, Toxicity and Resistance," 630–636.
81. Médecin Lt. Col Durieux to Pasteur Vallery-Radot, 23 March 1940; see also Pasteur Vallery-Radot to Lt. Col Durieux, 4 April 1940, and the circular to the Pasteur Institutes of AOF, AEF, Indochina, Madagascar and Shanghai, and Martinique, 12 April 1940, IP.DIR.1, AIP-Dakar.
82. Médecin Lt. Col Durieux to Pasteur-Vallery Radot, 19 April 1940, IP.DIR.1, AIP-Dakar.
83. Médecin Lt. Col Durieux to Pasteur-Vallery Radot, 11 December 1940, IP.DIR.1, AIP-Dakar.
84. Médecin Lt. Col Durieux to M. le Médecin Général, report, 30 July 1941, IP.DIR.5, AIP-Dakar.
85. "Vaccination mixte contre la fièvre jaune et la variole sur des populations indigènes du Sénégal," 15, IP.DIR.5, AIP-Dakar.
86. In particular the tables on 12, 31–32.
87. Médecin Lt. Col Durieux, "Rapport sur la mission de vaccinations effectué en Côte d'Ivoire," undated, IP.DIR.5, AIP-Dakar.
88. Médecin-Capitaine Bergouniou to Chef du Service de Santé à Abidjan, official report, 17 April 1940, IP.SER.3, AIP-Dakar; Arthur Vernes and René

Trautmann, *Observations générales à la suite d'une visite de prospection en AOF* (Dakar: Gouverment Général, 1940), 2013 ZK 005 161, SHD-Toulon.

89. Médecin-Capitaine Bergouniou to Chef du Service de Sante à Abidjan, official report, 17 April 1940, IP.SER.3, AIP-Dakar.

90. Médecin Lt. Col Durieux, "Rapport sur la mission de vaccinations effectué en Côte d'Ivoire," undated; M. Peltier, "Vaccination antiamarile, simple ou associée à la vaccination antivariolique . . . ," undated, IP.DIR.5, AIP.

91. "Vaccination antiamarile, simple ou associée à la vaccination antivariolique . . . ," undated, IP.DIR.5, AIP.

92. Latour, *Reassembling the Social*, 66.

93. Latour, *Reassembling the Social*, 70.

94. Bazin, *Vaccination*, 453–454.

Conclusion

1. Lachenal, "Lessons in Medical Nihilism," 107.

2. Adas, *Machines as the Measure of Men*; Guillaume Lachenal, *Le médecin qui voulut être roi: Sur les traces d'une utopie coloniale* (Paris: Seuil, 2017).

3. Rogaski, *Hygienic Modernity*.

4. Anderson, *Colonial Pathologies*.

5. Arnold, *Colonizing the Body*; Laura Briggs, *Reproducing Empire: Race, Sex, Science, and U.S. Imperialism in Puerto Rico* (Berkeley: University of California Press, 2003).

6. Discours de M. Darboux, Président du Conseil d'administration de l'Institut Pasteur, *L'Institut Pasteur, XXVe anniversaire de sa fondation, cérémoni du 15 Novembre 1913*, 8T7 2048, Bibliothèque Nationale de France.

7. Pasteur Vallery-Radot, Institut Pasteur—Cinquantième Anniversaire de sa Fondation—Cérémonie du 15 Mars 1939, DIR.CR7, AIP.

8. For example, Adas, *Machines as the Measure of Men*, 6–9.

9. The concept originates from European histories of technology; Thomas P. Hughes, "The Evolution of Large Technological Systems," in Bijker, Hughes, and Pinch, *The Social Construction of Technological Systems*, 51–81.

10. Fredrik Meiton, "The Radiance of the Jewish National Home," *Comparative Studies in Society and History* 57, no. 4 (December 2015): 975–1006, esp. 981–984. For other examples of imperial technological styles, see Richard Harry Drayton, *Nature's Government: Science, Imperial Britain, and the "Improvement" of the World* (New Haven, CT: Yale University Press, 2000); Claire Jean Cookson-Hills, "Engineering the Nile: Irrigation and the British Empire in Egypt, 1882–1914" (PhD diss., Queen's University, 2013).

11. J. P. Daughton, *Humanity So Far Away: Violence, Humanitarianism, and Rights in the Modern French Empire* (forthcoming).

12. Nicholas B. King, "Security, Disease, Commerce: Ideologies of Postcolonial Global Health," *Social Studies of Science* 32, nos. 5–6 (October–December 2002): 763–789; P. Wenzel Geissler, "What Future Remains?" and Vinh-Kim Nguyen, "Treating to

Prevent HIV: Population Trials and Experimental Societies," both in *Para-states and Medical Science*, 47–77; Biehl and Petryna, *When People Come First*. This is also what James C. Scott has termed the period of "high modernism"; *Seeing Like a State: How Certain Schemes to Improve the Human Condition Have Failed* (New Haven, CT: Yale University Press, 1998).

13. Randall Packard, "Visions of Postwar Health and Development and Their Impact on Public Health Interventions in the Developing World," in *International Development and the Social Sciences: Essays in the History and Politics of Knowledge*, ed. Randall Packard and Frederick Cooper (Berkeley: University of California Press, 1997), 93–117.

14. Pearson, *The Colonial Politics of Global Health*.

15. Packard, "Visions of Postwar Health and Development," 111–113.

16. Guillaume Lachenal, "The Dubai Stage of Public Health," *Revue Tiers Monde* 215 (July–September 2013): 54.

17. Andrew Lakoff, "Two Regimes of Global Health," *Humanity: An International Journal of Human Rights, Humanitarianism, and Development* 1, no. 1 (January 2010): 59–79.

18. For AIDS, see Joanna Crane, *Scrambling for Africa: AIDS, Expertise and the Rise of American Global Health Science* (Ithaca, NY: Cornell University Press, 2013); Didier Fassin, *Quand les corps se souviennent: Expériences et politiques du Sida en Afrique du Sud* (Paris: La Découverte, 2006); for Ebola, see Paul E. Farmer, "The Ebola Outbreak, Fragile Health Systems, and Quality as a Cure," *JAMA* 314, no. 18 (14 November 2014): 1859–1860; for drug trials, see Vinh-Kim Nguyen, "Government-by-Exception: Enrolment and Experimentality in Mass HIV Treatment Programmes in Africa," *Social Theory and Health* 7, no. 3 (October 2009): 196–217.

19. Lachenal, "The Dubai Stage of Global Health," 12–14.

20. King, "Security, Disease, Commerce," 775, 782; Lachenal, "The Dubai Stage of Global Health," 10; Warwick Anderson, "Making Global Health History: The Postcolonial Worldliness of Biomedicine," *Social History of Medicine* 27, no. 2 (February 2014): 383, 384.

21. In recent years, scholars have increasingly highlighted the continuities and rhymes between the colonial era and our own. See, for instance, Anderson, "Making Global Health History"; Keller, "Geographies of Power, Legacies of Mistrust."

22. Lachenal, "The Dubai Stage of Public Health," 4.

Bibliography

Archives

Archives de l'Institut Pasteur de Dakar, Dakar (AIP-Dakar)
Archives de l'Institut Pasteur, Paris (AIP)
Archives Départementales de la Seine-Maritime, Rouen (ADSM)
Archives Nationales de France, Paris (AN)
Archives Nationales d'Outre-Mer, Aix-en-Provence (ANOM)
Archives Nationales du Sénégal, Dakar (ANS)
Bibliothèque Nationale de France, Paris (BNF)
Centre National du Cinéma, Paris (CNC)
League of Nations Archives, Geneva (LNA)
New York Academy of Medicine, New York City (NYAM)
Rockefeller Archive Center, Sleepy Hollow, NY (RAC)
Service Historique de la Defense, Toulon (SHD-Toulon)
Trung tâm Lưu trữ quốc gia I, Hanoi (VNA-I)
Trung tâm Lưu trữ quốc gia II, Ho Chi Minh City (VNA-II)
Trung tâm Lưu trữ quốc gia IV, Da Lat (VNA-IV)

Newspapers and Journals

Newspapers

Courrier Colonial
Courrier de Saigon
La Dépêche de Toulouse
La Dépêche Coloniale
La France
La France Coloniale
La France Militaire
La Liberté
La Nation Annamite
La Race Nègre
Le Bien Public
Le Cri des Nègres
L'Écho Annamite
L'Écho de Paris
L'Ère Nouvelle
Le Gaulois
Le Jour

Le Madagascar
Le Matin
Le Nord-Économiste
Le Nouveau Cri
Le Petit Journal
Le Petit Parisien
Les Annales Coloniales
Les Échos
Le Siècle Médical
Le Temps
Le Temps Colonial
L'Oeuvre
L'Union Libéral
Presse Coloniale

Journals

Acta Pædiatrica
Annales de Chimie et de Physique
Annales de l'Institut Pasteur
Annales de Médecine et de Pharmacie Coloniales
Annales d'Hygiène et de Médecine Coloniales
Annals of Tropical Medicine and Parasitology
Archives de l'Institut Pasteur de Tunis
Archives de Médecine et Pharmacie Navales
British Medical Journal
Bulletin Administratif du Gouvernement Général de l'Afrique Occidentale Française
Bulletin de l'Académie Nationale de Médecine
Bulletin de la Société de Pathologie Exotique
Bulletin de la Société Médico-Chirurgicale l'Ouest-Africain
Bulletin du Comité d'Études Historiques et Scientifiques de l'Afrique Occidentale Française
Bulletin Officiel de l'Indochine Française
Journal Officiel de l'Afrique Occidentale Française
Journal Officiel de l'Indochine Française
La Nature
La Presse Médicale
L'Écho de la Semaine
Le Journal de Morges
Le Journal des Voyages
Le Monde Illustré
Les Nouvelles Littéraires
Patrie: Revue Mensuelle Illustrée de l'Empire
Revue des Deux Mondes
Revue Générale des Sciences Pures et Appliquées
Revue Scientifique

Published Sources

Abbatucci, S. *Les prisonniers de l'opium*. Paris: Fournier, 1934.

Ackerknecht, Erwin H. *History and Geography of the Most Important Diseases*. New York: Hafner, 1965.

Ackerknecht, Erwin H. *Rudolf Virchow: Doctor, Statesman, Anthropologist*. Madison: University of Wisconsin Press, 1953.

Adas, Michael. *Machines as the Measure of Men: Science, Technology, and Ideologies of Western Dominance*. Ithaca, NY: Cornell University Press, 1989.

Ambler, Charles, and Jonathan Crush, eds. *Liquor and Labor in Southern Africa*. Athens: Ohio University Press, 1992.

Amster, Ellen. *Medicine and the Saints: Science, Islam and the Colonial Encounter in Morocco, 1877–1956*. Austin: University of Texas Press, 2013.

Anderson, Warwick. *The Collectors of Lost Souls: Turning Kuru Scientists into Whitemen*. Baltimore: Johns Hopkins University Press, 2006.

Anderson, Warwick. *Colonial Pathologies: American Tropical Medicine, Race, and Hygiene in the Philippines*. Durham, NC: Duke University Press, 2006.

Anderson, Warwick. "Making Global Health History: The Postcolonial Worldliness of Biomedicine." *Social History of Medicine* 27, no. 2 (February 2014): 372–384.

Anderson, Warwick. "Where Is the Post-colonial History of Medicine?" *Bulletin of the History of Medicine* 72 (1998): 522–530.

Annabi Ben-Nefissa, Kmar. "L'Organisation Sanitaire en Tunisie à la veille de la création de l'Institut Pasteur de Tunis." *Archives de l'Institut Pasteur de Tunis* 71 (July 1994): 345–349.

Arnold, David. *Colonizing the Body: State Medicine and Epidemic Disease in Nineteenth-Century India*. Berkeley: University of California Press, 1999.

Aso, Mitchitake. "Forests without Birds: Science, Environment, and Health in French Colonial Vietnam." PhD diss., University of Wisconsin–Madison, 2011.

Balandier, Georges. "La situation coloniale: Approche théorique." *Cahiers Internationaux de Sociologie* 11 (1954): 44–79.

Baldwin, Peter. *Contagion and the State in Europe, 1830–1930*. Cambridge: Cambridge University Press, 1999.

Barnes, David S. *The Great Stink of Paris and the Nineteenth-Century Struggle against Filth and Germs*. Baltimore: Johns Hopkins University Press, 2006.

Barnes, David S. *The Making of a Social Disease: Tuberculosis in Nineteenth-Century France*. Berkeley: University of California Press, 1995.

Barry, Andrew. *Material Politics: Disputes along the Pipeline*. West Sussex: Wiley-Blackwell, 2014.

Barry, Andrew. *Political Machines: Governing a Technological Society*. London: Athlone Press, 2001.

Bauman, Zygmunt. *Liquid Modernity*. New York: Wiley, 2000.

Bayly, C. A. *The Birth of the Modern World, 1780–1914: Global Connections and Comparisons*. Malden, MA: Blackwell, 2004.

Bazin, Hervé. *Vaccination: A History. From Lady Montagu to Genetic Engineering*. Montrouge: John Libbey Eurotext, 2011.

Beaune, Jean-Claude, ed. *La philosophie du remède*. Paris: Éditions Champs-Vallon, 1993.

Berenson, Edward. *Heroes of Empire: Five Charismatic Men and the Conquest of Africa.* Berkeley: University of California Press, 2011.

Berenson, Edward. *The Trial of Madame Caillaux.* Berkeley: University of California Press, 1992.

Bernard, Claude. *An Introduction to the Study of Experimental Medicine.* Translated by Henry Copley Greene. New York: Henry Schuman, 1949 [1865].

Bernard, Étienne. *Tuberculose et médecine sociale.* Paris: Masson et Cie, 1938.

Bernard, Noël. *La vie et l'oeuvre de Albert Calmette, 1863-1933.* Paris: Éditions Albin Michel, 1961.

Bernard, Noël. *Yersin: Pionnier—Savant—Explorateur 1863-1943.* Paris: La Colombe, 1955.

Bibel, David J., and T. H. Chen. "Diagnosis of Plague: An Analysis of the Yersin-Kitasato Controversy." *Bacteriological Reviews,* September 1976, 633–651.

Biehl, João, and Adriana Petryna, eds. *When People Come First: Critical Studies in Global Health.* Princeton, NJ: Princeton University Press, 2013.

Bijker, Wiebe E., Trevor P. Hughes, and Trevor J. Pinch, eds. *The Social Construction of Technological Systems: New Directions in the Sociology and History of Technology.* Cambridge, MA: MIT Press, 1987.

Bision, Yvette. "Le monopole des stupéfiants." PhD diss., Université de Paris X-Nanterre, 1993.

Blake, Jody. "The Truth about the Colonies, 1931: *Art indigène* in the Service of the Revolution." *Oxford Art Journal* 25, no. 1 (January 2002): 35–58.

Bloom, Peter J. *French Colonial Documentary: Mythologies of Humanitarianism.* Minneapolis: University of Minnesota Press, 2008.

Boittin, Jennifer. *Colonial Metropolis: The Urban Grounds of Anti-imperialism and Feminism in Interwar Paris.* Lincoln & London: University of Nebraska Press, 2010.

Bonah, Christian. *Histoire de l'expérimentation humaine en France: Discours et pratiques, 1900–1940.* Paris: Belles Lettres, 2007.

Borowy, Iris. *Coming to Terms with World Health: The League of Nations Health Organization, 1921–1946.* Frankfurt am Main: Peter Lang, 2009.

Boudin, J. C. M. *Traité de géographie et de statistique médicales et des maladies endémiques.* London: J. B. Baillière et fils, 1857.

Boyd, Byron. *Rudolf Virchow: The Scientist as Citizen.* New York: Garland, 1991.

Briggs, Laura. *Reproducing Empire: Race, Sex, Science, and U.S. Imperialism in Puerto Rico.* Berkeley: University of California Press, 2003.

Brisou, B. "Naissance du Service de Santé des Colonies. Dix ans de drames." *Médecine et Armées* 24, no. 5 (1996): 423–432.

Brocheux, Pierre, and Daniel Hémery. *Indochina: An Ambiguous Colonization 1858–1954.* Translated by Ly-Lan Dill Klein. Berkeley: University of California Press, 2011.

Brook, Timothy, and Bob Tadashi, eds. *Opium Regimes: China, Britain, and Japan, 1839–1952.* Berkeley: University of California Press, 2000.

Bruno, G. *Le tour de la France par les deux enfants.* Paris: Belin Frères, 1922.

Bui, Louis. *La tuberculose en Indochine. Étude épidémiologique, clinique, prophylactique. Projet d'armement antituberculeux.* Paris: Vigot Frères, 1933.

Buu Lam, Truong, ed. and trans. *Colonialism Experienced: Vietnamese Writings on Colonialism, 1900–1930.* Ann Arbor: University of Michigan Press, 2000.

Bynum, W. F. "Policing the Hearts of Darkness: Aspects of the International Sanitary Conferences." *History and Philosophy of the Life Sciences* 15, no. 3 (1993): 421–434.

Callon, Michel. *Laws of the Markets*. London: Wiley-Blackwell, 1998.

Callon, Michel. *Market Devices*. New York: Wiley, 2007.

Calmette, Albert. *Infection bacillaire et la tuberculose chez l'homme et chez les animaux*. Paris: Masson et Cie, 1920.

Calmette, Albert. *L'effort nationale de défense contre la tuberculose*. Paris: Comité Nationale de Défense contre la Tuberculose, 1920.

Calmette, Albert, and M. Breton. *L'ankylostomasie. Anémie des mineurs*. Paris: Masson et Cie, 1905.

Calmette, Albert, and Dr. Hautefeuille. *Rapport sur la désinfection par le procédé Clayton à bord des navires*. Paris: Masson et cie, 1902.

Camiscioli, Elisa. *Reproducing the French Race: Immigration, Intimacy, and Embodiment in the Early Twentieth Century*. Durham, NC: Duke University Press, 2009.

Carter, K. Codell. *The Rise of Causal Concepts of Disease*. Burlington, VT: Ashgate, 2003.

Céline. *Journey to the End of the Night*. Translated by Ralph Manheim. New York: New Directions, 2009 [1932].

Céline. *L'Église*. Paris: Gallimard, 1952.

Chakrabarti, Pratik. *Bacteriology and British India: Laboratory Medicine in the Tropics*. Rochester, NY: University of Rochester Press, 2012.

Chapman, Herrick, and Laura Frader, eds. *Race in France: Interdisciplinary Perspectives on the Politics of Difference*. New York: Berghahn Books, 2004.

Cohen, Ed. *A Body Worth Defending: Immunity, Biopolitics, and the Apotheosis of the Modern Body*. Durham, NC: Duke University Press, 2009.

Collignon, René, and Charles Becker. *Santé et population en Sénégambie des origines à 1960: Bibliographie annotée*. Paris: Institut National d'Études Démographiques, 1989.

Commission de la Tuberculose, ed. *Moyens pratiques de combattre la propagation de la tuberculose*. Paris: Masson et Cie, 1900.

Conklin, Alice. *In the Museum of Man: Race, Anthropology, and Empire in France, 1850–1950*. Stanford, CA: Stanford University Press, 2014.

Conklin, Alice. *A Mission to Civilize: The Republican Idea of Empire in France and West Africa, 1895–1930*. Stanford, CA: Stanford University Press, 1997.

Cook Andersen, Margaret. "Creating French Settlements Overseas: Colonial Medicine and Familial Reform in Madagascar." *French Historical Studies* 33, no. 3 (Summer 2010): 417–444.

Cook Andersen, Margaret. *Regeneration through Empire: French Pronatalists and Colonial Settlement in the Third Republic*. Lincoln: University of Nebraska Press, 2015.

Cookson-Hills, Claire Jean. "Engineering the Nile: Irrigation and the British Empire in Egypt, 1882–1914." PhD diss., Queen's University, 2013.

Coomber, Ross, ed. *The Control of Drugs and Drug Users: Reason or Reaction?* Amsterdam: Harwood Academic Publishers, 1998.

Cooper, Frederick. *Colonialism in Question: Theory, Knowledge, History*. Berkeley: University of California Press, 2005.

Cooper, Frederick. *Decolonization and African Society: The Labor Question in French and British Africa*. Cambridge: Cambridge University Press, 1996.

Cooper, Frederick, and Jane Burbank. *Empires in World History: Power and the Politics of Difference*. Princeton, NJ: Princeton University Press, 2011.

Cooper, Frederick, and Ann Stoler, eds. *Tensions of Empire: Colonial Cultures in a Bourgeois World*. Berkeley: University of California Press, 1997.

Corbin, Alain. *The Foul and the Fragrant: Odor and the French Social Imagination.* Translated by Miriam Kochan Berg. Cambridge, MA: Harvard University Press, 1986.

Corbin, Alain. *Le miasme et la jonquille: L'odorat et l'imaginaire social, XVIIIe–XIXe siècles.* Paris: Aubier-Montaigne, 1982.

Courtwright, David T. *Forces of Habit: Drugs and the Making of the Modern World.* Cambridge, MA: Harvard University Press, 2001.

Crambs, J. *Contribution à la géographie médicale du Soudan occidental (région aurifère entre le haut Sénégal et le haut Niger).* Bordeaux: These de doctorat, 1887.

Crane, Joanna. *Scrambling for Africa: AIDS, Expertise and the Rise of American Global Health Science.* Ithaca, NY: Cornell University Press, 2013.

Cunningham, Andrew, and Perry Williams, eds. *The Laboratory Revolution in Medicine.* Cambridge: Cambridge University Press, 1992.

Dahl, Robert. "The Concept of Power." *Behavioral Science* 2, no. 3 (1957): 201–215.

Darenberg, Georges. *La phtisie pulmonaire.* Vol. 2. Paris: J. Rueff, 1892.

Daston, Lorraine. "Objectivity and the Escape from Perspective." *Social Studies of Science* 22, no. 4 (November 1992): 597–618.

Daston, Lorraine, and Peter Galison. *Objectivity.* Cambridge, MA: MIT Press, 2007.

Daston, Lorrain, and H. Otto Sibum. "Introduction: Scientific Personae and Their Histories." Special issue. *Science in Context* 16, nos. 1/2 (2003).

Daughton, J. P. *An Empire Divided: Religion, Republicanism, and the Making of French Colonialism, 1880–1914.* Oxford: Oxford University Press, 2006.

Debré, Patrice. *Louis Pasteur.* Translated by Elborg Forster. Baltimore: Johns Hopkins University Press, 1998.

Debré, Patrice. "Louis Pasteur et Claude Bernard: autour d'un conflit posthume." *Biologie aujourd'hui* 211, no. 2 (2017): 159–192.

Dedet, Jean-Pierre. *Les Instituts Pasteur d'outre-mer: Cent vingt ans de microbiologie francaise dans le monde.* Paris: L'Harmattan, 2001.

de Kruif, Paul. *Microbe Hunters.* Translated by Harry Greenwood Grover. New York: Harcourt, 1926.

De Lanessan, Jean-Marie. *La colonisation Francaise en Indochine.* Évreux: Imprimerie de Charles Hérissey, 1895.

De Lanessan, Jean-Marie. *L'expansion coloniale de la France.* Paris: F. Alcan, 1886.

Delaporte, François. *Disease and Civilization: The Cholera in Paris, 1832.* Translated by Arthur Goldhammer. Cambridge, MA: MIT Press, 1986.

De Saint-Mathurin, René. *La ferme de l'opium au Tonkin: Mémoire présenté a la Commission extraparlementaire.* Paris: L. Woestendieck, 1896.

Descours-Gatin, Chantal. *Quand l'opium finançait la colonisation en Indochine: L'élaboration de la régie generale de l'opium, 1860 à 1914.* Paris: L'Harmattan, 1992.

Dessertine, Dominique, and Olivier Faure. *Combattre la tuberculose.* Lyon: Presse Universitaire de Lyon, 1988.

Des Tournelles, F. *Procédés de préparation de l'alcool de riz de Cochinchine: Rapport de mission.* Paris: Challamel et Cie, 1888.

Dieng, Amady Aly. *Blaise Diagne, premier député africain.* Paris: Karthala, 1990.

Doumer, Paul. *Situation de l'Indochine francaise de 1897 à 1901.* Hanoi: F. H. Schneider, 1902.

Doumic, René. "Une biographie de savant." *Revue des Deux Mondes* 162 (1900): 457–468.

Drayton, Richard Harry. *Nature's Government: Science, Imperial Britain, and the "Improvement" of the World.* New Haven, CT: Yale University Press, 2000.

Dyer, Carol A. *Tuberculosis*. Santa Barbara, CA: Greenwood, 2010.

Echenberg, Myron. *Black Death, White Medicine: Bubonic Plague and the Politics of Public Health in Senegal, 1914–1945*. Portsmouth, NH: Heinemann, 2002.

Echenberg, Myron. "Pestis Redux: The Initial Years of the Third Bubonic Plague Pandemic, 1894–1901." *Journal of World History* 13, no. 2 (Fall 2002): 429–449.

Echenberg, Myron. *Plague Ports: The Global Urban Impact of the Bubonic Plague, 1894–1901*. New York: New York University Press, 2010.

Edwards, Paul N. *A Vast Machine: Computer Models, Climate Data and the Politics of Global Warming*. Cambridge, MA: MIT Press, 2010.

Eksteins, Modris. *Rites of Spring: The Great War and the Birth of the Modern Age*. Toronto: Vintage Canada, 2012.

Ellis, Heather. *Masculinity and Science in Britain, 1831–1918*. London: Palgrave Macmillan, 2018.

Ellis, Jack D. *The Physician-Legislators of France: Medicine and Politics in the Early Third Republic*. Cambridge: Cambridge University Press, 1990.

Espinosa, Mariola. "The Question of Racial Immunity to Yellow Fever in History and Historiography." *Social Science History* 38, nos. 3–4 (January 2014): 437–453.

Espinosa, Mariola. *Epidemic Invasions: Yellow Fever and the Limits of Cuban Independence, 1878–1930*. Chicago: University of Chicago Press, 2009.

Etzemüller, Thomas. *Alva and Gunnar Myrdahl: Social Engineering in the Modern World*. London: Lexington Books, 2014.

Ezra, Elizabeth. *The Colonial Unconscious: Race and Culture in Interwar France*. Ithaca, NY: Cornell University Press, 2000.

Farley, John. *To Cast Out Disease: A History of the International Health Division of the Rockefeller Foundation, 1913–1951*. Oxford: Oxford University Press, 2004.

Farmer, Paul E. "The Ebola Outbreak, Fragile Health Systems, and Quality as a Cure." *JAMA* 314, no. 18 (14 November 2014): 1859–1860.

Fassin, Didier. *Quand les corps se souviennent: Expériences et politiques du Sida en Afrique du Sud*. Paris: La Découverte, 2006.

Fee, Elizabeth, and Daniel Fox, eds. *AIDS: The Making of a Chronic Disease*. Berkeley: University of California Press, 1992.

Finch, Michael P. M. *A Progressive Occupation? The Gallieni-Lyautey Method and Colonial Pacification in Tonkin and Madagascar, 1885–1900*. Oxford: Oxford University Press, 2013.

Fishman, Alfred P. ed. *Pulmonary Diseases and Disorders*. 2nd ed. Vol. 3. New York: McGraw-Hill, 1988.

Fleck, Ludwik. *The Genesis and Development of a Scientific Fact*. Translated by F. Bradley and T. J. Trenn. Chicago: University of Chicago Press, 1979 [1935].

Forth, Christopher E. *The Dreyfus Affair and the Crisis of French Manhood*. Baltimore: Johns Hopkins University Press, 2006.

Forth, Christopher E., and Bertrand Taithe, eds. *French Masculinities: History, Culture and Politics*. Basingstoke: Palgrave Macmillan, 2007.

Forth, Christopher E., and Elinor Accampo, eds. *Confronting Modernity in Fin-de-Siècle France: Bodies, Minds and Gender*. New York: Palgrave Macmillan, 2009.

Fournieau, Charles. *Vietnam: Domination coloniale et résistance nationale 1858–1914*. Paris: Les Indes Savantes, 2002.

Frierson, J. Gordon. "The Yellow Fever Vaccine: A History." *Yale Journal of Biology and Medicine* 83, no. 2 (June 2010): 77–85.

Gaide, Laurent Joseph, and Henri Bodet. *La peste en Indochine*. Hanoi: Imprimerie d'Êxtreme-Orient, 1930.

Galison, Peter, Susan Haack, and Jerome Friedman, eds. *The Humanities and the Sciences*. ACLS Occasional Papers 14. 1999.

Geison, Gerald. "Louis Pasteur." In *The Dictionary of Scientific Biography*. Vol. 10. New York: Charles Scribner's Sons, 1974.

Geison, Gerald. *The Private Science of Louis Pasteur*. Princeton, NJ: Princeton University Press, 1995.

Geissler, P. Wenzel, ed. *Para-states and Medical Science: Making African Global Health*. Durham, NC: Duke University Press, 2015.

Geissler, P. Wenzel, Guillaume Lachénal, John Manton, and Noémi Tousignant, eds. *Traces of the Future: An Archaeology of Medical Science in Africa*. Chicago: Intellect, 2016.

Geoffray, G. *Reglementation des régies Indochinoises. Tome premier. Opium, alcools, sels*. Paris: Édition, 1936.

Gerth, H. H., and C. Wright Mills, ed. and trans. *From Max Weber: Essays in Sociology*. New York: New York University Press, 1948.

Gide, André. *Voyage au Congo*. Paris: Gallimard, 1928.

Gide, Paul. *L'opium—Thèse de doctorat*. Paris: Recueil Sirey, 1910.

Goebel, Michael. *Anti-imperial Metropolis: Interwar Paris and the Seeds of Third World Nationalism*. Cambridge: Cambridge University Press, 2015.

Goodman, Jordan, Paul Lovejoy, and Andrew Sherratt, eds. *Consuming Habits: Drugs in History and Anthropology*. London: Routledge, 1995.

Goswami, Manu. *Producing India: From Colonial Economy to National Space*. Chicago: University of Chicago Press, 2004.

Graboyes, Melissa. *The Experiment Must Continue: Medical Research and Ethics in East Africa*. Athens: Ohio University Press, 2015.

Gradmann, Christoph. *Laboratory Disease: Robert Koch's Medical Bacteriology*. Translated by Elborg Forster. Baltimore: Johns Hopkins University Press, 2009.

Grant, Kevin, Philippa Levine, and Frank Trentmann, eds. *Beyond Sovereignty: Britain, Empire and Transnationalism, c. 1880–1950*. London: Palgrave Macmillan, 2007.

Grellet, Isabelle, and Caroline Kruse. *Histoires de la tuberculose: Les fièvres de l'âme, 1800–1940*. Paris: Ramsay, 1983.

Guilliermond, Alexandre. *Yeasts: Culture, Identification, and Microbiology*. Boston: Stanhope Press, 1920.

Hacking, Ian. *Historical Ontology*. Cambridge, MA: Harvard University Press, 2002.

Hacking, Ian. *The Social Construction of What?* Cambridge, MA: Harvard University Press, 2000.

Hacking, Ian. *The Taming of Chance*. Cambridge, MA: Harvard University Press, 1990.

Hamlin, Christopher. *Public Health and Social Justice in the Age of Chadwick: Britain, 1800–1854*. Cambridge: Cambridge University Press, 1998.

Hardy, Anne. *The Epidemic Streets: Infectious Disease and the Rise of Preventive Medicine, 1856–1900*. Oxford: Oxford University Press, 1993.

Harrison, Mark. *Contagion: How Commerce Has Spread Disease*. New Haven: Yale University Press, 2013.

Harrison, Mark. "Disease, Diplomacy and International Commerce: The Origins of International Sanitary Regulation in the Nineteenth Century." *Journal of Global History* 1 (2006): 197–217.

Harrison, Mark. *Public Health in British India: Anglo-Indian Preventive Medicine, 1858–1914*. Cambridge: Cambridge University Press, 2014.

Headrick, Daniel. *Tentacles of Progress: Technology Transfer in the Age of Imperialism 1850–1950*. Oxford: Oxford University Press, 1988.

Hecht, Gabrielle. *Being Nuclear: Africans and the Global Uranium Trade*. Cambridge, MA: MIT Press, 2012.

Hecht, Gabrielle. "Interscalar Vehicles for an African Anthropocene: On Waste, Temporality, and Violence." *Cultural Anthropology* 33, no. 1 (January 2018): 109–141.

Hecht, Gabrielle. *The Radiance of France: Nuclear Power and National Identity after World War II*. Cambridge, MA: MIT Press, 1998.

Heckenroth, Ferdinand. "Traitement de la peste dans les colonies." *Congrès de la santé publique et de la prévoyance sociale, Marseille, 11–17 septembre 1922*. Paris, 1922.

Heidegger, Martin. *The Question Concerning Technology, and Other Essays*. Translated by William Lovitt. New York: Harper, 1977.

Héméry, Daniel. "Du patriotisme au marxisme: L'immigration vietnamienne en France de 1926 à 1930." *Le Mouvement Social* 90 (January–March 1970): 3–54.

Hérard, H., V. Cornil, and V. Hanot. *La phtisie pulmonaire*. 2nd ed. Paris: Felix Alsan, 1888.

Hirst, L. Fabian. *The Conquest of Plague: A Study of the Evolution of Epidemiology*. Oxford: Clarendon Press, 1953.

Hodeir, Catherine, and Michelle Pierre. *1931: L'Exposition Coloniale*. Paris: Éditions Complexe, 1991.

Howard-Jones, Norman. *The Scientific Background of the International Sanitary Conferences, 1851–1938*. Geneva: World Health Organization, 1975.

Huber, Valeska. "The Unification of the Globe by Disease? The International Sanitary Conferences on Cholera, 1851–1894." *Historical Journal* 42, no. 2 (Spring 2006): 453–476.

Huet, Maurice. *Le pommier et l'olivier: Charles Nicolle, une biographie (1866–1936)*. Paris: Sauramps Médical, 1995.

Hughes, Thomas. *Networks of Power: Electrification in Western Society, 1880–1930*. Baltimore: Johns Hopkins University Press, 1993.

Hunt, Nancy Rose. *A Colonial Lexicon: Of Birth Work, Medicalization, and Mobility in the Congo*. Durham, NC: Duke University Press, 1999.

Huss, Marie-Monique. "Pronatalism in the Inter-war Period in France." *Journal of Contemporary History* 25, no. 1 (January 1990): 39–68.

Jasanoff, Sheila, ed. *States of Knowledge: The Co-production of Science and the Social Order*. London: Routledge, 2004.

Jennings, Eric. *Imperial Heights: Dalat and the Making and Undoing of French Indochina*. Berkeley: University of California Press, 2011.

Johnson, G. Wesley. *The Emergence of Black Politics in Senegal: The Struggle for Power in the Four Communes, 1900–1920*. Stanford, CA: Stanford University Press, 1971.

Jones, David S. "Virgin Soils Revisited." *William and Mary Quarterly* 60, no. 4 (October, 2003): 703–742.

Jones, Hilary. *The Métis of Senegal: Urban Life and Politics in French West Africa*. Bloomington: Indiana University Press, 2013.

Keller, Richard C. "Geographies of Power, Legacies of Mistrust: Colonial Medicine in the Global Present." *Historical Geography* 34 (2006): 26–48

Kermorgant, Alexandre. *Instructions à nos colonies au sujet de mesures à prendre en cas de peste*. Paris: Imprimerie Nationale, 1900.

Kermorgant, Alexandre. *La tuberculose dans les colonies Francaises et plus particulierement chez les indigènes*. Paris: Imprimerie Nationale, 1906.

Kervran, Roger. *Albert Calmette et le B.C.G*. Paris: Librairie Hachette, 1962.

Khoi, Le Thanh. *Le Viet-Nam: Histoire et civilisation*. Paris: Les Éditions de Minuit, 1955.

King, Nicholas B. "Security, Disease, Commerce: Ideologies of Postcolonial Global Health." *Social Studies of Science* 32, nos. 5–6 (October–December 2002): 763–789.

Kohler, Robert. *Lords of the Fly: Drosophila Genetics and the Experimental Life*. Chicago: University of Chicago Press, 1993.

La Berge, Ann F. "Edwin Chadwick and the French Connection." *Bulletin of the History of Medicine* 62 (1988): 23–41.

La Berge, Ann F. *Mission and Method: The Early Nineteenth-Century French Public Health Movement*. Cambridge: Cambridge University Press, 1992.

Lachenal, Guillaume. "The Dubai Stage of Public Health." *Revue Tiers Monde* 215 (July–September 2013): 53–71.

Lachenal, Guillaume. *Le médecin qui voulut etre roi: Sur les traces d'une utopie coloniale*. Paris: Seuil, 2017.

Lachenal, Guillaume. *Le médicament qui devait sauver l'Afrique: Un scandale pharmaceutique aux colonies*. Paris: La Découverte, 2015.

Lakoff, Andrew. "Two Regimes of Global Health." *Humanity: An International Journal of Human Rights, Humanitarianism, and Development* 1, no. 1 (January 2010): 59–79.

Lâm, Truong Boo, ed, and trans. *Colonialism Experienced: Vietnamese Writings on Colonialism, 1900–1930*. Ann Arbor: University of Michigan Press, 2000.

Larkin, Brian. *Signal and Noise: Media, Infrastructure and Urban Culture in Nigeria*. Durham, NC: Duke University Press, 2008.

Latour, Bruno. "On Technical Mediation—Philosophy, Sociology, Genealogy." *Common Knowledge* 3, no. 2 (Fall 1994): 29–64.

Latour, Bruno. *The Pasteurization of France*. Translated by Alan Sheridan and John Law. Cambridge, MA: Harvard University Press, 1988.

Latour, Bruno. "Pasteur on Lactic Acid Yeast: A Partial Semiotic Analysis." *Configurations* 1, no. 1 (1993): 126–146.

Latour, Bruno. *Reassembling the Social: An Introduction to Actor-Network-Theory*. Oxford: Oxford University Press, 2005.

Latour, Bruno. *Science in Action: How to Follow Scientists and Engineers through Society*. Cambridge, MA: Harvard University Press, 1987.

Latour, Bruno. *We Have Never Been Modern*. Cambridge, MA: Harvard University Press, 1991.

Leavitt, Judith Walzer. *Typhoid Mary: Captive to the Public's Health*. Boston: Beacon Press, 1996.

Lee, Victoria. *The Arts of the Microbial World: A History of Japanese Fermentation Science*. Forthcoming.

le Failler, Philippe. *Monopole et prohibition de l'opium en Indochine: Le pilori des chimeres*. Paris: L'Harmattan, 2001.

Leichtman, Mara A. *Shi'i Cosmopolitanisms in Africa: Lebanese Migration and Religious Conversion in Senegal*. Bloomington: Indiana University Press, 2015.

Leigh Star, Susan, and Karen Ruhleder. "Steps toward an Ecology of Infrastructure: Design and Access for Large Information Spaces." *Information Systems Research* 7, no. 1 (March 1996): 111–134.

Lemaistre, Alexis. *L'Institut de France et nos grands établissements scientifiques.* Paris: Hachette, 1896.

Liauzu, Claude. *Aux origines des Tiers-Mondismes: Colonisés et anti-colonialistes en France (1919–1939).* Paris: L'Harmattan, 1981.

Lilienfield, David E., and Paul D. Stolley. *The Foundations of Epidemiology.* Oxford: Oxford University Press, 1994.

Livingston, Julie. *Debility and the Moral Imagination in Botswana.* Bloomington: Indiana University Press, 2005.

Livingston, Julie. *Improvising Medicine: An African Oncology Ward in an Emerging Cancer Epidemic.* Durham, NC: Duke University Press, 2012.

Loir, Adrien. "Prophylaxie sanitaire internationale: La question des quarantaines et mesures sanitaires contre la peste". *Congrès maritime international de Copenhague, 1902* (Paris: Assocation Internationale de la Marine, 1902).

Løkke, Anne. "Creating the Social Question: Imagining Society in Statistics and Political Economy in Late Nineteenth-Century Denmark." *Histoire Sociale/Social History* 35, no. 70 (2002): 393–422.

Longuenesse, Elisabeth, ed. *Santé, médecine et société dans le monde Arabe.* Paris: L'Harmattan, 1995.

Lorin, Amaury. *Paul Doumer, gouverneur general de l'Indochine.* Paris: L'Harmattan, 2004.

Lot, Germaine. *Charles Nicolle et la biologie conquérante.* Paris: Éditions Seghers, 1961.

Löwy, Ilana. *Virus, moustiques et modernité: La fièvre jaune au Brésil entre science et politique.* Paris: Éditions des Archives Contemporaines, 2001.

Lumiere, Auguste. *Tuberculose: Contagion, hérédité.* Lyon: Joannès Desvigne et Cie, 1931.

Lynteris, Christos. *Ethnographic Plague: Configuring Disease on the Chinese-Russian Frontier.* London: Palgrave Macmillan, 2016.

MacKenzie, Donald, Fabian Muniesa, and Lucia Siu, eds. *Do Economists Make Markets?* Princeton, NJ: Princeton University Press, 2007.

MacNamara, F. N. "Reactions Following Neurotropic Yellow Fever Vaccine Given by Scarification in Nigeria." *Transactions of the Royal Society of Tropical Medicine and Hygiene* 47, no. 3 (May 1953): 199–208.

Marr, J. S., and J. T. Cathey. "The 1802 Saint-Domingue Yellow Fever Epidemic and the Louisiana Purchase." *Journal of Public Health Management and Practice* 19, no. 1 (January–February 2013): 77–82.

Martin, L., and G. Brouardel. *Traité d'hygiène.* Vol. 23. Paris: Baillière, 1929.

Martinez, Francisco Javier. "Double Trouble: French Colonialism in Morocco and the Early History of the Pasteur Institutes of Tangier and Casablanca (1895–1932)." *Dynamis* 36, no. 2 (2016): 317–339.

Mathis, Constant. *Oeuvre des Pastoriens en Afrique Noire, Afrique Occidentale Francaise.* Paris: Presses Universitaires de France, 1946.

Mathis, Maurice. *Contribution a l'étude du virus amaril et à la vaccination de la fièvre jaune.* Paris: Imprimierie P. et A. Davy, 1934.

McGoey, Linsey. *No Such Thing as a Free Gift.* New York: Verso, 2015.

Meiton, Fredrik. *Electrical Palestine: Capital and Technology from Empire to Nation.* Berkeley: University of California Press, 2019.

Meiton, Fredrik. "The Radiance of the Jewish National Home." *Comparative Studies in Society and History* 57, no. 4 (December 2015): 975–1006

Mendelsohn, J. Andrew. "'Like All That Lives': Biology, Medicine and Bacteria in the Age of Pasteur and Koch." *History and Philosophy of the Life Sciences* 24, no. 1 (November 1996): 3–36

Mellemgaard, Signe. "Bourgeois Ideals in Nineteenth-Century Hygiene: The Evidence of a Danish Medical Topography." *Ethnologia Scandinavica: A Journal for Nordic Ethnology* 22 (1992): 27–35.

Milam, Erika Lorraine, and Robert Nye. "Scientific Masculinities." Special issue. *Osiris* 30 (2015).

Miller, Clark A., and Paul N. Edwards, eds. *Changing the Atmosphere: Expert Knowledge and Environmental Governance.* Cambridge, MA: MIT Press, 2001.

Mirowski, Philip. *Science-Mart: Privatizing American Science.* Cambridge, MA: Harvard University Press, 2011.

Mischel, Theodore, ed. *The Self: Psychological and Philosophical Issues.* Oxford: Blackwell, 1977.

Mitchell, Timothy. *Rule of Experts: Egypt, Techno-politics, Modernity.* Berkeley: University of California Press, 2002.

Mol, Annemarie. *The Body Multiple: Ontology in Medical Practice.* Durham, NC: Duke University Press, 2003.

Mollaret, Henri H., and Jacqueline Brossollet. *Alexandre Yersin, 1863–1943: Un Pasteurien en Indochine.* Paris: Bellin, 1985.

Monier, René. *La question du monopole de l'alcool au Tonkin et dans le Nord-Annam.* Paris: Émile Larose, 1914.

Monnais, Laurence. "Uses of the BCG Vaccine in French Colonial Vietnam between the Two World Wars." *International Journal of Asia-Pacific Studies* 2, no. 1 (May 2006): 40–66.

Monnais-Rousselot, Laurence. *Medecine et colonisation: L'aventure indochinoise, 1860–1939.* Paris: CNRS Éditions, 1999.

Morton, Patricia. *Hybrid Modernities: Architecture and Representation at the 1931 Colonial Exhibition, Paris.* Cambridge, MA: MIT Press, 2000.

Mosse, George L. *The Image of Man: The Creation of Modern Masculinity.* Oxford: Oxford University Press, 1996.

Moulin, Anne-Marie, and Alberto Cambroisio, eds. *Singular Selves: Historical Issues and Contemporary Debates in Immunology.* New York: Elsevier, 2000.

Moulin, Anne-Marie, Patrick Petitjean, and Catherine Jami, eds. *Science and Empires: Historical Studies about Scientific Development and European Expansion.* Berlin: Springer, 1992.

Mukerji, Chandra. *Impossible Engineering: Technology and Territoriality on the Canal Du Midi.* Princeton, NJ: Princeton University Press, 2015.

Murard, Lion, and Patrick Zilberman. "L'autre guerre (1914–1918): La santé publique en France sous l'œil de l'Amérique." *Revue Historique* 276, no. 2 (October–December 1986): 367–398.

Murard, Lion, and Patrick Zilberman. "Les fondations indestructibles: La santé publique en France et la Fondation Rockefeller." *Médicine/Sciences* 18, no. 5 (2002): 625–632.

Musto, David F. *The American Disease: Origins of Narcotics Control.* New Haven, CT: Yale University Press, 1973.

Nash, Linda. "The Nature of Agency or the Agency of Nature?" *Environmental History* 10, no. 1 (January 2005): 67–69.

Neill, Deborah. *Networks in Tropical Medicine: Internationalism, Colonialism, and the Rise of a Medical Specialty, 1890–1930*. Stanford, CA: Stanford University Press, 2012.

Nguyen, Vinh-Kim. *The Republic of Therapy: Triage and Sovereignty in West Africa's Time of AIDS*. Durham, NC: Duke University Press, 2010.

Nguyen, Vinh-Kim. "Government-by-Exception: Enrolment and Experimentality in Mass HIV Treatment Programmes in Africa." *Social Theory and Health* 7, no. 3 (October 2009): 196–217.

Nicolle, Pierre. "Un événement historique dans la vie de Charles NICOLLE: l'inauguration officielle, il y aura 70 ans cette année, de l'Institut Pasteur de Tunis (d'après des lettres de Charles Nicolle, retrouvées et commentées par Pierre Nicolle)." *Archives de l'Institut Pasteur de Tunis* 69. 1975: 193–202.

Niemi, Marjaana. *Public Health and Municipal Policy Making: Britain and Sweden, 1900–1940*. London: Routledge, 2016.

Niollet, Dominique. *L'épopée des douaniers en Indochine 1874–1954*. Paris: Éditions Kailash, 1998.

Nora, Pierre, ed. *Realms of Memory: The Construction of the French Past*. Vol. 2. *Traditions*. New York: Columbia University Press, 1997.

Nye, Robert A. *Masculinity and Male Codes of Honor in Modern France*. Berkeley: University of California Press, 1998.

Nye, Robert A. "Medicine and Science as Masculine 'Fields of Honor.'" *Osiris* 12 (1996): 60–79.

Ogle, Vanessa. *The Global Transformation of Time*. Cambridge, MA: Harvard University Press, 2015.

Ortolano, Guy. *Thatcher's Progress: From Social Democracy to Market Liberalism through an English New Town*. Cambridge: Cambridge University Press, 2019.

Osborne, Michael A. *The Emergence of Tropical Medicine in France*. Chicago: University of Chicago Press, 2014.

Osterhammel, Jürgen. *The Transformation of the World: A Global History of the Nineteenth Century*. Princeton, NJ: Princeton University Press, 2014.

Packard, Randall M. *White Plague, Black Labor: Tuberculosis and the Political Economy of Health and Disease in South Africa*. Berkeley: University of California Press, 1989.

Packard, Randall, and Frederick Cooper, eds. *International Development and the Social Sciences: Essays in the History and Politics of Knowledge*. Berkeley: University of California Press, 1997.

Pasteur, Louis. *Études sur la bière: Ses maladies, causes qui les provoquent, procédé pour la rendre inaltérable; Avec une théorie nouvelle de la fermentation*. Paris: Gauthier-Villars, 1876.

Pasteur, Louis. "Mémoire sur la fermentation appelée lactique." *Annales de Chimie et de Physique*, 3rd ser., 52 (1858): 404–418.

Pearson, Jessica Lynne. *The Colonial Politics of Global Health: France and the United Nations in Postwar Africa, 1945–1960*. Cambridge, MA: Harvard University Press, 2018.

Peckham, Robert, and David M. Pomfret, eds. *Imperial Contagions: Medicine, Hygiene, and Cultures of Planning in Asia*. Hong Kong: Hong Kong University Press, 2013.

Pedersen, Susan. *Family, Dependence and the Origins of the Welfare State, Britain and France, 1914–1945*. Cambridge: Cambridge University Press, 1993.

Pedersen, Susan. *The Guardians: The League of Nations and the Crisis of Empire*. Oxford: Oxford University Press, 2015.

Pelis, Kim. *Charles Nicolle, Pasteur's Imperial Missionary: Typhus and Tunisia.* Rochester, NY: Rochester University Press, 2006.

Peters, Erica J. "Taste, Taxes, and Technologies: Industrializing Rice Alcohol in Northern Vietnam, 1902–1913." *French Historical Studies* 27, no. 3 (Summer 2003): 569–600.

Peters, Erica J. "What the Taste Test Showed: Alcohol and Politics in French Vietnam." *Social History of Alcohol and Drugs* 19 (2004): 94–110.

Petryna, Adriana. *Life Exposed: Biological Citizens after Chernobyl.* Princeton, NJ: Princeton University Press, 2002.

Petryna, Adriana. *When Experiments Travel: Clinical Trials and the Global Search for Human Subjects.* Princeton, NJ: Princeton University Press, 2009.

Peyrouton, Bernard-Marcel. *Étude sur les monopoles en Indo-Chine. Thèse pour le doctorat.* Paris: Émile Larose, 1913.

Pick, Daneil. *Faces of Degeneration: A European Disorder, c. 1848–1918.* Cambridge: Cambridge University Press, 1993.

Pierre, José, ed. *Tracts Surréalistes et déclarations collectives, 1922–1969.* Vol. 1. Paris: La Terrain Vague, 1980.

Porter, Dorothy. *Health, Civilization and the State: A History of Public Health from Ancient to Modern Times.* London: Routledge, 1999.

Porter, Dorothy, ed. *The History of Public Health and the State.* London: Routledge, 1996.

Porter, Dorothy, and Roy Porter. "What Was Social Medicine? An Historiographical Essay." *Journal of Historical Sociology* 1 (January 1989): 90–106.

Porter, Theodore M. *The Rise of Statistical Thinking, 1820–1900.* Princeton, NJ: Princeton University Press, 1986.

Pritchard, Sara. *Confluence: The Nature of Technology and the Remaking of the Rhône.* Cambridge, MA: Harvard University Press, 2011.

Proust and Faivre. *Rapport général sur les maladies pestilentielles exotiques en 1901.* Melun: Imprimerie Administrative, 1902.

Rabinow, Paul. *French Modern: Norms and Forms of the Social Environment.* Chicago: University of Chicago Press, 1989.

Raj, Kapil. "Beyond Postcolonialism . . . and Postpositivism: Circulation and the Global History of Science." *Isis* 104, no. 2 (June 2013) 337–347.

Ranger, Terence, and Paul Slack, eds. *Epidemics and Ideas: Essays on the Historical Perception of Pestilence.* Cambridge: Cambridge University Press, 1992.

Rauch, André. *Le premier sexe: Mutations et crise de l'identité masculine.* Paris: Hachette, 2000.

Reggiani, Andres Horacio. "Procreating France: The Politics of Demography, 1919–1945." *French Historical Studies* 19, no. 3 (Spring 1996): 725–754.

Reichman, Lee B., and Earl S. Hershfield. *Tuberculosis: A Comprehensive International Approach.* 2nd ed. New York: Marcel Dekker, 2005.

Renan, Ernest. *The Future of Science: Ideas of 1848.* Translated by Albert D. Vandam and C. B. Pitman. London: Chapman and Hill, 1891 [1890].

Revel, Jacques, ed. *Jeux d'échelles: La micro-analyse à l'expérience.* Paris: Gallimard, 1996.

Roberts, Mary Louise. *Civilization without Sexes: Reconstructing Gender in Postwar France, 1917–1927.* Chicago: University of Chicago Press, 1994.

Roelcker, V., and M. Giovanni, eds. *Twentieth Century Ethics on Human Subjects Research: Historical Perspectives on Values, Practices and Regulations.* Stuttgart: Steiner, 2004.

Rogaski, Ruth. *Hygienic Modernity: Meanings of Health and Disease in Treaty-Port China.* Berkeley: University of California Press, 2004.

Rosen, George. *A History of Public Health.* New York: MD Publications, 1954.

Rosenberg, Charles. "Cholera in Nineteenth-Century Europe: A Tool for Social and Economic Analysis." *Comparative Studies in Society and History* 8, no. 4 (July 1966): 452–462.

Rosenberg, Clifford. "The International Politics of Vaccine Testing in Interwar Algiers." *American Historical Review* 117, no. 3 (June 2012): 671–697.

Rosenberg, Emily, ed. *A World Connecting, 1870–1945.* Cambridge, MA: Harvard University Press, 2012.

Saada, Emmanuelle. *Empire's Children: Race, Filiation, and Citizenship in the French Colonies.* Chicago: University of Chicago Press, 2012.

Salomon-Bayet, Claire, et al. *Pasteur et la révolution Pastorienne.* Paris: Payot, 1986.

Sasges, Gerard H. "Contraband, Capital, and the Colonial State: The Alcohol Monopoly in Northern Viet Nam, 1897–1933." PhD diss., University of California, Berkeley, 2006.

Schaffer, Simon. "The Eighteenth Brumaire of Bruno Latour." *Studies in the History and Philosophy of Science* 22, no. 1 (March 1991): 175–192.

Schich, Thomas, and Ulrich Thöler, eds. *The Risks of Medical Innovation: Risk Perception and Assessment in Historical Context.* London: Routledge, 2006.

Schmidt, Lars-Henrik, and Jens Erik Kristensen. *Lys, luft og renlighed: Den moderne socialhygiejnes fødsel.* Copenhagen: Akademisk Forlag, 1986.

Schneider, William. *Quality and Quantity: The Quest for Biological Regeneration in Twentieth-Century France.* Cambridge: Cambridge University Press, 1990.

Scott, James C. *Seeing Like a State: How Certain Schemes to Improve the Human Condition Have Failed.* New Haven, CT: Yale University Press, 1998.

Searle, John R. *Intentionality: An Essay in the Philosophy of Mind.* Cambridge: Cambridge University Press, 1983.

Sewell, William H. "Historical Events as Transformations of Structures: Inventing Revolution at the Bastille." *Theory and Society* 25, no. 6 (December 1996): 841–881.

Shapin, Steven. *The Scientific Life: A Moral History of a Late Modern Vocation.* Chicago: University of Chicago Press, 2008.

Shapin, Steven. *A Social History of Truth: Civility and Science in Seventeenth-Century England.* Chicago: University of Chicago Press, 1994.

Shyrock, Richard H. *American Medical Research, Past and Present.* New York: Commonwealth Fund, 1947.

Simon, Jonathan. *Diphtheria Serum as a Technological Object: A Philosophical Analysis of Serotherapy in France 1894–1900.* Lanham, MD: Lexington Books, 2016.

Skran, Claudena M. *Refugees in Interwar Europe: The Emergence of a Regime.* Oxford: Clarendon Press, 1995.

Sluga, Glenda. *Internationalism in the Age of Nationalism.* Philadelphia: University of Pennsylvania Press, 2013.

Solomon, Tom. "Hong Kong, 1894: The Role of James A. Lowson in the Controversial Discovery of the Plague Bacillus." *Lancet,* 5 July 1997, 60.

Stepan, Nancy. *Beginnings of Brazilian Science: Oswaldo Cruz, Medical Research and Policy, 1890–1920.* New York: Science History Publications, 1976.

Stoler, Ann Laura. *Along the Archival Grain: Epistemic Anxieties and Colonial Common Sense.* Princeton, NJ: Princeton University Press, 2009.

Stoler, Ann Laura. *Carnal Knowledge and Imperial Power: Race and the Intimate in Colonial Rule*. Berkeley: University of California Press, 2002.

Stones, P. B., and F. N. MacNamara. "Encephalitis Following Neurotropic Yellow Fever Vaccine Administered by Scarification in Nigeria: Epidemiological and Laboratory Studies." *Transactions of the Royal Society of Tropical Medicine and Hygiene* 49, no. 2 (March 1955): 176–186.

Strachan, John. "The Pasteurization of Algeria?" *French History* 20, no. 3 (August 2006): 260–275.

Sturrock, John. *Céline: Journey to the End of the Night*. Cambridge: Cambridge University Press, 1990.

Stutchey, Benediky, ed. *Science across the European Empires—1800-1950*. Oxford: Oxford University Press, 2005.

Sunder Rajan, Kaushik. *Lively Capital: Biotechnologies, Ethics and Governance in Global Markets*. Durham, NC: Duke University Press, 2012.

Sunder Rajan, Kaushik. "Pharmaceutical Crises and Questions of Value: Terrains and Logics of Global Therapeutic Politics." *South Atlantic Quarterly* 111, no. 2 (Spring 2012): 321–346.

Sutphen, Mary P. "Not What, but Where: Bubonic Plague and the Reception of Germ Theories in Hong Kong and Calcutta, 1894-1897." *Journal of the History of Medicine and the Allied Sciences* 52, no. 1. (January 1997): 81–113.

Thévenot, J. P. F. *Traité des maladies des Européens dans les pays chauds et spécialement au Sénégal*. Paris: J-B Baillière, 1840.

Thirion, André. *Revolutionaries without Revolution*. Translated by Joachim Neugroschel. New York: Macmillan, 1975.

Thomas, Martin. *The French Empire between the Wars: Imperialism, Politics, and Society*. Manchester: Manchester University Press, 2005.

Tilley, Helen. *Africa as a Living Laboratory: Empire, Development, and the Problem of Scientific Knowledge*. Chicago: University of Chicago Press, 2011.

Tomes, Nancy. *The Gospel of Germs: Men, Women, and the Microbe in American Life*. Cambridge, MA: Harvard University Press, 1998.

Tomes, Nancy J., and John Harley Warner, eds. "Rethinking the Reception of the Germ Theory of Disease: Comparative Perspectives." Special issue. *Journal of the History of Medicine and Allied Sciences* 51, no. 1 (January 1997).

Tousignant, Noémi. *Edges of Exposure: Toxicology and the Problem of Capacity in Postcolonial Senegal*. Durham, NC: Duke University Press, 2018.

Tousignant, Noémi. "Trypanosomes, Toxicity and Resistance: The Politics of Mass Therapy in French Colonial Africa." *Social History of Medicine* 25, no. 3 (August 2012): 625–643.

Treille, Georges. *Besoins et organisation de l'enseignement de la médecine et de l'hygiène coloniales*. Paris: Jean Gainche, 1903.

Treille, Georges. *De l'acclimatisation des Européens dans les pays chauds*. Paris: Octave Doin, 1888.

Treille, Georges. *Organisation sanitaire des colonies: Progrès réalisés—Progrès à faire*. Marseille: Barlatier, 1906.

Tsang, Steve. *A Modern History of Hong Kong*. London: Palgrave Macmillan, 2007.

Tsing, Anna. *Friction: An Ethnography of Global Connection*. Princeton, NJ: Princeton University Press, 2005.

Tumblety, Joan. *Remaking the Male Body: Masculinity and the Uses of Physical Culture in Interwar and Vichy France*. Oxford: Oxford University Press, 2012.

Vallery-Radot, René. *La vie de Pasteur*. Paris: Hachette, 1911.

Vann, Michael. "Of Rats, Rice, and Race: The Great Hanoi Rat Massacre, an Episode in French Colonial History." *French Colonial History* 4 (2003): 191–203.

van Onselen, Charles. "Randlords and Rotgut 1886–1903: An Essay on the Role of Alcohol in the Development of European Imperialism and Southern African Capitalism." *History Workshop Journal* 1, no. 2 (Autumn 1976): 33–89.

Vaughan, Megan. *Curing Their Ills: Colonial Power and African Illness*. Stanford, CA: Stanford University Press, 1991.

Velmet, Aro. "Beauty and Big Business: Race and Civilizational Decline in French Beauty Pageants, 1920–37." *French History* 28, no. 1 (March 2014): 66–91.

Viet, Vincent. *La santé en guerre, 1914–1918: Une politique pionnière en univers incertain*. Paris: Presses de Sciences Po, 2015.

Vilhelmsson, Andreas. "Folkhälsoarbetets historia i socialmedicinsk belysning." *Socialmedicisnk Tidskrift* 89, no. 1 (2012): 44–53.

Wailoo, Keith. *Drawing Blood: Technology and Disease Identity in Twentieth-Century America*. Baltimore: Johns Hopkins University Press, 1999.

Warwick, Andrew. *Masters of Theory: Cambridge and the Rise of Mathematical Physics*. Chicago: University of Chicago Press, 2003.

Weindling, Paul, ed. *International Health Organisations and Movements, 1918–1939*. Cambridge: Cambridge University Press, 1995.

Weisz, George. *The Medical Mandarins: The French Academy of Medicine in the Nineteenth and Early Twentieth Centuries*. Oxford: Oxford University Press, 1995.

Worboys, Michael. *Spreading Germs: Disease Theories and Medical Practice in Britain, 1865–1900*. Cambridge: Cambridge University Press, 2000.

Worboys, Michael. "Was There a Bacteriological Revolution in Late Nineteenth-Century Medicine?" *Studies in History and Philosophy of Biological and Biomedical Sciences* 38, no. 1 (March 2007): 20–42.

Zuschlag, Emil. *Le rat migratoire et sa destruction rationnelle*. Copenhagen: Fr. Bagge, 1903.

Zuschlag, Emil, and Harald Goldschmitt. *Rotterne samt deres Forhold til det moderne Samfundsliv: Et Agitationsskrift for Rottesagen*. Copenhagen: Fr. Bagge, 1900.

Index

Figures are indicated by *f* following the page number

For the benefit of digital users, indexed terms that span two pages (e.g., 52-53) may, on occasion, appear on only one of those pages.